Contributors

BARBARA A. ARANEO, Ph.D.

Research Associate Professor, Department of Pathology, University of Utah Medical Center, Salt Lake City, Utah
Mechanisms of Allograft Rejection

MARGARET E. BILLINGHAM, M.B., B.S., F.R.C.Path.

Professor of Pathology (Cardiovascular), Stanford University School of Medicine, Stanford, California; Attending Staff, Stanford University Medical Center, Stanford, California
Cardiac Transplant Pathology

JOHN F. CARLQUIST, Ph.D.

Research Assistant Professor, Division of Cardiology, Department of Medicine, University of Utah School of Medicine, Salt Lake City, Utah; Research Associate, Departments of Cardiology and Pathology, LDS Hospital, Salt Lake City, Utah
Application of Transplant Biopsy Culture Techniques to the Understanding of Allograft Rejection

DAVID C. CLASSEN, M.D., M.S.

Assistant Professor of Medicine, University of Utah School of Medicine, Salt Lake City, Utah; Attending Physician, Infectious Disease Department, LDS Hospital, Salt Lake City, Utah
Infections in Transplant Patients

ROBERT B. COLVIN, M.D.

Benjamin Castleman Professor of Pathology, Harvard Medical School, Boston, Massachusetts; Chief, Pathology Service, Massachusetts General Hospital, Boston, Massachusetts
Differential Diagnosis of Renal Allograft Biopsies

MARIA ROSA COSTANZO, M.D.

Associate Professor of Medicine, Loyola University, Chicago, Illinois; Medical Director, Hines Veterans Administration/Loyola University Medical Center Heart Failure/Cardiac Transplant Program, Chicago, Illinois
Actions, Interactions, and Toxicities of Immunosuppressive Drugs and Techniques: New and Old

W. PAGE FAULK, M.D., F.R.C.Path.

Professor, Department of Medicinal Chemistry, Purdue University, West Lafayette, Indiana; Director, Experimental Pathology, Methodist Hospital, Indianapolis, Indiana
Fibrinolytic and Anticoagulant Control of Hemostasis in Human Cardiac and Renal Allografts

ROBERT L. FLINNER, M.D.

Clinical Professor of Pathology, University of Utah School of Medicine, Salt Lake City, Utah; Director of Surgical Pathology, LDS Hospital, Salt Lake City, Utah
Liver Transplant Pathology; Infections in Transplant Patients; Neoplasms Occurring in Solid Organ Transplant Recipients

ELIZABETH H. HAMMOND, M.D.

Professor of Pathology, University of Utah School of Medicine, Salt Lake City, Utah; Chairman of Pathology, LDS Hospital, Salt Lake City, Utah
Pathology of Cardiac Vascular (Microvascular) Rejection; Liver Transplant Pathology

CARLOS A. LABARRERE, M.D.

Head Immunopathologist, Methodist Hospital of Indiana, Indianapolis, Indiana; Transplant Immuno-pathologist, Methodist Hospital of Indiana, Indianapolis, Indiana
Fibrinolytic and Anticoagulant Control of Hemostasis in Human Cardiac and Renal Allografts

CHARLES C. MARBOE, M.D.

Associate Professor of Pathology, University of Southern California School of Medicine, Los Angeles, California; Director, Anatomic Pathology, USC–University Hospital, Los Angeles, California
Cardiac Transplant Vasculopathy

THOMAS M. McINTYRE, Ph.D.

Professor of Biochemistry and Medicine, University of Utah School of Medicine, Salt Lake City, Utah
The Role of Endothelial Cells in Transplant Rejection

SHANE M. MEEHAN, M.D.

Renal Pathology Fellow, Department of Pathology, Harvard Medical School, Boston, Massachusetts; Massachusetts General Hospital, Boston, Massachusetts
Differential Diagnosis of Renal Allograft Biopsies

DOUGLAS J. NORMAN, M.D.

Professor of Medicine, Oregon Health Sciences University, Portland, Oregon; Director, Transplant Medicine and Director, Laboratory of Immunogenetics and Transplantation, Portland, Oregon
Actions, Interactions, and Toxicities of Immunosuppressive Drugs and Techniques: New and Old

STEPHEN M. PRESCOTT, M.D.

Professor of Internal Medicine and Director, Program in Human Molecular Biology and Genetics, University of Utah School of Medicine, Salt Lake City, Utah; Attending Staff, University of Utah Medical Center, Salt Lake City, Utah
The Role of Endothelial Cells in Transplant Rejection

ROBERT E. SHADDY, M.D.

Associate Professor of Pediatrics, University of Utah School of Medicine, Salt Lake City, Utah; Medical Director, Heart Transplantation Program, Primary Children's Medical Center, Salt Lake City, Utah
The Role of Endothelial Cells in Transplant Rejection

SUSAN STEWART, B.A., M.A., M.B., B.Ch., M.R.C.Path.

Associate Lecturer, Department of Pathology, University of Cambridge, Cambridge, England; Consult-ant Histopathologist, Papworth Hospital, Cambridgeshire, England; Honorary Consultant Histopathol-ogist, Addenbrookes Hospital, Cambridge, England
Lung Transplant Pathology

ROBERT L. YOWELL, M.D.

Clinical Assistant Professor, Department of Pathology, University of Utah School of Medicine, Salt Lake City, Utah; Director, Electron Microscopy Laboratory, LDS Hospital, Salt Lake City, Utah
Mechanisms of Allograft Rejection

GUY A. ZIMMERMAN, M.D.

Professor of Medicine, University of Utah School of Medicine, Salt Lake City, Utah; Attending Physician, University Hospital and Salt Lake Veteran's Administration Medical Center, Salt Lake City, Utah
The Role of Endothelial Cells in Transplant Rejection

Solid Organ Transplantation Pathology

MPP

30

ELIZABETH H. HAMMOND, M.D.
Professor of Pathology
University of Utah School of Medicine
Chairman of Pathology
LDS Hospital
Salt Lake City, Utah

Solid Organ Transplantation Pathology

Volume 30 in the Series

MAJOR PROBLEMS IN PATHOLOGY

W.B. SAUNDERS COMPANY
A Division of Harcourt Brace & Company
PHILADELPHIA LONDON TORONTO MONTREAL SYDNEY TOKYO

W. B. SAUNDERS COMPANY
A Division of
Harcourt Brace & Company

The Curtis Center
Independence Square West
Philadelphia, Pennsylvania 19106

Library of Congress Cataloging-in-Publication Data

Solid organ transplantation pathology / [edited by] Elizabeth H. Hammond.—1st ed.

    p. cm.—(MPP ; v. 30)

ISBN 0–7216–4482–1

1. Transplantation of organs, tissues, etc.—Complications.   2. Graft rejection.   I. Hammond, Elizabeth H.   II. Series: Major problems in pathology;   v. 30.

[DNLM: 1. Organ Transplantation—pathology.   W1 MA492X v. 30 1994 WO 660 S686   1994]

RD120.78.S65 1994

617.9′5—dc20

DNLM/DLC   93–36143

Solid Organ Transplantation Pathology   ISBN 0–7216–4482–1

Last digit is the print number: 9   8   7   6   5   4   3   2   1

Foreword

This MPP monograph on *Solid Organ Transplantation Pathology* diverges slightly from the emphasis of these books on single organ pathology. However, it summarizes the pathologic changes of rejection and complications affecting individuals with transplanted organs and affecting the graft itself.

Dr. Hammond has brought together recognized experts in the field. This monograph will serve as a frequent reference for the practicing pathologist, who is seeing a growing caseload of pathology specimens from transplanted organs. I am pleased that this work is an integral part of the MPP series.

VIRGINIA A. LIVOLSI, M.D.
SERIES EDITOR

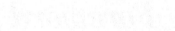

Preface

This book was conceived as a resource for pathologists and other medical specialists dealing with pathologic tissue specimens from solid organ allograft recipients. It is the product of many authors, all of whom were selected because of their knowledge of their subject. The book approaches transplant pathology in the context of other related basic and clinical disciplines. It is organized into three sections. In the first section, fundamental processes that affect allograft pathology are addressed: immunologic mechanisms of allograft rejection, expression of these allograft responses in the context of culture of allograft biopsy fragments, aspects of endothelial biology that are important in allograft responses, and the impact of coagulation and fibrinolysis on allografted tissue. The second section deals with the specific pathologic features of allograft rejection involving solid organ allografts. The chapters are written by pathologists who have dealt with and written about these pathologic problems. Practical diagnostic criteria are emphasized. Three chapters deal with cardiac transplant rejection, reflecting my own special interest in this allograft. The chapter on chronic cardiac vasculopathy contains information and references that are also relevant to the evaluation of chronic allograft vasculopathy in other solid organ allografts. In the third section, aspects of transplantation common to all solid organ allografts are discussed. Immuno-suppression is addressed by two very experienced clinicians, and the discussion includes the most well known as well as the most recently used therapeutic agents. Other chapters deal with serious potential complications of transplantation—infections and neoplasms. Thus, within this range of chapters, physicians and other health care personnel can gain a better and more complete understanding of the pathologic processes involving solid organ allografts and their recipients.

ELIZABETH H. HAMMOND, M.D.

Acknowledgments

I have major debts of gratitude to many individuals. First, I owe my interest in the subject of immunopathology to my sister, Kathleen Hale Webb, who, through her friendship and courageous response to her illness, has strongly motivated me to search for better understanding of immunologic processes such as allograft rejection. Second, I am indebted to my teachers in immunology: George and Eva Klein, and Harold Dvorak. Third, I am deeply indebted to my colleagues and collaborators: to Robert L. Flinner, with his uncompromising desire for clinical excellence in surgical pathology; to Margaret Billingham, a wonderful example of what a transplant pathologist and physician should be; and to my technicians, Janet Hansen, Louise Spencer, Donna Riddell, and Ann Jensen—individuals who have given consistent competent service. The book would never have been completed without the dedication and excellence of my secretarial assistant, Sherree Terry. My family, Jack, Jonathan, Thomas, and Kathleen, have given me unqualified love and support.

I am also grateful to the editors and technical personnel at W. B. Saunders, who provided excellent professional help in producing this volume; to John B. O'Connell for helpful suggestions and comments at the initiation of the project; and to Virginia LiVolsi, who believed that this subject would be a valuable addition to the series. I am very thankful for the continued financial support of the A. Lee Christensen Fund of the Deseret Foundation, LDS Hospital, which has made this and many other projects financially feasible.

Contents

PART I
PATHOGENIC MECHANISM OF SOLID ORGAN
ALLOGRAFT REJECTION 1

Chapter 1
MECHANISMS OF ALLOGRAFT REJECTION 4
Robert L. Yowell, MD, PhD, and Barbara A. Araneo, PhD

Chapter 2
APPLICATION OF TRANSPLANT BIOPSY CULTURE TECHNIQUES
TO THE UNDERSTANDING OF ALLOGRAFT REJECTION 19
John F. Carlquist, PhD

Chapter 3
THE ROLE OF ENDOTHELIAL CELLS IN TRANSPLANT
REJECTION 35
Robert E. Shaddy, MD, Stephen M. Prescott, MD, Thomas M. McIntyre, PhD, and
Guy A. Zimmerman, MD

Chapter 4
FIBRINOLYTIC AND ANTICOAGULANT CONTROL OF HEMOSTASIS
IN HUMAN CARDIAC AND RENAL ALLOGRAFTS 49
W. Page Faulk, MD, FRCPath, and Carlos A. Labarrere, MD

PART II
PATHOLOGY OF REJECTION OF SOLID ORGAN ALLOGRAFTS 67

Chapter 5
CARDIAC TRANSPLANT PATHOLOGY 69
Margaret E. Billingham, MB, BS, FRCPath

Chapter 6
PATHOLOGY OF CARDIAC VASCULAR
(MICROVASCULAR) REJECTION 92
Elizabeth H. Hammond, MD

Chapter 7
CARDIAC TRANSPLANT VASCULOPATHY 111
Charles C. Marboe, MD

Chapter 8
LUNG TRANSPLANT PATHOLOGY 133
Susan Stewart, BA, MA, MB, BCh, MRCPath

Chapter 9
DIFFERENTIAL DIAGNOSIS OF RENAL ALLOGRAFT BIOPSIES 159
Shane M. Meehan, MD, and Robert B. Colvin, MD

Chapter 10
LIVER TRANSPLANT PATHOLOGY 186
Robert L. Flinner, MD, and Elizabeth H. Hammond, MD

PART III
PROCESSES COMMON TO ALL SOLID ORGAN ALLOGRAFTS 215

Chapter 11
ACTIONS, INTERACTIONS, AND TOXICITIES OF
IMMUNOSUPPRESSIVE DRUGS AND TECHNIQUES:
NEW AND OLD 217
Douglas J. Norman, MD, and Maria Rosa Costanzo, MD

Chapter 12
INFECTIONS IN TRANSPLANT PATIENTS 239
David C. Classen, MD, MS, and Robert L. Flinner, MD

Chapter 13
NEOPLASMS OCCURRING IN SOLID ORGAN TRANSPLANT
RECIPIENTS 262
Robert L. Flinner, MD

INDEX 275

Pathogenic Mechanisms of Solid Organ Allograft Rejection

For the past several years, I have been the instructor for the portion of a pathology course dealing with immunopathology. My section of pathology is taught at the same time that the sophomore medical students are learning basic immunology, a comprehensive course taught by basic scientists, delving into the newest developments in the understanding of immunology. Each year I begin by explaining the differences between our understanding of immunopathology in humans and basic immunology in laboratory animal models: one discipline deals with outbred animals in non-controlled, in vivo experiments, whereas the other deals with carefully controlled inbred animal studies.

As I have worked on this volume, I have been struck by other important differences between immunology and immunopathology: while immunology tries to understand individual elements of complex processes that can be studied in dissected models, immunopathology in humans is complicated by other important pathologic mechanisms operative in an in vivo situation: inflammation, repair, effects of altered blood supply, nutrition, infection, and so on. Thus, evaluation of alterations in allografts in humans, the subject of this book, can be understood only in the context of other fundamental processes.

The first section of this book deals with some of these fundamental processes of major importance in allograft pathology: immunology as applied to solid organ allograft rejection (Chapter 1), immunologic responses of hu-

man solid allografts as understood in the context of culture of allograft biopsy fragments (Chapter 2), aspects of endothelial biology important in allograft responses (Chapter 3), and the impact of coagulation and fibrinolysis on allograft responses (Chapter 4). Other important processes that could be included in this section have been excluded because of the constraints of space or the lack of pertinent information.

Foremost among the latter is the topic of inflammation and repair as modulators of allograft pathology. Although the inciting events in allograft rejection are most certainly immunologic, as described in Chapter 1 by Yowell and Araneo, these responses are certainly amplified in various ways by inflammatory stimuli. All the cells, plasma proteins, and vascular constituents of inflammation are present in the allograft.[1-3] Many of the vascular and cellular responses of inflammation are mediated by chemical factors derived from the action of the inflammatory stimulus.[2-5]

Early after transplantation, a potent inflammatory stimulus is always present—ischemia, induced by the necessary removal from the donor, delay, and reimplantation. Such ischemia is of variable extent depending on circumstances; however, there is always some parenchymal cell necrosis that triggers elaboration of inflammatory mediators.[4] In all solid organ allografts in the early post-transplant period, hallmarks of acute inflammation can be seen; frequently there is vasodilation and vascular permeability, slowing of the circulation and leukocyte margination, adhesion, and emigration. These changes are protean in the first few biopsies and are not seen as manifestations of allograft rejection.

Chapter 3 by Shaddy and coworkers discusses the role of the vascular endothelium in allograft rejection. The endothelium assumes a central role in immune mechanisms as both stimulator and target cell and also plays a central effector function in inflammatory responses, including production of adhesion molecules and inflammatory mediators such as interleukin 1 (IL-1), tumor necrosis factor (TNF), and platelet-activating factor (PAF).[5-8]

The endothelium also promotes amplification and prolongation of the inflammatory response by facilitating adhesion and emigration by neutrophils and macrophages. These cells, especially the long-lived macrophages, have the potential to secrete additional mediators into the extracellular spaces of the allograft, including neutral proteases, chemotactic factors for other leukocytes, reactive oxygen metabolites, products of arachidonic acid metabolism—especially prostaglandins and leukotrienes, complement components, coagulation factors, growth-promoting factors, PAF, interferon, and cytokines such as IL-1 and TNF.[9-11] These substances are potent amplifiers of tissue damage in the allograft, and their effects are regulated by the interaction of the macrophage with its environment.

The role of macrophages in the expression of allograft rejection is difficult to quantify separately, since these cells are also important in the inflammatory responses and in the subsequent reparative phase. In chapters concerning the pathology of allograft rejection in each solid organ, the reader may note the dearth of comments specifically directed toward the contribution of macrophages. Careful investigations of populations of inflammatory cells in allografts usually ignore the contribution of these cells, probably because they are always present. Some recent publications have described the importance of macrophage activation markers in predicting kidney, liver, and cardiac allograft rejection, as well as inflammation in native hearts with myocarditis.[12-15] These cells are abundant, difficult to study or quantify in routine histologic sections, and act as nonspecific effectors of delayed hypersensitivity in addition to their role in inflammation and repair.

The other important compartment active in inflammation is the blood plasma with its complement kinin and coagulation systems. The complement system functions in inflammation by mediating biologic events that lead to chemotaxis of inflammatory cells (C5a, C5a des Arg), increased vascular permeability (C3a), opsonization (C3b, C3bi), and cell lysis (C5b-9).[16-19] Complement activation can be triggered by antigen-antibody complexes or aggregated IgG, plasmin, endotoxin, or necrotic cells such as myocytes. The kinin and clotting systems can be triggered by activation of Hageman factor (factor XII) because of interaction with collagen or basement membrane, a situation potentiated by ischemic necrosis. Activation of Hageman factor leads to release of bradykinin, a potent mediator of vascular permeability, which amplifies inflammation. Activated Hageman factor also initiates the clotting and fibrinolytic systems, which can lead to further chemotaxis of inflammatory cells, activation of complement components, and recurrent Hageman factor activation that leads to further cyclic inflammatory stimuli.[3, 18]

The coagulation and fibrinolysis systems are tightly regulated by endothelial cell anticoagulant and procoagulant activities. The natural expression of these regulatory substances and their alteration by allograft rejection is the subject of Chapter 4 by Faulk and Labarrere. Alteration of the coagulation and fibrinolytic systems provides a common pathway for both acute and chronic tissue damage regardless of whether the response is initiated by immunologic or inflammatory stimuli.

Another important part of the coagulation system is the platelet.[20] Platelets are inhibited from aggregation by endothelial mechanisms, including elaboration of prostacyclin. Platelets are altered by interaction with injured endothelium, something commonly observed in inflammation, ischemia, and allograft rejection. At such sites, platelets adhere to collagen in the subendothelium, release mediators stored in granules, including adenosine diphosphate (ADP) and fibrinogen, and secrete thromboxane A_2, which promotes further aggregation and activation of intrinsic and extrinsic coagulation pathways.

The foregoing briefly described aspects of inflammation occur during early post-transplant ischemia and are controlled by normal regulatory mechanisms of the host. During later episodes of allograft rejection, other potent activators of inflammation become important, including potentiation of leukocyte adhesion by immune endothelial activation (described in Chapters 1 and 3). Endothelial injury by cytotoxic lymphocyte-mediated reactions, by antibody to HLA or other antigens expressed on the endothelium, or by nonspecific effector macrophage-induced injury during delayed hypersensitivity reaction (DTH) will also potentiate inflammation.[21, 22] Complement activation is an expected part of such allograft reactions: it is facilitated by antigen-antibody complex formation and by macrophage activation occurring as part of delayed hypersensitivity.

Fortunately, inflammation is mitigated by current immunosuppression, especially by the use of corticosteroids; however, few specific therapeutic attempts have been directed at these inflammatory mechanisms that amplify allograft damage. Therapeutic drugs are available to alter coagulation and fibrinolysis (Chapter 4), control reactive oxygen compounds, and inhibit the action of platelets, complement activation, and arachidonic acid metabolites.[3, 4, 7, 20] These strategies, which exert specific effects on aspects of inflammation, are attractive options for future use.

REFERENCES

1. Ryan G, Majno G. Acute inflammation: A review. Am J Pathol 86:185, 1977.
2. Harlan JM. Consequences of leukocyte vessel wall interactions in inflammatory and immune reactions. Semin Thromb Hemost 13:434, 1987.
3. Gallin JI, et al (eds). *Inflammation; Basic Principles and Clinical Correlates.* New York, Raven Press, 1988.
4. Cochrane CG, Gimbrone MA (eds). *Biological Oxidants: Generation and Injurious Consequences.* New York, Academic Press, 1992.
5. Cotran RS. New roles for the endothelium in inflammation and immunity. Am J Pathol 129:407, 1987.
6. McManus LM. Pathobiology of platelet activating factor. Pathol Immunopathol Res 5:104, 1986.
7. Braquet P, Hosford D, Braquet M, Bourgain R, Bussolino R. Role of cytokines and platelet activating factor in microvascular immune injury. Int Arch Allergy Immunol 88:88, 1989.
8. Le J, Vilcek J. TNF and IL1: Cytokines with multiple overlapping biological activities. Lab Invest 56:234, 1987.
9. Unanue ER, Allen PM. The basis for the immunoregulatory role of macrophages and other accessory cells. Science 236:551, 1987.
10. Nathan CF. Secretory products of macrophages. J Clin Invest 79:319, 1987.
11. Johnston RB. Monocytes and macrophages. N Engl J Med 318:747, 1988.
12. Bogman MJT, et al. Diagnosis of renal allograft rejection by macrophage immunostaining with a CD14 monoclonal antibody, WT14. Lancet, 1:255, 1989.
13. Steinhoff G, Wonigeit K, Sorg C, et al. Patterns of macrophage immigration and differentiation in human liver grafts. Transplant Proc 21:398, 1989.
14. Gassel AM, Hansmann ML, Radzun HJ, Weyland M. Human cardiac allograft rejection: Correlation of grading with expression of different monocyte/macrophage markers. Am J Clin Pathol 94:274, 1990.
15. Mues B, Brisse B, Zwadlo G, et al. Phenotyping of macrophages with monoclonal antibodies in endomyocardial biopsies as a new approach to diagnosis of myocarditis. Eur Heart J 11:1, 1990.
16. Ross GD (ed): *Immunobiology of the Complement System.* New York, Raven Press, 1988.
17. Muller-Eberhard HJ. The membrane attack complex of complement. Annu Rev Immunol 4:503, 1986.
18. Samuelsson B, et al. Leukotrienes and lipotoxins: Structure, biosynthesis and biologic effects. Science 237:1171, 1987.
19. Schafer H, Mathey D, Hugo F, Bhakdi S. Deposition of the terminal C5b-C9 complex in infarcted areas of human myocardium. J Immunol 137:1945, 1986.
20. Roth GJ. Platelets and blood vessels: The adhesion event. Immunol Today 13:100, 1992.
21. Cines DB. Disorders associated with antibodies to endothelial cells. Rev Infect Dis 11:705, 1989.
22. Dvorak HF, Galli SJ, Dvorak AM. Cellular and vascular manifestations of cell-mediated immunity. Hum Pathol 17:122, 1986.

1

MECHANISMS OF ALLOGRAFT REJECTION

Robert L. Yowell, MD, PhD, and Barbara A. Araneo, PhD

The advances that have been made in cellular and molecular immunology have led to a better understanding of the biology of solid organ transplantation. Although many controversies remain unresolved, our understanding of the events involved in immunologic recognition at the molecular level and our insight into the requirements for cellular activation have altered our perceptions of allograft rejection. An understanding of current concepts of graft rejection is aided by a knowledge of the structure of lymphocyte antigen receptors and related cell surface antigens. Antigen processing requirements for recognition and activation of graft-reactive lymphocytes must be appreciated. Lymphocyte recirculation pathways and the effector functions of graft reactive cells must be understood.

Following placement of a vascularized organ graft, the host immune system is confronted with foreign antigens that stimulate the humoral and cellular arms of the immune response through genetically related cellular antigen receptors. B cells recognize antigen through well-characterized surface immunoglobulin, which has an antigen-combining site identical to the secreted immunoglobulin effector molecules of that particular clone,[1, 2] associated in the membrane with two additional transmembrane proteins to form the functional B cell antigen receptor complex.[3]

The recognition of antigen by T cells is not as simple; it involves recognition of small peptides of foreign antigens that are "held in place" on the surface of antigen-presenting cells by recipient-encoded cell membrane molecules. The "holder" (on the surface of antigen-presenting cells) is a product of major histocompatibility complex (MHC) genes of the recipient. In allograft immunity, the "antigen being held" (foreign graft antigen) may be a product of major histocompatibility complex (MHC) genes of the donor.[4–6] The presence of foreign antigen, presented in the context of the proper "holder," can then be recognized by T cells bearing receptor molecules specific for the combined "antigen holder plus held antigen" complex (Fig. 1–1).

Our current understanding of transplantation immunity is based on our knowledge of the structure and functions of major histocompatibility antigens, as well as the characterization of T cell antigen receptors. Therefore we present here a brief description of the human MHC and summarize what is known about the T cell antigen receptor.

MAJOR HISTOCOMPATIBILITY COMPLEX

The MHC is a region containing multiple genes that encode the expression of cell surface antigens recognized as foreign on an allograft. In 1936, Gorer described a group of antigens on mouse cells that greatly affected allograft survival.[7] In 1958, Dausset recognized a remarkably similar set of antigens in humans;[8] since these early descriptions,[9] the characterization of the MHC region has been accomplished in many species. However, only recently have immunologists appreciated the

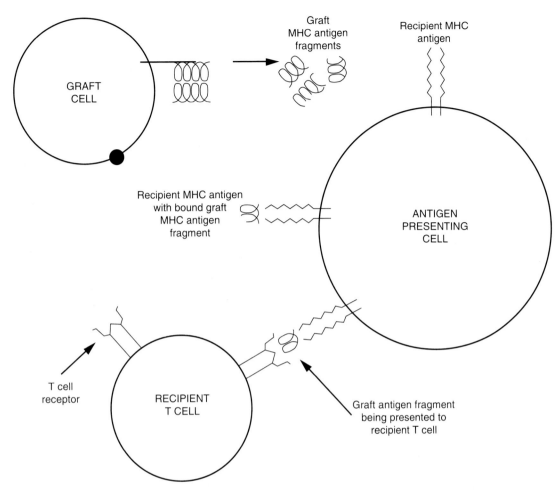

Figure 1–1. Antigen recognition by T cells. Fragments of host cell surface proteins are bound to MHC molecules on host antigen presenting cells. Antigen associated with MHC class I molecules stimulates CD8+ T cells, whereas antigen associated with MHC II cells stimulates CD4+ T cells.

vital role that these molecules serve in cell cooperation, immune response regulation, and antigen recognition by T cells.[10, 11]

In humans, the MHC is termed *human leukocyte antigen* (HLA), and it is located on the short arm of chromosome 6. Six separate loci that code for cell surface antigens have been mapped: beginning from the centromere, these are DP, DQ, DR, B, C, and A. These six loci are highly polymorphic, with as many as 26 different alleles described for the A locus, greater than 40 for the B locus, at least 14 proposed for the C locus, and 56, 30, and 25 alleles proposed for the DR, DQ, and DP loci, respectively.[12] The HLA region also contains several genes encoding soluble proteins involved in the immune system, as well as several genes encoding nonimmune-related proteins[13] (Fig. 1–2). Antigens encoded by the B, C, and

A loci share a common structure and function and are termed class I antigens, whereas DP, DQ, and DR gene products are termed class II antigens. Both class I and class II antigens are transmembrane glycoproteins and are members of the immunoglobulin gene superfamily.[14] Molecules of this family share several interesting properties, including extensive sequence homology and similar three-dimensional structure.[15]

All class I antigens are composed of two polypeptide chains. The α, or heavy, chain is encoded in the MHC, and the light chain of class I antigens is β$_2$-microglobulin[16] (Fig. 1–3). Class I molecules normally bind and present fragments (that is, act as "holders") of antigens to CD8+ cytotoxic T cells (see later). Class I molecules normally present peptides derived from endogenously produced proteins

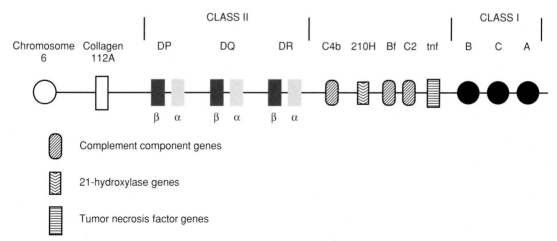

Figure 1–2. The human MHC complex. The HLA complex is found on the short arm of chromosome 6. The number of α and β genes in each MHC class II locus varies among different alleles.

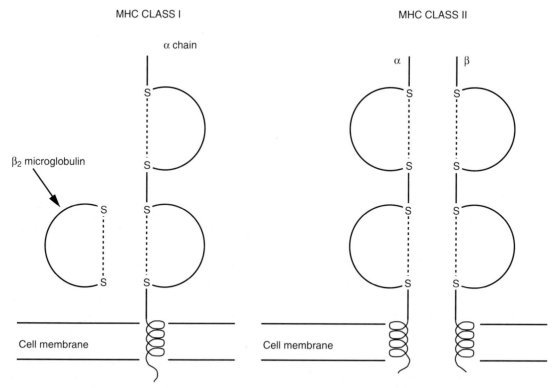

Figure 1–3. Diagram of human MHC class I and MHC class II molecules. MHC molecules span the cell membrane and project into the extracellular space.

and thus offer a mechanism to present samples of intracellular proteins at the cell surface.[17] This allows cytotoxic T cells to check for the expression of nonself peptides, such as virus-derived peptides from infected cells or aberrant peptides from mutated and potentially tumorigenic cells. Class I antigen is expressed on most cell types, but the amount expressed on different cells varies, depending on the degree of differentiation and state of activation; the amount can be regulated up or down by different inflammatory mediators and cytokines.[18] For example, in most cell types studied, interferon-γ (IFN-γ) increases the level of class I molecules expressed on the cell surface. Upregulation of MHC class I potentially can increase the immunogenicity of grafts during episodes of rejection or viral infection. Class I expression is also upregulated by interferon-α and -β, tumor necrosis factor (TNF), and lymphotoxin.[18]

Class II MHC molecules are also composed of two separate polypeptide chains, α and β, which are noncovalently associated within the cell membrane (see Figure 1–3). Both chains are encoded by polymorphic MHC genes. Class II molecules have been shown primarily to present extrinsically derived peptides (foreign antigens) to CD4+ "helper/inducer" T cells.[19, 20] In contrast to MHC class I antigen, class II antigens are constitutively expressed in relatively few cell types. Lymphoid dendritic cells express high levels of class II antigen while circulating mononuclear phagocytes express only low levels.[21] Several cell types, including Langerhans' cells of the epidermis, mononuclear cells, and vascular endothelium, readily express increased levels of MHC class II in response to IFN-γ.[22] MHC class II antigens have been shown to be strong antigens, thus the upregulation of these antigens in a graft as a result of viral infection or a rejection episode also could potentially increase the immunogenicity of the graft and thus trigger or exacerbate rejection episodes.[22] It has been shown immunohistologically that renal tubular epithelial cells, which normally do not express HLA-DR (class II), are induced to express class II during acute rejection episodes.[23] This finding can be useful in distinguishing rejection from cyclosporin toxicity (in which increased class II expression is not seen) in human renal allografts.[23] Irreversible rejection is associated with persistent expression of HLA-DR by tubular epithelial cells.[24] Similar upregulation of class II antigens has been described for graft endothelial cells in human cardiac allografts.[25]

T CELL RECEPTORS

Although CD4+ helper/inducer T cells recognize antigen presented in the context of MHC class II and CD8+, cytotoxic/suppressor T cells recognize antigen presented in association with MHC class I. Both cell subpopulations possess a similar antigen receptor.[26–28] T cell precursors arise in the bone marrow and mature in the thymus. Precursor cells committed to the T cell lineage enter the thymic cortex via the blood vessels. The most immature thymocytes do not express antigen receptors or surface markers characteristic of peripheral T cells; however, during maturation these cells acquire antigen receptors, specific differentiation antigens, and functional capability.[29–31] Concurrent with the maturation process in the thymus, self-reactive clones of thymocytes are eliminated, and MHC restriction is imposed.[27] Thus mature T cells possess clonally expressed T cell antigen receptors (TCR) made up of α and β TCR chains (Fig. 1–4). The α chain of the TCR is a 40- to 50-kD acidic glycoprotein that is covalently linked via a single disulfide bond to the 40- to 45-kD uncharged or slightly basic β chain.[32, 33] There is striking structural similarity between the TCR and immunoglobulin (Ig). Both α and β chains have variable and constant regions separated by a separately encoded J region, as seen in both light and heavy Ig chains. Both α and β chains possess positively charged lysine residues in their transmembrane domains, which are important in the association of the TCR with the CD3 complex[32, 33] (see later).

The hypothesis that the αβ heterodimer recognizes the complex of processed peptide bound to self MHC molecules has been validated by several experimental approaches. The key feature of T cell specificity is linked antigen recognition and MHC restriction; a single receptor confers specificity for both antigen and MHC—that is, the T cell receptor recognizes a "held antigen-antigen holder" complex.[34]

The TCR endows T cells with recognition specificity; however, the cell surface expression of TCR and the ability of T cells to respond to stimulation depends on the presence of associated cell membrane proteins comprising the CD3 molecular complex.[35] The CD3 complex is composed of five distinct polypeptides; γ, δ, ε, η, and ζ (Fig. 1–5). The CD3 complex is thought to transduce activating signal to the T cell cytoplasm. The CD3 complex and the TCR are mutually dependent for cell surface expression, and these molecules are physically associated in the cell membrane.[32]

The CD3 complex is the component against which the therapeutic monoclonal antibody OKT-3 is directed. In humans, this antibody depletes mature T cells from the circulation and is an effective agent for the treatment of acute rejection; however, the initial hopes of inducing graft tolerance with prophylactic OKT-3 administration have not been realized. Recent work in a mouse model[36, 37] has demonstrated that different classes of antibodies directed against cell surface antigens have different immunomodulating effects: the possibility that antibodies to different components of the CD3 complex either preferentially deplete or stimulate T cells is suggested. These studies raise the hope that tolerance-inducing anti-CD3 (or, alternatively, anti-CD4) antibodies may yet be achieved.

The two nonoverlapping subpopulations of mature T cells that possess CD3-TCR complex are distinguished by the expression of either CD4 or, alternatively, CD8 surface antigens. These antigens reflect functional differences in these cell populations.[38] Approximately two thirds of peripheral T cells express CD4 antigen on their surface, recognize peptide antigens in association with MHC class II, and have primarily helper/inducer cell function. The second mutually exclusive subpopulation express CD8 antigen on their surface, recognize peptide antigens in association with MHC class I, and have primarily cytotoxic/suppressor cell function.[38]

The CD4 molecule is a 55-kD, nonpolymorphic monomer possessing four Ig-like domains, a hydrophilic transmembrane sequence, and a 38-residue cytoplasmic tail. CD4 apparently binds to MHC class II molecules and functions as a cell-cell adhesion molecule to stabilize the interaction of CD4 + T cells and antigen-presenting cells[38] (Fig. 1–5).

The CD8 antigen in humans is expressed as

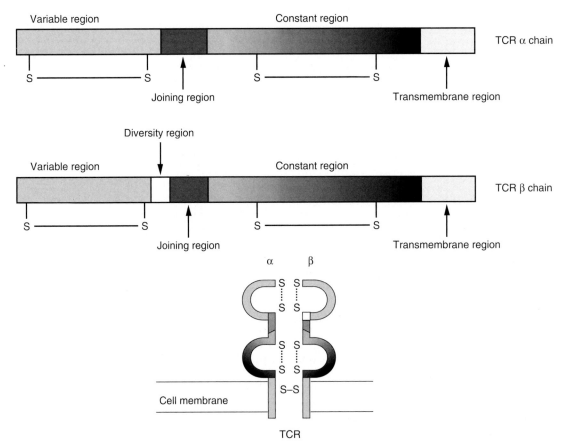

Figure 1–4. Diagram of the structure of the human T cell receptor. The TCR β chain possesses an additional segment between the variable region and the joining region, termed the diversity region.

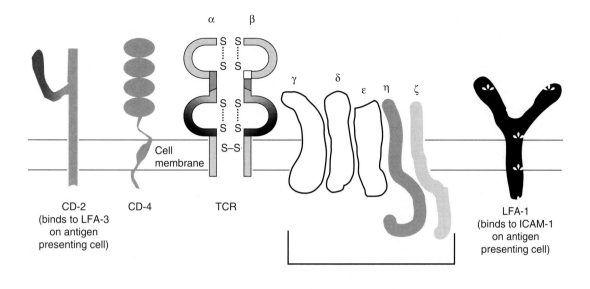

Figure 1–5. T cell surface antigen molecules. In addition to the T cell antigen receptor–CD3 antigen complex, T cells also express LFA-1, CD2, and either CD4 (as shown) or CD8 antigens on the surface. This family of surface molecules is important in cell-cell interactions, cell tissue interactions, and cell antigen interactions.

both a dimer of 34-kD α-polypeptides and as a higher molecular-weight multimer possessing distinct β chains. CD8 apparently binds to MHC class I molecules and functions as a stabilizing cell-cell adhesion molecule.[38]

In addition to CD4/CD8 molecules expressed by T cells, these cells possess accessory membrane proteins that function as cell-cell adhesion molecules and are important in the recirculation patterns of T cells.[39, 40] These molecules are differentially expressed in unprimed versus memory T cells, as well as during different phases of activation[41] (Fig. 1–5).

ALLOGRAFT REJECTION

Since the first descriptions of allograft rejection responses, a vast amount of data from many experimental models have revealed a remarkably precise understanding of the potential immunologic mechanisms involved in acute allograft rejection. Many early controversies have been resolved, and investigators and clinicians appreciate the complexity of interdependent host-graft interactions. The immunology, cell biology, and physiology of chronic rejection are much less clear; attention has been increasingly focused on immunologically triggered inflammatory damage to graft vessels and the reparative responses of these damaged

vessels.[42–44] Alterations of the normal protective anticoagulant and fibrinolytic pathways within allograft vessels and proliferative responses of mural smooth muscle cells are implicated in chronic graft damage[45, 46] (see Chapter 4, page 58).

Allograft rejection is a complex process involving both antigen-specific and nonspecific mechanisms, and both cell-mediated and antibody-mediated effectors can be involved in graft rejection episodes.[47–52] The ultimate goal of clinical monitoring of transplant patients is to determine the relative importance of each mechanism during specific rejection episodes in order to direct treatment effectively. It is clear that the responses seen are influenced by the particular organ grafted, the immune status of the host, and the length of time the graft has been present.

Following placement of a vascularized transplant, a complex series of events is initiated. Graft-derived antigens are released from the graft as a result of ischemia and transplantation (Fig. 1–6). Increasing ischemic time is thought to result in increased graft damage and increased antigen release. This has been especially well studied in kidney grafts and has been correlated with poorer graft survival in both kidney[53] and liver transplants[54] (see Chapter 9, page 160 and Chapter 10, page 187). Released antigen is presented to host CD4 +

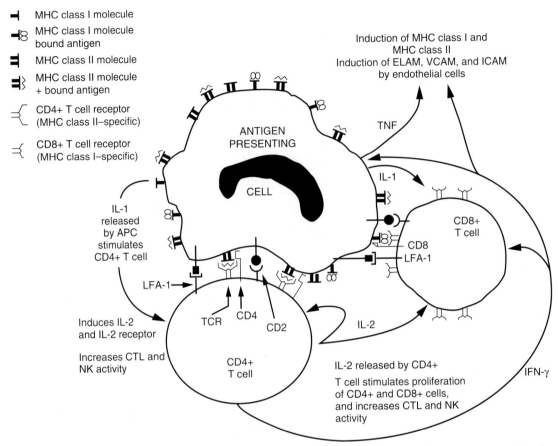

Figure 1–6. T cell activation. T cell antigen presenting cell interactions in T cell activation involve multiple cell surface molecule interactions.

lymphocytes by antigen-presenting cells of both graft and host origin, including macrophages and dendritic cells. This activates specific CD4+ cells, resulting in their initial secretion of IL-2 and subsequent production of IL-3, IL-4, IL-5, IL-6, and interferon-γ. In addition, there is induction of increased expression of IL-2 receptor and proliferation of both CD4+ and CD8+ cells. The release of interferon-γ increases the expression of MHC on graft endothelium,[22] while the later lymphokines induce expansion of antigen-reactive B cell clones.[55, 56]

Cell-mediated responses include antigen-specific cytotoxic T cells (CD8+ cytotoxic/suppressor cells, or cytotoxic T lymphocytes (CTLs), which require cell-to-cell contact between the killer cell and its target (graft parenchymal cell).[57] Cytotoxic T cells secrete substances onto target cells that damage the cell membrane of the target cell and cause its destruction.[57] The main morphologic manifestation of this mechanism is the peritubular lym-

phocytic infiltrates seen in rejecting kidney biopsies (see Chapter 9, page 162), the perimyocytic lymphoid infiltrates seen in rejecting hearts (see Chapter 5, page 74), and the portal infiltrates seen in rejecting liver biopsies (see Chapter 10, page 194).

CD4+ helper/inducer T cells, which do not bind directly to graft cells, are also involved in rejection.[52, 58] Helper/inducer T cells release substances (lymphokines) into surrounding tissues, which, in addition to promoting the proliferation and differentiation of cytotoxic T cells[51] and B cells,[59] recruit nonspecific inflammatory cells, increase vascular permeability, and activate recruited cells[60] (a delayed-type hypersensitivity response, or DTH; Fig. 1–7). DTH responses are manifested as perivascular and interstitial edema, red cell extravasation, and increased numbers of interstitial macrophages in graft biopsies. The resulting graft dysfunction is probably related to impaired tissue perfusion and relative ischemia.

Antibody responses can include specific

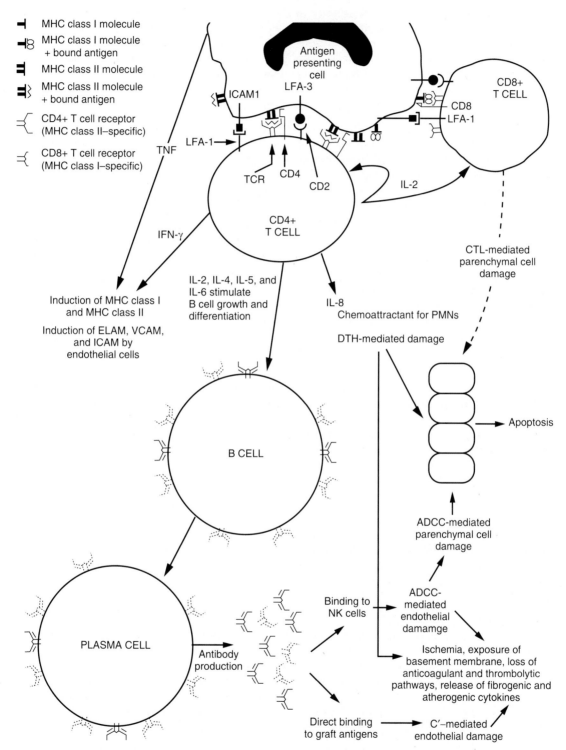

Figure 1–7. Schematic illustration of immunologic mechanisms in allograft rejection.

complement-activating antibody responses to graft cell antigens. The clearest example of this mechanism is hyperacute rejection, in which preformed circulating antibodies present in the host bind to specific graft endothelial antigens and activate complement.[61-63] Histologically, one sees margination of neutrophils and extensive graft vessel thrombosis. Antibody can also enhance graft damage by natural killer (NK) cells.[64] These NK cells are also known as large granular lymphocytes: one important attribute is their membrane receptor for IgG (Fc receptor). Allograft-specific antibody can enhance the binding of NK cells to graft tissues via Fc receptors. Significant numbers of NK cells infiltrating human allografts have been reported during episodes of acute rejection in both renal[65] and cardiac[66] transplants.

Antibody deposition has been implicated in both acute[67] and chronic[68, 69] allograft rejection; however, the pathogenesis of this deposition is unclear; it may result from direct antibody-mediated endothelial damage or, alternatively, may reflect altered vascular permeability mediated by delayed-type hypersensitivity (DTH) reaction.

T Cell Arm of Allograft Rejection

Early studies of immunologically naive[70] and subsequently T cell–deficient mice (thymectomized or congenitally athymic mice) established the critical role of T cells in graft rejection.[71] Reconstitution experiments demonstrated restoration of graft rejection responses with T cells but not with antibodies (serum). Further animal experiments led to the recognition of two functionally distinct subpopulations of T cells. The obvious question to be answered is, what role does each T cell subpopulation serve in graft rejection? Are both subpopulations necessary, or can one or both function independently? Studies designed to answer this basic question generated a great deal of controversy in the transplantation field.[reviewed in 72] Adoptive transfer experiments of different T cell subpopulations and studies of the surface markers (CD4 versus CD8) of graft-infiltrating cells gave often contradictory results and fueled the dispute over the relative importance of cytotoxic versus DTH mechanisms.[reviewed in 73] Results depended on the animal model used, the organ transplanted, and the specific methods used for eliminating differing T cell populations. Fur-

ther confusion arose from differences in subpopulations required for the initiation versus the effector phases of immunity and was compounded by different subset requirements for primary versus secondary responses.

Extensive work from several groups has resolved many of the controversies and explained discrepancies of results. Insights from cell biology, immunogenetics, and transplantation have converged, resulting in a general consensus regarding salient features of cell-mediated acute allograft rejection:[74-78]

1. There is support for involvement of both specific CTL-mediated graft damage and classic DTH responses where effector T cells release cytokines that activate macrophages and induce them to cause tissue damage.

2. The initiation of rejection responses following transplantation of a vascularized organ graft requires helper/inducer cells that support the proliferation and differentiation of cytotoxic T cells through the elaboration of the lymphokine IL-2.

3. In addition to providing helper function for cytotoxic T cells (IL-2-mediated proliferation and differentiation of CD8+ cells), the lymphokines released from CD4+ helper T cells also stimulate B cell proliferation and differentiation and thus augment antibody-mediated damage.

4. CD4-mediated DTH responses have a primary role in allograft damage early in rejection episodes (see DTH responses following).

5. Graft-infiltrating cytotoxic T lymphocytes usually express CD8; although CD8+ cytotoxic cells are often the predominant cell type in graft cytotoxic responses, they are not absolutely essential for graft rejection.

6. Non-CTL–mediated graft rejection has been observed in human kidney and heart rejection, and in these cases vascular damage is the common attribute.

Delayed-Type Hypersensitivity in Allograft Rejection

The activation of CD4 cells by graft-antigens also instigates DTH responses. Early in DTH responses the effector cell is the activated macrophage. Thus DTH responses are highly specific in *initiation phase* but are nonspecific in *effector phase*.[73, 79] The release of IL-2 by CD4+ T cells recruits macrophages and other leukocytes to sites of antigen recognition and results in activation of macrophages, which then secrete IL-1 and TNF.[57] Activated T cells also secrete interferon-γ, which also activates macrophages and induces the upregulation of HLA class II molecules on antigen-presenting cells, including macrophages and graft endothelial cells.[80] In addition, upregulation of MHC antigen expression by endothelial cells induced by interferon-γ and TNF results in increased expression of endothelial adhesion molecules[81]—initially endothelial leukocyte adhesion molecule-1 (ELAM-1), which binds polymorphonuclear cells (PMNs), and subsequently intercellular adhesion molecule-1 (ICAM-1) and vascular cell adhesion molecule-1 (VCAM-1), which bind lymphocytes and monocytes.[82–84]

Thus DTH responses have two profound effects on graft endothelium; first, antigen presentation is enhanced, and second, leukocyte adhesion to vessels at the site of antigen release is promoted. The presence of activated macrophages triggers further inflammatory changes, with increase of vascular permeability, migration of leukocytes out of vessels, leakage of serum components into the interstitium, and red cell extravasation. The resultant edema and poor tissue perfusion cause acute ischemic graft damage.[85]

In studies of human skin grafts,[86] the predominant cell type in perivascular infiltrates was CD4+ cells, consistent with an important DTH component. The relative importance of DTH responses can only be inferred from the histologic appearance of biopsy specimens, characterized as perivascular infiltrates, interstitial edema, and endothelial cell activation, and indirectly from immunophenotyping of graft infiltrating cells.[86] The fact that DTH responses result in the release of many soluble mediators that can affect surrounding bystander cells suggests that DTH responses may be as important in chronic rejection as in acute rejection (see the following).

T Cell–Mediated Cytotoxicity in Allograft Rejection

The differentiation of CTL precursors into functional cytotoxic cells requires two signals.[87] The first signal consists of antigenic peptide fragments bound to class I MHC, presumably on graft cells. The binding of relevant antigen to precursor CD8 cells induces the synthesis of the p55 subunit of the IL-2 receptor and thus results in the expression of a complete IL-2 receptor on CD8 cells. As a consequence, these CD8+ cells acquire responsiveness to CD4 helper cell–derived IL-2. Under the influence of IL-2, IL-6, and interferon-γ released by CD4+ helper cells, graft-specific CD8+ cytotoxic cell precursors undergo proliferation, clonal expansion, and differentiation. Differentiation involves acquisition of cytolytic granules and the ability to transcribe and secrete cytokines, including IL-2. The amount of IL-2 produced by CTLs is insufficient to support the differentiation of naive CTL precursors but may be sufficient to support secondary CTL responses.[72] This may explain the observation in animal adoptive transfer experiments that primed cytotoxic responses are much less dependent on CD4 cells.

CD8+ T cells then infiltrate the graft, specifically bind to target cells bearing foreign peptides bound to foreign class I MHC molecules, and cause specific graft damage. Cytotoxic cell lysis of target cells is antigen specific, requires cell-cell contact, and does not result in the killing of the cytotoxic cell. At least two separate mechanisms are operative in target cell destruction.[(reviewed in 88)] In a calcium ion dependent mechanism, pore-forming molecules are released from CTL granules and in the presence of extracellular concentrations of calcium polymerize in target cell plasma membranes to form ion channels. If present in sufficient numbers, these pores induce osmotic damage of target cells. A second pathway involves release of lymphotoxin. This molecule is a serine protease that activates target cell enzymes that cleave target cell DNA, leading to apoptosis of target cells. CTLs apparently escape damage because of increased expression of membrane proteins that depolymerize the pore-forming protein and inactivate the lymphotoxin serine esterase.

Antibody-Mediated Responses in Allograft Rejection

Antibody-mediated rejection has been clearly demonstrated in renal allografts and more recently in cardiac allografts.[62, 89–95] The most dramatic demonstration of antibody-mediated rejection occurs in the face of preformed antidonor antibodies and is recognized as hyperacute rejection. This form of rejection is usually clinically obvious, with impaired graft function immediately or very soon after re-establishment of graft blood flow. Histologically, this form of rejection is recognized by vascular damage, with capillary thrombosis proceeding to necrosis. In hyperacute rejection of the kidney, there is cortical necrosis with glomerular thrombosis, often with neutrophil infiltrate of the graft and arterial necrosis. In heart biopsies, capillary congestion, with thrombosis of venules and arterioles and margination and infiltration of the myocardium by neutrophils and interstitial hemorrhage, is accompanied by hypereosinophilia of myocytes, contraction band formation, and disruption of intercalated discs, leading to separation of myocytes.[63] Liver allografts have shown a resistance to cytotoxic antibody-mediated rejection; however, evidence is emerging that there is significantly decreased liver allograft survival in cross-match–positive recipients compared with cross-match–negative recipients.[93] Histologically, failed liver allografts demonstrated vascular damage in five of six grafts characterized as coagulative necrosis of the hepatic parenchyma, venular or arterial thrombosis, and neutrophilic infiltration.[93]

The ability of preformed MHC class I antibodies to cause hyperacute rejection is well recognized.[89] With modern histocompatibility testing, this complication is rare; however, hyperacute rejection resulting from preformed antibody to vascular endothelial cell antigens has been described in both renal and cardiac transplantation.[90, 96] In these cases direct immunofluorescence stains demonstrate the presence of antibodies on the surface of vascular endothelial cells, accompanied by vascular deposition of C3, C1q, and fibrin. Acute vascular rejection with vascular immune complexes has been described in human renal allografts and more recently cardiac allografts.[63, 92]

Mechanisms of Chronic Allograft Rejection (Vasculopathy)

As the short-term results with transplantation have improved, attention has been focused on understanding the mechanisms involved in chronic rejection. Steady improvement in 1-year survival rates in both renal and cardiac transplantation, resulting from enhancements in organ preservation, surgical techniques, and treatment of acute rejections and infection, has not been matched in success in decreasing the annual rate of graft loss after the first year post-transplant. Chronic rejection is the major factor responsible for late graft loss in renal and cardiac transplants.[86, 87]

Chronic rejection in kidney and heart allografts is characterized primarily by manifestations of vascular damage, whereas in liver transplants progressive loss of bile ducts is the major determinant of long-term prognosis.[49] Bile duct loss is associated with large vessel changes similar to those of heart and kidney grafts.[96] The histopathologic findings characteristic of chronic rejection in renal transplants are concentric narrowing of arteries and arterioles (vasculopathy), with resultant interstitial fibrosis and tubular atrophy and loss secondary to chronic ischemia.[97] Glomeruli commonly show evidence of ischemia characterized by atrophy and sclerosis, with collapse of capillary tufts. Some kidneys demonstrate transplant glomerulopathy, which is manifest as two distinct histopathologic patterns that may reflect different mechanisms of injury.[98] Segmental sclerosis, which can be a reflection of altered perfusion, is one pattern recognized in chronic rejection. A second pattern demonstrates mesangial expansion, with thickening of capillary walls and simplification of lobularity. This pattern is characterized ultrastructurally by lucent subendothelial widening similar to the appearance in hemolytic uremic syndrome.

Chronic rejection in heart allografts is characterized by diffuse coronary artery vasculopathy.[99–101] In contrast to the eccentric atherosclerosis affecting major epicardial vessels of native hearts, graft atherosclerosis in heart transplants is usually concentric and diffusely affects graft vessels from major epicardial branches down through penetrating arteries to smaller intramyocardial arteries and arterioles. Ultrastructurally, one sees evidence of myocyte ischemia, with loss of myofilaments and compensatory hypertrophic changes and interstitial fibrosis, as well as evidence of small vessel disease with endothelial alteration and reduplication of external lamina.[102]

The diffuse involvement of graft vasculature has been taken as evidence to support the hypothesis that vasculopathy results from diffuse immunologic injury in response to graft endothelial antigens.[44] Both endothelial cells and smooth muscle cells become activated following vessel wall injury, and both respond to immunologically derived cytokines and produce additional growth factors.[103–105]

The immunologic mechanisms involved in chronic rejection remain controversial. Humoral immunity is implicated from studies of immunoglobulin deposits within vessel walls. Donor-specific antibody has been shown to induce atherosclerosis in susceptible animals,[106] and the risk of developing graft vasculopathy is increased in cardiac allograft patients shown to have vascular deposition of immunoglobulin; however, it is likely that additional mechanisms may be important. DTH responses to vascular alloantigens with release of inflammatory cytokines are likely contributors. Upregulated class II antigen on endothelial cells is often found in chronically rejected allografts, supporting the hypothesis that DTH is playing a role. The finding that CD8+ cells are strong inducers of class II antigen on endothelium suggests that CD8+ cells may serve an important role.[107, 108]

It is known that heparin sulfate proteoglycan matrix surrounding vascular smooth muscle cells inhibits smooth muscle cell proliferation. Rejection results in a loss of heparin sulfate matrix, and this may be important in allowing the proliferation of vascular smooth muscle cells[109] seen in graft vasculopathy.

The local release of IL-1 and TNF-α can induce the production of platelet-derived growth factor–like (PDGF) protein by endothelial cells and vascular smooth muscle cells,[110] as well as induce the expression of PDGF receptors.[111] PDGF can have mitogenic and fibrogenic effects within the vessel wall.[112]

Thus, there are many specific and nonspecific mechanisms that may play a role in allograft rejection.

REFERENCES

1. Kehry A. The immunoglobulin μ chains of membrane-bound and secreted IgM molecules differ in their C-terminal segments. Cell 21:393, 1980.
2. Alzari PM, Lascombe M, Poljak RJ. Three-dimensional structure of antibody. Annu Rev Immunol 6:555, 1988.
3. Reth M. Antigen receptors on B lymphocytes. Annu Rev Immunol 10:97, 1992.
4. Lechler RI, Lombardi G, Batchelor JR, Reinsmoen N, Bach FH. The molecular basis of alloreactivity. Immunol Today 11:83, 1992.
5. Duquesnoy RJ, Trager JDK, Zeevi A. Propagation and characterization of lymphocytes from transplant biopsies. Crit Rev Immunol 10:455, 1991.
6. Zeevi A, Fung J, Zerbe TR, Kaufman C, Rabin BS, Griffith BP, Hardesty RL, Dusquenoy RJ. Allospecificity of activated T cells grown from endomyocardial biopsies from heart transplant patients. Transplantation 41:620, 1986.
7. Gorer PA. The detection of antigenic differences to mouse erythrocytes by the employment of immune sera. Br J Exp Pathol 17:42, 1936.
8. Dausset J. Iso-leukoanticorps. Acta Haematologica 20:156, 1958.
9. Medawar PB. The immunology of transplantation. In The Harvey Lectures 1956–1957. New York, Academic Press, 1957, p 144.
10. Strominger JL. Structure of products of the major

11. histocompatibility complex in man and mouse. Prog Immunol 4:541, 1980.
11. Silver J. Genetic and structural organization of murine IA and human DR antigens. Crit Rev Immunol 2:225, 1981.
12. Committee Report. Nomenclature for factors of the HLA system, 1990. Hum Immunol 31:186, 1991.
13. Trowsdale J, Campbell RD. Physical map of the human HLA region. Immunol Today 9:34, 1988.
14. Williams AF. A year in the life of the immunoglobulin superfamily. Immunol Today 8:298, 1987.
15. Abbas AK, Lichtman AH, Pober JS. Cellular and Molecular Immunology. Philadelphia, WB Saunders, 1991, p 144.
16. Bjorkman PJ, Saper MA, Samouri B, Bennett WS, Strominger JL, Wiley DC. Structure of the human class I histocompatibility antigen HLA-A2. Nature 329:506, 1987.
17. Monaco JJ. A model of MHC class-I-restricted antigen processing. Immunol Today 13:173, 1992.
18. Pober JS, Lapierre LA, Stolpin AH, Brock TA, Springer TA, Fier W, Bevilacqua MP, Mendrick DL, Gimbrone MA Jr. Activation of cultured human endothelial cells by recombinant lymphotoxin; Comparison with tumor necrosis factor and interleukin-1 species. J Immunol 138:3319, 1987.
19. Neefjes JJ, Ploegh HL. Intracellular transport of MHC class II molecules. Immunol Today 13:179, 1992.
20. Babbitt BP, Allen PM, Matsueda G, Haber E, Unanue E. Binding of immunogenic peptides to Ia histocompatibility molecules. Nature 317:359, 1985.
21. Klein J. Natural History of the Major Histocompatibility Complex. New York, John Wiley, 1986.
22. Skoskiewicz MJ, Colvin RB, Schneeberger EE, Russell PS. Widespread and selective induction of MHC-determined antigens in vitro by interferon-gamma. J Exp Med 162:1645, 1985.
23. Hall BM, Bishop GA, Duggin GG, Horvath JS, Phillips J, Tiller DJ. Increased expression of HLA-DR antigens on renal tubular cells in renal transplants; relevance to the rejection response. Lancet 2:247, 1984.
24. von Willebrand E, Salmela K, Isoniemi H, Krogerus L, Taskinen E, Hayry P. Induction of HLA class II antigen and interleukin-2 receptor expression in acute vascular rejection of human kidney allografts. Transplantation 53:1077, 1992.
25. Rabin BS, Griffith BP, Hardesty RL. Vascular endothelial cell HLA-DR antigen and myocyte necrosis in human allograft rejection. Heart Transplant 4:293, 1985.
26. Marrack P, Kappler JW. The antigen specific, major histocompatibility complex-restricted receptor on T cells. Adv Immunol 38:1, 1986.
27. Davis MM, Bjorkman PJ. T-cell antigen receptor genes and T-cell recognition. Nature 334:395, 1988.
28. Davis MM. T cell receptor gene selection. Annu Rev Biochem 59:475, 1990.
29. Adkins B, Mueller C, Okada CY, Reichert R, Weisman IL, Spangrude GJ. Early events of T cell maturation. Annu Rev Immunol 5:325, 1987.
30. Fowlkes BJ, Pardoll DM. Molecular and cellular events of T cell development. Adv Immunol 44:207, 1989.
31. von Boehmer H. Developmental biology of T cell receptor transgenic mice. Annu Rev Immunol 8:531, 1990.
32. Clevers H, Alarcon B, Wileman T, Terhorst C. The T

cell receptor/CD-3 complex: A dynamic protein ensemble. Annu Rev Immunol 6:629, 1988.

33. Allison JP, Lanier LL. Structure, function and serology of the T cell antigen receptor complex. Annu Rev Immunol 5:503, 1987.

34. Marrack P, Kappler J. The antigen-specific, major histocompatibility complex-restricted receptor on T cells. Adv Immunol 38:1, 1986.

35. Alcover A, Ramarli D, Richardson NE, Chang H-C, Reinherz EL. Functional and molecular aspects of human T lymphocyte activation via T3, Ti and T11 pathways. Immunol Rev 95:5, 1987.

36. Darby CR, Morris PJ, Wood KJ. Evidence that long-term cardiac allograft survival induced by anti-CD4 monoclonal antibody does not require depletion of CD4+ T cells. Transplantation 54:483, 1992.

37. Morris PJ, Wood KJ, Dallman MJ. Antigen-induced tolerance to organ allografts. Ann NY Acad Sci 670:295, 1992.

38. Parnes JR. Molecular biology and function of CD4 and CD8. Adv Immunol 44:265, 1989.

39. Springer TA, Dustin ML, Kishimoto TK, Marlin SD. The lymphocyte function associated LFA-1, CD-2 and LFA-3 molecules: Cell adhesion receptors of the immune system. Annu Rev Immunol 5:223, 1987.

40. Shimizu Y, Newman W, Tanaka Y, Shaw S. Lymphocyte interactions with endothelial cells. Immunol Today 13:106, 1992.

41. Mackay CR. T-cell memory: The connection between function, phenotype and migration pathways. Immunol Today 12:189, 1991.

42. Sedmak DD, Orosz CG. The role of vascular endothelial cells in transplantation. Arch Pathol Lab Med 115:260, 1991.

43. Colvin RB. Cellular and molecular mechanisms of allograft rejection. Annu Rev Med 41:361, 1990.

44. Paul LC, Fellstrom B. Chronic vascular rejection of the heart and the kidney—have rational treatment options emerged? Transplantation 53:1169, 1992.

45. Labarrere CA, Pitts D, Halbrook H, Faulk WP. Natural anticoagulant pathways in normal and transplanted human hearts. J Heart Lung Transplant 11:342, 1992.

46. Faulk WP, Gargiulo P, McIntyre JA, Bang NU. Hemostasis and fibrinolysis in renal transplantation. Semin Thromb Hemost 15:88, 1989.

47. Mason DW, Morris PJ. Effector mechanisms in allograft rejection. Annu Rev Immunol 4:119, 1986.

48. Donnelly P, Henderson R, Fletcher K, Stratton A, Lennard T, Wilson R, Proud G, Taylor R. Specific and non-specific immunoregulatory factors and renal transplantation. Transplantation 44:523, 1987.

49. Tilney NL, Whitley WD, Diamond JR, Kupiec-Weglinski JW, Adams DH. Chronic rejection—an undefined conundrum. Transplantation 52:389, 1991.

50. Lafferty KJ, Prowse SJ, Simeonovic CJ. Immunobiology of tissue transplantation: A return to the passenger leukocyte concept. Annu Rev Immunol 1:143, 1983.

51. Winn HJ. Antibody mediated rejection. *In* Williams GM, Burdick JF, Solez K (eds). *Kidney Transplantation Rejection.* New York, Marcel Dekker, 1986.

52. Hall BM, Dorsch SE. Cells mediating allograft rejection. Immunol Rev 77:31, 1984.

53. Cho YW, Terasaki PI, Graver B. Fifteen-year kidney graft survival. *In* Terasaki P (ed). *Clinical Transplants 1989.* Los Angeles, UCLA Tissue Typing Laboratory, 1989, p 325.

54. Howard TK, Klintmalm GBG, Cofer JB, Husberg BS,

Goldstein RM, Gonwa TA. The influence of preservation injury on rejection in the hepatic transplant recipient. Transplantation 49:103, 1990.

55. Arai K, Lee F, Miyajima A, Miyatake S, Arai N, Yokota T. Cytokines: Coordinators of immune and inflammatory responses. Annu Rev Biochem 59:783, 1990.

56. Smith KA. The interleukin-2 receptor. Annu Rev Cell Biol 5:397, 1989.

57. Kupfer A, Singer SJ. Cell biology of cytotoxic and helper T-cell functions. Annu Rev Immunol 7:309, 1989.

58. Bishop DK, Shelby J, Eichwald EJ. Mobilization of T lymphocytes following cardiac transplantation: Evidence that CD4-positive cells are required for cytotoxic T lymphocyte activation, inflammatory endothelial development, graft infiltration, and acute allograft rejection. Transplantation 53:849, 1992.

59. Bradley JA, Sarawar SR, Porteous C, Wood PJ, Card S, Ager A, Bolton EM, Bell EB. Allograft rejection in CD4+ T cell–reconstituted athymic nude rats—the nonessential role of host-derived CD8+ cells. Transplantation 52:477, 1992.

60. Paul WE, Ohara J. B-cell stimulatory factor/interleukin 4. Annu Rev Immunol 5:429, 1987.

61. Kissmeyer-Nielsen F, Olsen S, Peterson VP, Fjeldborg O. Hyperacute rejection of kidney allografts associated with pre-existing humoral antibodies against donor cells. Lancet 2:662, 1966.

62. Patel R, Terasaki PI. Significance of the positive cross-match test in kidney transplantation. N Engl J Med 280:735, 1969.

63. Trento A, Hardesty RL, Griffith BP, Zerbe T, Kormos RL, Bahnson HT. Role of the antibody to vascular endothelial cells in hyperacute rejection in patients undergoing cardiac transplantation. J Thorac Cardiovasc Surg 95:37, 1988.

64. Perussia B, Trinchieri G, Jackson A, Warner NL, Faust J, Rumpold H, Kraft D, Lanier LL. The Fc receptor for IgG on human natural killer cells: Phenotypic, functional, and comparative studies with monoclonal antibodies. J Immunol 133:180, 1984.

65. Blancho G, Buzelin F, Dantal J, Hourmant M, Catarovich D, Baatard R, Bonneville M, Vie H, Bugeon L, Soulillou JP. Evidence that early acute renal failure may be mediated by CD3−/CD16+ cells in a kidney graft recipient with large granular lymphocyte proliferation. Transplantation 53:1242, 1992.

66. Marboe CC, Knowles DM II, Chess L, Reemtsma K, Fenoglio JJ Jr. The immunologic and ultrastructural characterization of the cellular infiltrate in acute cardiac allograft rejection; Prevalence of cells with natural killer (NK) phenotype. Cell Immunol Immunopathol 27:141, 1983.

67. Morris PJ, Williams GM, Hume DM, Mickey MR, Terasaki PI. Serotyping for homotransplantation. XII. Occurrence of cytotoxic antibodies following kidney transplantation in man. Transplantation 6:392, 1968.

68. Hammond EH, Yowell RL, Price GD, Menlove RL, Olsen SL, O'Connell JB, Bristow MR, Doty DB, Millar RC, Karwande SV, Jones KW, Gay WA Jr, Renlund DG. Vascular rejection and its relationship to allograft coronary artery disease. J Heart Transplant 11(part II):S111, 1992.

69. Petrossian GA, Nichols AB, Marboe CC, Sciacca R, Rose EA, Smith CR, Canno PJ, Reemtsma K, Powers ER. Relation between survival and development of coronary artery disease and anti-HLA antibodies after cardiac transplantation. Circulation 80Suppl III:122, 1989.

70. Billingham RE, Brent L, Medawar PB. Quantitative studies on tissue transplantation immunity. II. The origin, strength and duration of actively and adoptively acquired immunity. Proc R Soc Lond (Biol) 143:58, 1954.
71. Miller JFAP. Role of the thymus in transplantation tolerance and immunity. *In* Wolstenholme GEW, Cameron MP (eds). *Transplantation.* London, Churchill, 1962, p 397.
72. Hall BM. Cells mediating allograft rejection. Transplantation 51:1141, 1991.
73. Rosenberg AS, Singer A. Cellular basis of skin allograft rejection: An in vivo model of immune-mediated tissue destruction. Annu Rev Immunol 10:333, 1992.
74. Mintz B, Silvers WK. Histocompatibility antigens on melanoblasts and hair follicle cells. Cell localized homograft rejection in allophenic skin grafts. Transplantation 9:497, 1970.
75. Waldmann H. Manipulation of T cell responses with monoclonal antibodies. Annu Rev Immunol 7:407, 1989.
76. Tyler JD, Galli SJ, Snider ME, Dvorak AM, Steinmuller D. Cloned cytolytic T lymphocytes destroy allogeneic tissue in vivo. J Exp Med 159:234, 1984.
77. Hancock WW, Thompson NM, Adkins RC. Composition of interstitial cellular infiltrate identified by monoclonal antibodies in renal biopsies of rejecting human allografts. Transplantation 35:458, 1983.
78. Kolbeck PC, Tatum AH, Sanfilippo F. Relationships among the histologic pattern, intensity and phenotypes of T cells infiltrating renal allografts. Transplantation 38:709, 1984.
79. Mason DW, Dallman MJ, Arthur RP, Morris PJ. Mechanisms of allograft rejection: The role of cytotoxic T cells and delayed-type hypersensitivity. Immunol Rev 77:167, 1984.
80. Pober JS, Collins T, Gimbrone MA, Libby P, Reiss CS. Inducible expression of class II major histocompatibility complex antigens and the immunogenicity of vascular endothelium. Transplantation 41:141, 1986.
81. Pober JS, Cotran RS. Cytokines and endothelial cell biology. Physiol Rev 70:427, 1990.
82. Butcher EC. Cellular and molecular mechanisms that direct leukocyte traffic. Am J Pathol 136:1, 1990.
83. Osborn L. Leukocyte adhesion to endothelium in inflammation. Cell 62:3, 1990.
84. Duijvestin A, Hamann A. Mechanisms and regulation of lymphocyte migration. Immunol Today 10:23, 1989.
85. Forbes RDC, Gomersall M, Lowry RP, Blackburn J. Cellular mechanisms of cardiac allograft rejection. Heart Transplant 3:300, 1984.
86. Bhan AK, Mihm MC Jr, Dvorak HF. T cell subsets in allograft rejection: *In situ* characterization of T cell subsets in human skin allografts by the use of monoclonal antibodies. J Immunol 129:1579, 1982.
87. Wilson DB, Howard JC, Nowell PC. Some biological aspects of lymphocytes reactive to strong histocompatibility alloantigens. Transplant Rev 12:3, 1972.
88. Cerotini JC, MacDonald HR. 17th Forum in Immunology: Molecular mechanisms of T-cell mediated cytotoxicity. Ann Inst Past Immunol 138:287, 1987.
89. Halloran PF, Schlaut J, Solez K, Srinivasa N. The significance of the anti-class I response. Transplantation 53:550, 1992.
90. Cerilli J, Brasile L, Galousis T, Lempert N, Clarke J. The vascular endothelial cell antigen system. Transplantation 39:286, 1985.
91. Sibley RK, Payne W. Morphologic findings in the renal allograft biopsy. Semin Nephrol 5:294, 1985.
92. Hammond EH, Yowell RL, Nunoda S, Menlove RL, Renlund DG, Bristow MR, Gay WA Jr, Jones KW, O'Connell JB. Vascular (humoral) rejection in heart transplantation: Pathologic observations and clinical implications. J Heart Transplant 8:430, 1989.
93. Takaya S, Bronsther O, Iwaki Y, Nakamura K, Abu-Elmagd K, Yagihashi A, Demetris AJ, Kobayashi M, Todo S, Tzakis AG, Fung JJ, Starzl TE. The adverse impact on liver transplantation of using positive cytotoxic crossmatch donors. Transplantation 53:400, 1992.
94. Smith JD, Danskine AJ, Rose ML, Yacoub MH. Specificity of lymphocytotoxic antibodies formed after cardiac transplantation and correlation with rejection episodes. Transplantation 53:1358, 1992.
95. Wray DW, Baldwin WM, SanFilippo F. IgM and IgG alloantibody responses to MHC class I and II following rat renal allograft rejection. Transplantation 53:167, 1992.
96. Fennell RH. Ductular damage in liver transplant rejection. Pathol Annu 16(part II):289, 1981.
97. Kasiske BL, Kalil RSN, Lee HS, Rao KV. Histopathologic findings associated with a chronic, progressive decline in renal allograft function. Kidney Int 40:514, 1991.
98. Maryniak RK, First MR, Weiss MA. Transplant glomerulopathy: Evolution of morphologically distinct changes. Kidney Int 27:799, 1985.
99. Uys CJ, Rose AG. Pathologic findings in long-term cardiac transplants. Arch Pathol Lab Med 108:112, 1984.
100. Gao SZ, Schroeder JS, Alderman EL, Hunt SA, Silverman JF, Wiederhold V, Stinson EB. Clinical and laboratory correlates of accelerated coronary artery disease in the cardiac transplant patient. Circulation 76(Suppl 5):V56, 1987.
101. DeCampli WM, Johnson DE, Gao SZ, Schroeder JS, Billingham M, Stinson EB, Shumway NE. Transplant coronary vascular disease: Histomorphometric properties and clinical correlations. Curr Surg 45:477, 1988.
102. Hammond EH, Hansen JK, Spenser LS, Jensen A, Riddell D, Craven CM, Yowell RL. Vascular rejection in cardiac transplantation: Histologic, immunopathologic, and ultrastructural features. Cardiovasc Pathol 2:1, 1993.
103. Busch GJ, Galvanek EG, Reynolds ES Jr. Human renal allografts: Analysis of lesions in long-term survivors. Hum Pathol 2:253, 1971.
104. Libby P, Salomon DD, Payne FJ, Schoen FJ, Pober JS. Functions of vascular wall cells related to development of transplantation-associated coronary arteriosclerosis. Transplant Proc 21:3677, 1989.
105. Pober JS. Cytokine-mediated activation of vascular endothelium. Am J Pathol 133:426, 1988.
106. Friedman RJ, Moore S, Singal DP. Repeated endothelial injury and induction of atherosclerosis in normolipemic rabbits by human serum. Lab Invest 32:404, 1975.
107. Doukas J, Pober JS. Lymphocyte-mediated activation of cultured endothelial cells (EC); CD4+ T cells inhibit EC class II MHC expression despite secreting IFN-γ and increasing EC class I MHC and intercellular adhesion molecule-1 expression. J Immunol 145:1088, 1990.
108. Bender JR, Pardi R, Kosek J, Engelman EG. Evidence that cytotoxic lymphocytes alter and traverse alloge-

neic endothelial cell monolayers. Transplantation 47:1047, 1989.

109. Clowes AW, Clowes MM, Kocher O, Ropraz P, Chaponnier C, Gabbiani G. Arterial smooth muscle cells in vivo: Relationship between actin isoform expression and mitogenesis and their modulation by heparin. J Cell Biol 107:1939, 1988.

110. Hajjar KA, Hajjar DP, Silverstein RL, Nachman RL. Tumor necrosis factor–mediated release of platelet-derived growth factor from cultured endothelial cells. J Exp Med 166:235, 1987.

111. Fellstrom B, Klareskog L, Larsson E, Tufveson G, Wahkberg J, Ronnstrand L, Heldin CH, Terracia L, Rubin K. Tissue distribution of macrophages, class II, transplantation antigens and receptors for platelet-derived growth factor (PDGF) in normal and rejected human kidneys. Transplant Proc 19:3625, 1987.

112. Williams LT, Antoniades HN, Goetzl EJ. Platelet-derived growth factor stimulates 3T3 cell mitogenesis and leucocyte chemotaxis through different structural determinants. J Clin Invest 72:1759, 1983.

Chapter

APPLICATION OF TRANSPLANT BIOPSY CULTURE TECHNIQUES TO THE UNDERSTANDING OF ALLOGRAFT REJECTION

2

JOHN F. CARLQUIST, PHD

Since the early work of Medewar and Billingham established the involvement of cells as mediators of graft rejection,[1-3] an understanding of its underlying cellular mechanisms has been an eagerly sought after—and occasionally elusive—goal. Much of the effort to elucidate these mechanisms has been driven by the need to develop specifically directed immunosuppressive therapy. The result has been the progression of transplantation from the era of corticosteroid immunosuppression (with its attendant risk for infection) to the present, with the availability of immunosuppressive agents that specifically interfere with T cells (cyclosporine, FK506, OKT3) or with the function of T cell subsets (OKT4). However, with advancing knowledge came the additional awareness of the complexities that attend graft rejection and the variety of forms in which it can appear; organ recipients may experience a broad spectrum of antigraft responses, from mild self-limiting rejection to rapidly life-threatening vascular or cellular rejection. Thus, the present challenge is to continue to unravel the mysteries that surround the interrelationship between the immune system and foreign tissue. With this added understanding, it is foreseen that there will also come an improvement in diagnostic, prognostic, and therapeutic abilities.

EARLY STUDIES OF CELLULAR EFFECTORS OF GRAFT REJECTION

The examination of cellular changes in the peripheral blood following transplantation was the point of departure for many studies of organ rejection. Since the cells responsible for graft rejection gain access to the grafted tissue via the circulation, this approach is founded in logic; it has, however, met with only limited success. In one reported study,[4] the investigators concluded that morphologic evaluation of peripheral blood and the monitoring of the proportions of lymphocyte subpopulations and subsets (CD4 and CD8) was an effective means of differentiating between graft rejection and infection. Infections could be further subdivided into viral versus bacterial or fungal infections based on the cellular contents of the peripheral blood. Despite the apparent optimism generated by such a report, substantiation of these observations has been slow to appear.

Using morphologic and phenotypic criteria, Hanson and colleagues found that 83 per cent of patients experiencing rejection had an increase in the number of activated peripheral blood lymphocytes.[5] Unfortunately, the same blood findings were observed for 81 per cent of patients without rejection. Likewise, quantification of CD4 and CD8 T cells was not found to be diagnostic of rejection. In a similar study, shifts in the proportions of CD4 to CD8 T cells were found to occur in conjunction with cytomegalovirus and *Pneumocystis carinii* infections, but no association was noted between subset alterations and graft rejection.[6] Thus, the authors of both of these reports concluded that the peripheral blood markers identifiable by currently available techniques are not sufficiently specific to aid in the diagnosis of acute rejection.

The apparent lack of correlation between peripheral blood findings and graft rejection appears to be based on physiologic mechanisms. Functional studies have shown that graft-derived T cells are highly cytolytic to donor target cells whereas simultaneously obtained peripheral blood lymphocytes are not.[7] This functional discrepancy between peripheral blood and graft-derived T cells is presumably the result of the migration pattern of T cell subsets. Memory T cells are programmed to migrate into tissues in which they were originally stimulated and into other tissues under conditions of inflammation. Likewise, inflammation stimulates the entry of naive T cells into lymph nodes.[8] Thus, lymphocyte activation in response to a graft may not necessarily be reflected in the peripheral blood.

An alternative approach is the staining of graft-infiltrating cells in situ in an attempt to demonstrate the cells most commonly associated with rejection.[9-13] Most of the studies using this approach have described only the graft infiltrate observed during acute rejection. Under these conditions, the infiltrate is predominantly of the CD8+ phenotype; although these reports are of value, they fail to address the issue that graft rejection is a dynamic process involving multiple cell types at different stages.

Hancock and coworkers used in situ staining to examine serially obtained renal biopsy specimens.[9] This study showed that the number of activated lymphocytes (expressing the interleukin-2 (IL-2) receptor) was maximal at 10 to 12 days post-transplant (14.6 per cent of cells) and decreased significantly beyond that time interval (2.2 per cent of cells). This indicates that, at a maximum, less than one third of the T cells present within these specimens were functionally mature T cells. As discussed by the investigators, this observation raises questions about the actual contribution to the rejection process of the remainder of these precursor T cells.

Thus, this method for examining the cell types involved in rejection can be misleading: many cell types may be present (particularly in the presence of inflammation), but the principal elements with respect to initiation and mediation of rejection may be difficult to ascertain against the background "noise" present in the cellular infiltrate. An additional problem with this approach is that for those patients receiving OKT3 therapeutically, mouse immunoglobulin can be present in the perivascular spaces during periods of inflammation. Extravasated mouse immunoglobulin has been found to interfere with the antimouse second antibodies used for the indirect staining of cells and to cause problems with interpretation.[14]

INTERLEUKIN-2 (IL-2) AND THE IL-2 RECEPTOR: REGULATION OF THE IMMUNE RESPONSE

The immune system has evolved a complex system of regulatory mechanisms through which control of immune functions is maintained. This control is accomplished through many receptor-ligand pairs that act cooperatively in producing stimulatory or suppressive signals as they are needed for host survival. One of the first described and most extensively examined immunologic regulatory mechanisms is the interleukin-2 (IL-2) system. IL-2 (originally named T cell growth factor) is produced and secreted predominantly by activated CD4+ T helper lymphocytes and is required—along with antigen stimulation—to induce T lymphocyte proliferation.[15] The action of IL-2 is mediated through its binding to its high affinity receptor that is expressed by T lymphocytes following the contact with foreign antigen. This high affinity receptor is composed of two glycoproteins, each of which individually possesses low-intermediate IL-2 binding affinity. The first described IL-2 binding molecule is the p55 (55 kD) or T activating (TAC) receptor (dissociation constant [K_d] of approximately 10^{-8} M). A later discovered IL-2 receptor is the p70 (70 to 75 kD) glycoprotein, which has a K_d of approximately 10^{-9} M.[16-18]

Upon T cell activation by ligation of the T cell receptor by foreign peptide (or alloantigen), the p55 and p70 protein chains form a noncovalently associated heterodimeric complex that exhibits high affinity ($K_d = 10^{-11}$ M) binding of IL-2.[19] Additionally, the cell undergoes a transition from the G_0 to the G_1 state, but further progression through the cell cycle does not occur without IL-2. Subsequent to IL-2 binding to the high affinity IL-2 receptor (IL-2R), however, the T cell will undergo mitosis and clonal proliferation.[20, 21] In this manner, IL-2 can stimulate division of the cell from which it was released (autocrine stimulation) or can act as a growth factor for nearby antigen-activated T cells (paracrine stimulation).

This interplay between antigen and cytokine affords the host a system of checks and balances through which the level and duration of immune activation can be controlled. The requirement for antigen binding prior to expression of the IL-2R precludes the nonspecific activation of the entire T cell population by a cascade of IL-2 release. Further, this system specifically directs the attention of the immune system to an invading microorganism or allogeneic tissue through the clonal expansion of only those T cells with receptors capable of recognizing the foreign epitopes (see Chapter 1, pages 8, 9).

Finally, negative regulation of a specific immune response has been shown to correspond to a reduction in the surface density of IL-2R that occurs rapidly upon removal of the activating signal.[21] This control of ongoing clonal proliferation can also be facilitated by other lymphocyte subsets through the release of another cytokine (IL-10) that suppresses IL-2 production and T cell proliferation.[22] Thus, the evolution of this complex regulatory scheme appears to have been directed by the need for control of the immune responses to prevent overwhelming T cell activation that would prove detrimental to the host.

USE OF IL-2 IN VITRO TO EXPAND CLONES OF IN VIVO ANTIGEN-ACTIVATED T CELLS; APPLICATIONS TO GRAFT REJECTION

Several investigators have explored the potential of exploiting the two signal requirements (antigen plus IL-2) to obtain quantities of in vivo–activated T cells. This approach is based on the assumption that only T cells expressing the high affinity IL-2 receptor (as a result of antigen activation) will proliferate in vitro when provided with a physiologic concentration of IL-2. The presence of activated T cells is readily detected microscopically as dividing cells and growth clusters (Fig. 2–1B), and large quantities of these cells can be ob-

tained for experimental purposes. In contrast, no proliferative response is seen when no activated T cells are present (Fig. 2–1A).

This approach has received much attention as a means for isolating tumor-specific activated T cells from solid tumors.[23] These cells have been used for experimental immunotherapy[24] or to study the biology of the T cell response to tumor growth.[25] In addition to these applications of this method, IL-2 expansion of activated lymphocytes has been applied successfully to the study of the rejection of a number of solid organ grafts, including kidney,[7] heart,[14] pancreas,[26] cornea,[27] and liver.[28]

Several independent studies have shown that there is a strong correlation between increasing severity of rejection, as determined histologically, and the percentage of specimens positive for T cell growth. In our investigation, we examined 271 specimens from 44 heart recipients. The percentages of culture positivity for each of the histologic grades are presented in Figure 2–2. The histologic grading has been described elsewhere.[14] Briefly, the grading is as follows: grade 1, *no evidence of rejection*, and grade 2, *cannot rule out mild rejection*—these two grades are considered as ISHLT 0; grade 2.5, *focal mild rejection*—ISHLT 1A; grade 3, *mild rejection*—ISHLT 1B and 2; grade 4, *moderate rejection*—ISHLT 3A and B; grade 5, *severe rejection*—ISHLT 4.

T cell proliferation was observed for 70.9 per cent of specimens obtained during rejection, 51.9 per cent from biopsies graded as equivocal (grade 2, ISHLT 0), and 28.9 per cent of histologically negative specimens (grade 1, ISHLT 0). There was an overall highly significant association between histologic diagnosis of rejection and culture positivity ($p < 0.001$, chi-square).

Weber and colleagues obtained remarkably similar findings with respect to the correlation between culture positivity and histologic findings.[29] In their study, T cell growth was seen for 80 per cent of specimens histologically graded as mild-severe rejection, approximately 50 per cent of specimens graded as "minimal" rejection, and approximately 30 per cent of specimens without cellular infiltrates. These observations indeed support the premise that culture positivity is associated with graft rejection.

PHENOTYPES OF LYMPHOCYTES CULTURED FROM ALLOGRAFTS

One approach to furthering our understanding of graft rejection has been the study

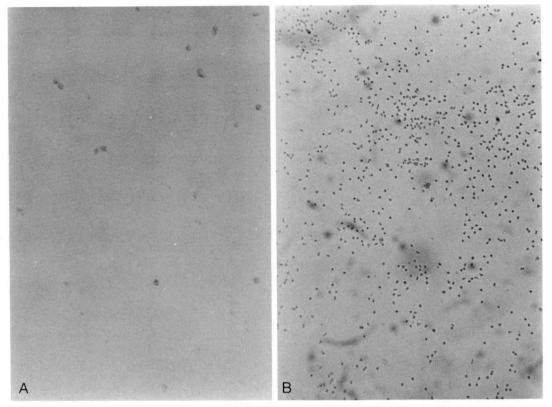

Figure 2–1. *A*, Negative, and *B*, positive IL-2-induced lymphocyte growth from tissue obtained from cardiac allografts. (× 40)

of cells that infiltrate an allograft before and during acute rejection. The intent of these studies has been to identify the processes and events that ultimately lead to graft loss, with the hope of identifying elements that may be

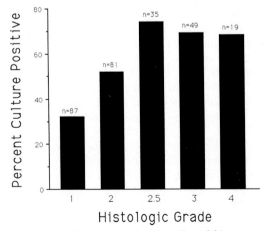

Figure 2–2. The percent of cardiac allograft biopsy specimens (n = 271) within each histologic grade positive for lymphocyte growth.

amenable to therapeutic intervention. The phenotypes of cells infiltrating solid organ grafts have been examined both in situ and in IL-2 expanded lymphocyte cultures. The findings suggest that acute rejection involves a multitude of cell types, but certain phenotypic patterns can be discerned.

One prevailing issue that has been repeatedly addressed is the extent of correlation between the types of cells that can be identified immunohistologically in tissue sections and populations of cells expanded in tissue culture. Two independent studies of acutely rejecting kidneys, one performing phenotype analysis of cells in frozen sections (n = 8)[30] and the other for cultures of IL-2 expanded lymphocytes (n = 4),[31] found similar proportions of CD4+ T cells (20 ± 37 per cent and 15 ± 3 per cent, respectively) and CD8+ T cells (48 ± 7 per cent and 61 ± 8 per cent, respectively). Thus, there appears to be overall concordance between the two methods. In a third study, however, in which parallel comparisons of the two methods for identifying phenotypes of graft-infiltrating cells were made, individual variations were seen. The T cell phenotypes infiltrating six acutely rejecting renal allografts were determined as noted: in situ and in culture. No difference was found with respect to the overall mean percentage of CD8 + T cells detected by the two methods (in situ: 66 per cent; culture: 53 per cent; p = 0.32). However, for three of the six kidney allografts (50 per cent), the predominant phenotype (CD4 or CD8) alternated, depending upon the method used.[32]

A possible explanation for this discrepancy is the inherent differences between the methods. Culture identifies only activated T cells in tissue specimens, as opposed to in situ identification, which does not discriminate between alloactivated mediators of rejection and nonspecifically accumulating cells. In this regard, IL-2 expansion acts as a "filter" eliminating nonspecific inflammatory infiltrate. This difference between methods may be increasingly important during severe rejection, when the nonspecific component of the infiltrate becomes large.[33, 34]

Phenotypic information pertaining to the T cell subsets that can be recovered from allograft biopsies by IL-2 stimulation has been obtained, but firm conclusions regarding the significance of these subsets are lacking. We characterized phenotypically 28 T cell cultures obtained from heart allograft biopsies. Of the 28, 17 were predominantly CD4+, and 11 were predominantly CD8+; the mean percentage of CD4+ T cells identified in all cultures was 48.8 ± 7 per cent and 41.9 ± 8 per cent for CD8+. No correlation was apparent between phenotype and severity of rejection; HLA matching studies failed to show a correlation between culture phenotype and the degree of mismatch.

We were able to conclude, however, that there appears to be consistency with respect to the T cell phenotype of multiple cultures obtained serially from the same individual. We followed six heart recipients and obtained a mean of three cultures (range: 2 to 5) from each recipient. Biopsies from four of the six patients consistently gave rise to T cell cultures of the same phenotype (three were CD4+, one was CD8+), even when the biopsies were obtained as far apart as 60 days.

A confounding factor in the attempt to identify a clinical correlation for T cell subsets is the effect of different immunosuppressive protocols. Certain immunosuppressants have been shown to favor differentially the recovery in culture of certain T cell phenotypes. In one study, for example, CD8 cells were the predominant phenotype recovered from patients treated with azathioprine/prednisone, but for patients receiving cyclosporine and azathioprine, CD8 and CD4 T cells were found in equal numbers.[32]

Although the information presently available regarding the phenotype(s) of graft-derived T cell cultures is somewhat intriguing, conclusions regarding the significance of these subsets are generally difficult to obtain in the clinical setting. Less confusing information relative to the significance of the individual T cell subsets has come from the use of animal models of transplantation and is discussed later.

DONOR HLA SPECIFICITY OF GRAFT-DERIVED LYMPHOCYTES

The most compelling evidence implicating graft-derived lymphocytes in the rejection process has come from the demonstration of the donor HLA-specific alloreactivity of these cells. In one study, Moreau and colleagues obtained 55 clones of T cells (22 CD8+ and 33 CD4+) from a rejected human kidney by culturing graft tissue in IL-2.[31] Testing of these clones in a cell-mediated cytotoxicity assay revealed that 14 of 33 (42 per cent) of the CD4+ T cells and 21 of 22 (95 per cent) of the CD8 T cell clones were cytotoxic against donor-derived target cells. In addition, all 55 clones demonstrated proliferative responses when stimulated with donor B cells; all clones were nonreactive when stimulated with autologous B cells. Finally, five of the CD4+ clones (15 per cent) were found to be IL-2 producers; the production of this cytokine was deemed specific in that IL-2 was not produced in the absence of donor antigen stimulation.

Mayer and associates generated bulk T cell cultures from needle biopsy specimens from transplanted kidneys undergoing rejection.[7] They tested these cultures for a proliferative response against a panel of stimulator cells that shared from 0 to 4 HLA antigens with the respective organ donors. To assess the proliferative response, the amount of tritiated thymidine incorporated into newly synthesized DNA was measured in T cells cocultured with stimulator cells. The results were reported as a stimulation index. The median stimulation index in response to donor HLA antigens was 14 (14-fold increase over control levels); the median stimulation index observed for stimulator cells unrelated to the graft donors was 1.5. Thus, in these experiments, the specificity of these graft-derived T cells for HLA antigens of the graft donor was clearly established.

In a similar study, investigators employed cultures of graft-infiltrating lymphocytes (GIL) grown from heart biopsies obtained serially post-transplantation to study changes in the HLA specificity of the GIL cultures as a function of time.[35] In this report, the investigators describe the use of the primed lymphocyte test (PLT) to assess the reactivity of the cultured T cells in response to a panel of stimulator cells. The PLT is a short-term (3-day) blastogenesis (DNA synthesis) assay measuring tritiated thymidine uptake. The HLA phenotypes for the donor-recipient combinations and the HLA specificities of the PLT are presented in Table 2–1. The first culture isolated from recipient 1 at 4 days post-transplantation (heart biopsy 1.4) showed minimal activity when challenged with a panel of 11 stimulator cells expressing a variety of HLA specificities. However, cultures of GIL isolated from the same recipient on days 17, 43, and 62 following transplantation all showed HLA DR1 (donor)–specific proliferation.

The second heart recipient in their study showed an interesting pattern of response. A culture grown from a biopsy specimen obtained 13 days following transplantation responded in the PLT assay to the donor A11 antigen. A second biopsy specimen 9 days later (day 22 post-transplantation) gave rise to a culture that reacted with Bw4, a public specificity encoded at the HLA B locus. A third biopsy specimen, on day 29 post-transplantation, possessed alloreactivity that was specific for both donor DR antigens—DR1 and DR4. The unusual feature of these findings is the sequential generation of GIL cultures that identify disparities at all three HLA loci—A, B, and DR. This is clearly in contrast to the other three patients for whom serial GIL cultures showed alloreactivity directed to a single HLA specificity.

The third patient in this series experienced a moderate-severe rejection episode 8 days after transplantation. This was the highest grade rejection episode in the study and, paradoxically, the GIL-generated T cell cultures had very weak PLT activity; no specificity for any HLA antigen could be identified. Cultures derived from histologically normal biopsy specimens taken at days 14 and 22 post-transplantation were reactive with the donor DR3 and DR4 antigens.

With respect to patient 3, it is of interest that T cells isolated at the peak of a rejection episode should show weak reactivity when tested against the panel of stimulator cells. However, it has previously been shown that at the time of maximal cellular infiltration and inflammation, there is a nonspecific cellular component for which target specificity is unknown.[33, 34] It is possible that the HLA specificity of graft-infiltrating T cells is most easily demonstrated during the induction phase of a rejection episode, and that a dilution of the HLA-specific T

Table 2–1. Relation of T Cell Phenotype and PLT Specificity of Cultured Lymphocytes to Biopsy Histology

HLA Phenotype			Heart Biopsy	T Cell Phenotype			PLT Specificity
A	B	DR		Leu4	Leu3	Leu2	
R: 2, —	44, 60	2, 5	1.4	98	93	4	No activity
D: 2, —	35, 57	1, —	1.17	96	80	15	DR1
			1.43	—	13	70	DR1
			1.62	—	—	—	DR1
R: 3, 23	7, 18	2, 6	2.13	—	37	49	All
D: 11, 23	44, 51	1, 4	2.22	96	55	25	Bw4
			2.29	—	—	—	DR1, DR4
R: 3, 26	7, 14	—, —	3.8	98	10	77	Weak activity
D: 2, 11	8, 62	3, 4	3.14	—	—	—	DR4 (DRw53)
			3.22	95	89	1	DR4 (DRw53), DR3
R: 2, 3	27, 44	7, —	4.9	—	—	—	DR5
D: 3, 26	14, 51	1, 5	4.25	—	—	—	DR5 (+w6)
			4.38	97	6	93	DR5 (+w6), DR1

From Zeevi A, Fung J, Zerbe TR, Kaufman C, Rabin BS, Griffith BP, Hardesty RL, Duquesnoy RJ. Allospecificity of activated T cells grown from endomyocardial biopsies from heart transplant patients. Transplantation 41:620, 1986.

cells by this nonspecific infiltrate occurs as inflammation increases. This hypothesis offers an explanation for the noted results but remains to be tested.

Finally, GIL cultures obtained from the fourth graft recipient on days 9, 25, and 38 post-transplantation (corresponding to histologically normal, minimal rejection, and mild rejection, respectively) were all specific for DRw5; the culture generated from the day 38 biopsy specimen also had specificity for the second donor DR antigen—DR1. Thus, this study confirms other reports of HLA specificity of graft-derived T cell cultures.

An additional feature of interest in this particular investigation was the phenotypic characterization of the GIL cultures as to the relative percentages of CD4+ and CD8+ T cells (Table 2–1). This is of interest because, for the case of nominal antigen (e.g., foreign peptide) recognition, the CD8 T lymphocyte subset interacts with MHC class I (HLA A, B, and C) expressing antigen-presenting cells (APC). CD4-expressing T cells share a similar relationship with MHC class II (HLA DR, DQ, and DP) expressing APC.[36, 37] The question has been raised whether these rules for nominal antigen recognition also apply to allorecognition. These studies revealed a noted departure from these rules. Patient 1 showed consistent reactivity of GIL cultures with the donor-specific DR1 antigen. However, one DR1-reactive T cell culture was predominantly CD4+ (80 per cent), and another was predominantly CD8+ (70 per cent). A CD8+ T cell response to DR antigens was also seen for patient 4 (day 38 culture). These cells were 93 per cent CD8+, but the PLT reactivity was directed to both the DR3 and DR5 antigens of the donor. These findings suggest that additional factors may be operative that can influence the cellular response to donor antigens, and that CD8+ T cells can, under certain circumstances, have recognition capability for class II–bearing target cells.

In a companion study, the same investigators concluded that the HLA specificity of the alloreactive cells grown in culture correlated with the histologic pattern of cellular infiltrate observed in tissue sections.[38] They showed that reactivity with class II–bearing target cells was associated with low histologic grades and a focal pattern of cellular infiltrate. By contrast, isolation of MHC class I–reactive T cells from biopsy material corresponded to the occurrence of cellular infiltrates of higher grade histologically characterized as a diffuse pattern.

The foregoing studies illustrate that IL-2–responsive T cells isolated from transplanted solid organs possess reactivity directed (in general) to MHC antigens of the organ donor. The appearance of these cells in culture indicates a graft-directed immune response mediated by the recipient. Thus, this method has potential for diagnostic and prognostic applications and provides a window through which the initiation and progression of graft rejection can be viewed.

RELATIONSHIP BETWEEN IL-2–INDUCED LYMPHOCYTE PROLIFERATION AND DONOR MHC ANTIGEN EXPRESSION

The correlation between the isolation of IL-2–responsive T cells from biopsy material, the occurrence of graft rejection, and the specificity of these T cells for HLA antigens of the graft donor has been discussed. It remains, however, to examine the sequence of events and signalling mechanisms that lead to the appearance of IL-2–responsive T cells within the graft.

Allograft rejection is initiated by the interaction of immunocompetent lymphocytes of the recipient with donor MHC antigens expressed on passenger mononuclear cells and the cells of the grafted organ. The inducible expression of class II antigens on the surface of vascular endothelium of the graft and its constitutive expression on passenger mononuclear cells suggests an important role for class II expression in the generation of a rejection episode. Thus, we hypothesized a relationship between class II expression and the appearance of IL-2–responsive T cells within the graft.

For this study, the intensity and distribution of HLA DR antigen were assessed in serial sections of cardiac allograft biopsy specimens stained with a mouse monoclonal antibody directed against a nonpolymorphic epitope of all human DR antigens.[39] Visualization was accomplished by staining with a fluorescein isothiocyanate (FITC)-conjugated goat antimouse second antibody. The staining for HLA DR was semiquantitatively graded independently from 1+ to 5+ by two readers. Two patterns of HLA DR distribution were identified: DR expressed on the vascular endothelium of graft and DR molecules expressed on interstitial (intermyocytic and perivascular) infiltrating mononuclear cells. We were able to analyze relationships retrospectively between the pattern and quantity of DR expression, the isolation of IL-2–responsive (activated) T cells, and the histologic diagnosis for 212 biopsies. The results suggest that these variables are interrelated.

T cell proliferation and DR expression (both patterns) were maximal for those specimens that were histologically judged as normal but retrospectively were found to precede an episode of acute rejection by a mean ($\pm$ SE) of 6 $\pm$ 0.4 days (prerejecting specimens). These data are shown in Figure 2–3. Thus, upregulation of DR expression on the vascular endothelium of the graft and infiltration of the myocardium with activated T cells (and other DR-expressing mononuclear cells) are events that take place early in the rejection process and may be useful as an early diagnostic indicator.

It is of interest that there was a slight decrease in the per cent positivity for DR expression (both patterns) and T cell proliferation for specimens that were obtained during rejection. The contribution of immunosuppressive therapy to this observation is probably significant, but other factors should be considered. It has been shown, for example, that IL-2 can effect the downregulation of its own receptors as a negative regulatory control.[21] Moreover, interferon-γ, a T cell product that causes upregulation of DR expression, can be antagonized by E series prostaglandins,[40] glucocorticosteroids,[41] and intracellular increases in cAMP.[42, 43] Finally, IL-10, a product of a subpopulation of CD4+ T cells, can suppress interferon-γ and IL-2 production, and antigen-specific proliferation.[44] Experience has shown that mild (and occasionally severe) rejection episodes can be self-limited and resolve without treatment. Therefore, it is probable that the observed decrease in DR expression and T cell growth coincident to a rejection episode are responses to negative regulatory control mechanisms.

Vascular and interstitial DR expression appear to be independently regulated. The mean scores for these two patterns as a function of histologic grade are shown in Figure 2–4. The vascular pattern was maximal for specimens graded as focal mild rejection—ISHLT 1A—and decreased thereafter. The interstitial pattern, by contrast, was at its lowest level of expression for ISHLT 1A specimens and was highest for ISHLT 3A and B specimens (i.e., correlates with histologic assessment). Statistical analysis of the mean score/grade for the two patterns indicated that these two variables

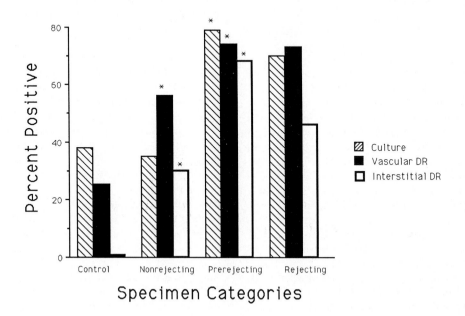

* Significantly elevated over previous category

Figure 2–3. Comparison of cardiac allograft specimen categories with respect to the percent positive for culture growth, vascular DR staining, and interstitial DR staining. (From Carlquist JF, Hammond ME, Yowell RL, O'Connell JB, Anderson JL. Correlation between class II antigen (CDR) expression and interleukin-2–induced lymphocyte proliferation during acute cardiac allograft rejection. Transplantation 50:582, 1990.)

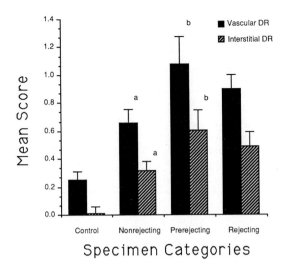

a p<0.002 (compared to previous category).

b p<0.05 (compared to previous category).

Figure 2–4. Comparison of mean scores for vascular and interstitial DR staining for different categories of specimens for cardiac allografts. (From Carlquist JF, Hammond ME, Yowell RL, O'Connell JB, Anderson JL. Correlation between class II antigen (CDR) expression and interleukin-2–induced lymphocyte proliferation during acute cardiac allograft rejection. Transplantation 50:582, 1990.)

are not correlated (p = 0.87, Spearman correlation).

A correlation was established, however, between increased expression of vascular DR and culture positivity. As shown in Table 2–2, the mean vascular fluorescence score was higher for culture-positive specimens than for culture-negative specimens in each histologic grade (p < 0.02, Mann-Whitney). No correlation was noted between interstitial fluorescence scores and culture growth. Thus, the coincident occurrence of vascular DR upregulation and T cell activation suggests (not unexpectedly) that these events are functionally linked.

Other investigators similarly demonstrated that increased MHC class II expression correlated with the percentage of heart biopsy specimens that produced T cell growth.[45] They also reported that increased class II expression could be demonstrated in advance of histologically recognizable rejection.

It is clear that the increased expression of donor MHC antigens and T cell activation are important early events in the onset of acute rejection. Activation of CD4+ T cells in response to alloantigens results in the release of interferon-γ, which further upregulates MHC class II expression on a number of cell types, including endothelium. Whereas this can

cause further T cell activation, DR expression on capillary endothelium has also been shown to facilitate exit of lymphocytes from the circulation into the surrounding tissues by promoting lymphocyte-endothelial adhesion.[46] Lymphocyte adhesion to vascular endothelium is greatly increased following priming of T cells against the allotypic HLA antigens expressed on the endothelial surface of a foreign capillary.[47] Thus, although the initiating factors may be variable, it appears that once begun, these events form a "vicious cycle" leading to recruitment and accumulation of a cellular infiltrate in the grafted organ. MHC class II expression and the acquisition of the IL-2 receptor are key elements in the initiation and maintenance of this cycle.

DIAGNOSTIC APPLICATIONS OF T CELL CULTURES FROM ALLOGRAFTS

Early studies, our own and elsewhere, discovered the seemingly paradoxic growth of T cells from specimens histologically graded as either negative or equivocal. It is now recognized that this observation indicates early immunologic activity within the graft occurring before progression to a stage that can be recognized microscopically. Thus, the appearance of activated, IL-2–responsive T cells within the graft provides the potential for early diagnosis of graft rejection and has been applied in this manner by a number of transplant centers. For example, to assess the predictive significance of a positive culture, we followed the clinical course of 64 heart transplant patients with ISHLT 0, Utah grade 2 biopsies, 33 of which had positive cultures and 29 of which were culture negative. The histologic gradings for the next scheduled biopsy for these patients are given in Figure 2–5. Of those patients with positive cultures, 51.1 per cent progressed to a rejection episode; only 9 per cent of patients with a positive culture showed histologic improvement (to Utah grade 1) by the next scheduled biopsy. In contrast, follow-up of culture-negative patients revealed that 24.1 per cent progressed to rejection, versus 34.5 per cent of whom improved to a Utah grade 1 status (p < 0.03). Thus, the growth of T cells from graft tissue can be used prognostically.

Cultures of graft-infiltrating lymphocytes can also be used to predict success of treatment for acute rejection.[48] This was demonstrated in a study performed at our institution in which patients with histologically diagnosed

Table 2–2. Comparison of Mean Fluorescence Scores (Both Vascular and Interstitial) Between Culture-Positive and Culture-Negative Specimens

	Vascular (n)		Interstitial (n)	
Grade	Culture-Positive	Culture-Negative	Culture-Positive	Culture-Negative
1	0.83 ± 0.2 (18)	0.43 ± 0.1 (37)	0.22 ± 0.1 (18)	0.27 ± 0.1 (37)
2	0.73 + 0.1 (41)	0.61 ± 0.1 (35)	0.35 ± 0.1 (41)	0.42 ± 0.1 (35)
2.5	1.00 ± 0.2 (12)	ND*	0.29 ± 0.1 (12)	ND*
3	0.94 ± 0.2 (23)	0.75 ± 0.2 (14)	0.52 ± 0.2 (23)	0.46 ± 0.2 (14)
4	0.93 ± 0.2 (14)	0.71 ± 0.2 (7)	0.72 ± 0.2 (14)	0.72 ± 0.1 (7)
Means	0.87 ± 0.1 (108)	0.59 ± 0.1 (93)	0.41 ± 0.1 (108)	0.36 ± 0.1 (93)
		p < 0.02†		p = NS‡

*Not done due to small sample size (n = 3).
†By Mann-Whitney U-test.
‡Not significant.
From Carlquist JF, Hammond ME, Yowell RL, O'Connell JB, Anderson JL. Correlation between class II antigen (CDR) expression and interleukin-2–induced lymphocyte proliferation during acute cardiac allograft rejection. Transplantation 50:582, 1990.

rejection (Utah grades 3 to 4, ISHLT 1B and 2—i.e., requiring treatment) were grouped as to culture-positive or culture-negative at the time of diagnosis of rejection. These two groups were followed and the cumulative incidence of a second rejection following therapy determined. These results are shown in Figure 2–6. There was a greater than twofold increase in the incidence of rejection in the culture-positive group (72 per cent compared with 35 per cent for culture-negative patients) at day 14 following initiation of therapy. The rate of rejection for the culture-positive group was still increased (97 per cent versus 71 per cent) at the termination of the study at 60 days after first diagnosis of rejection. The biologic implications of these results are as yet unknown;

however, the observation that immunosuppressive therapy does not abrogate the risk for rejection associated with T cell growth implies that additional factors may be operative.

We have also observed that the cultures grown from cardiac allografts have broad variability in their in vitro susceptibility to antithymocyte globulin (ATG). Using a viability assay to test the sensitivity of graft-derived T cells to ATG, we found a range of concentrations from 0.01 to 0.09 mg/ml that were able to effect a 50 per cent reduction in viability of the culture (LD_{50}). It is of interest that the highest LD_{50} values were associated with prolonged rejection episodes.[14] Thus, this method holds promise as a means of detecting sensitivity to this and possibly other immunosuppressive drugs.

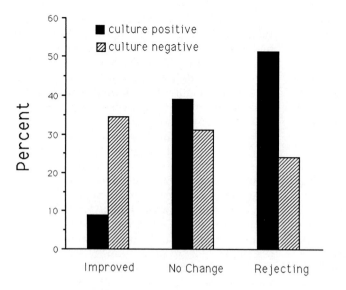

Figure 2–5. The use of lymphocyte culture as a predictor of histologic changes for cardiac allografts. The data presented are the histologic findings for the next scheduled biopsy following a grade 2 (cannot rule out mild rejection) biopsy. Culture results are for the first (grade 2) biopsy.

Histologic Evaluation of Next Biopsy

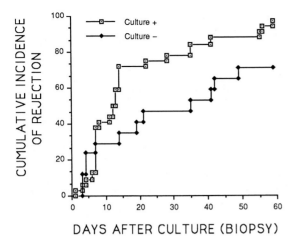

Figure 2–6. A comparison of the incidence of rejection for cardiac transplant patients with positive and negative lymphocyte cultures. All patients (both groups) were begun on treatment for acute rejection at day 0. There was a significant increase in the incidence of rejection following positive cultures as compared to negative cultures (p < 0.05).

Weber and colleagues at the University of Pittsburgh were able to subdivide those patients at increased risk for rejection (culture-positive) into an even higher risk group (high-high) or a slightly decreased risk group (low-high) by virtue of whether or not the cultures that were derived from the allograft possessed reactivity specific for the HLA antigens of the organ donor.[49] The cultures were assayed for donor antigen–specific proliferation using the primed lymphocyte test (PLT). Of 32 positive cultures, 18 demonstrated donor-specific activity in the test; 14 cultures did not. The incidence of rejection among the PLT-positive group was 17 of 18 (94 per cent) within 50 days following culture. The rejection incidence was approximately 50 per cent for cultures without organ-donor specificity.

The Pittsburgh group also reported a progressive decline with time post-transplantation in the percentage of culture-positive biopsies. In their study (which included 520 biopsies from 73 heart recipients), the percentage of culture-positive biopsies was maximal in the first 50 days following transplantation (45 per cent) and decreased thereafter (15 per cent culture positivity at times greater than 180 days). This pattern was consistent with the progressive decrease these workers observed in the frequency of positive biopsies. It is of interest that the most marked decline in culture positivity was noted for the specimens with a significant cellular infiltrate. The authors spec-

ulate that this loss of ability to stimulate growth of cells from heavily infiltrated myocardial tissue may result from immunosuppressive therapy or possibly the activation of suppressor mechanisms.

With respect to this latter possibility, a recently published report described the progressive decline of the cytolytic response to donor alloantigens mediated by peripheral blood lymphocytes (PBL) from a long-surviving kidney recipient.[50] At the time of transplantation, the recipient's PBL had normal ability to mediate killing of donor-derived target cells, but at 1 year post-transplantation, this activity had been reduced three- to fourfold and was completely absent at 2 years following transplantation. In contrast, third party alloreactivity exhibited by the same patient's PBL steadily increased in this time interval. The lack of donor-specific cytolytic potential was not found to be due to the elimination of donor-specific clones; a high frequency of cytotoxic T lymphocytes (CTL) specific for donor HLA antigens could be generated from the PBL of the recipient (9 years post-transplantation) by nonspecific activation of these cells with phytohemagglutinin prior to the CTL assay. Thus, it appears that suppressor mechanisms are present in organ recipients with long-surviving grafts that do not eliminate donor-specific CTL but, rather, functionally impede the cytolytic potential of these cells. It can be argued that similar mechanisms cause the steady decrease in culture positivity.

Consistent with the foregoing hypothesis, Weber and coworkers identified a group of patients for whom lymphocyte cultures remained consistently negative.[29] In their experience, with each successive negative culture the risk for rejection became correspondingly less: a single negative specimen was associated with a rejection rate of 55 per cent, and three negative cultures corresponded to a rejection rate of 13 per cent. Based on these observations, it appears that progressive culture negativity may correlate with increased graft stability. Whether this graft stability actually reflects a state of peripheral tolerance awaits direct demonstration.

The single most important conclusion that can be drawn from these various investigations is that the infiltration of an allograft by IL-2–responsive cells is an antecedent event to histologically demonstrable rejection. The clinical applicability of this method is somewhat diminished by the 7 to 10 days required for positive cultures to appear. However, a preliminary report in which a positive finding could be determined in 5 to 7 days potentially increases the usefulness of this method.[51] Additionally, the application of this method for identification of individuals at risk for rejection or for assessing response to therapy is quite apparent.

Association of Lymphocyte Growth from Cardiac Allografts and the Development of Coronary Artery Vasculopathy

One of the leading complications associated with cardiac transplantation is the development of obstructive coronary artery vasculopathy. Although the etiology is not known, it has been proposed that it may represent a vascular response to chronic graft rejection with the involvement of cytokines and growth factors.[52] Kaufman and colleagues studied the frequency of the development of coronary artery disease among cardiac graft recipients with positive lymphocyte cultures.[53] They found that 15 of 39 recipients (41 per cent) with persistent T cell growth developed coronary artery vasculopathy, compared with 1 of 15 (6 per cent) of those negative for T cell growth. In their experience, those patients with persistent T cell proliferation who nonetheless did not develop vasculopathy received more immunosuppressive therapy (and thus depressed immunologic activity) than those ultimately developing disease. These observations are consistent with the hypothesis setting forth a chronic immune response to foreign antigens as a factor in the etiology of this disease.

Effects of Immunosuppressive Therapy on the Outgrowth of IL-2–Responsive T Cells

Different immunosuppressive protocols have been found to affect the ability to induce growth of graft-derived T cells and also the phenotypes of the recovered cells. Kaufman and associates compared histologic findings and T cell growth for cardiac transplant patients randomized to either rabbit anti-thymocyte globulin (RATG) or OKT3 immunoprophylaxis.[54] They found an interesting difference between groups in the number of histologically normal specimens from which positive lymphocyte growth was seen. For the OKT3 group, 68 per cent of histologically non-

rejecting biopsies were positive for T cell proliferation, compared with 30 per cent for the patients assigned to the RATG protocol.

The cultures grown from these specimens were examined for in vitro donor-specific cytolytic activity to determine the effects of the different immunosuppressive protocols. For the OKT3 group, six of six cultures were cytolytic for spleen cells from the heart donor. This was in contrast to one of six tested from the RATG group. The investigators concluded that for patients receiving OKT3 (compared with RATG), there was a higher degree of graft infiltration with activated T cells that respond to Il-2 in culture and that are cytolytic for donor antigens. In their opinion, this was predictive of a higher frequency of rejection episodes upon withdrawal of therapy among the OKT3 group, which in fact was the case (27 per cent positive biopsies for the RATG group compared with 44 per cent positive biopsies for the OKT3 group).

The opposite result was observed in a study of liver allografts at the same institution.[55] In this study, liver recipients were maintained on a prophylactic immunosuppressive regimen of cyclosporine A and steroids. Rejection episodes were treated with either increased steroids or OKT3. Liver biopsies from OKT3-treated patients had less than one half the growth rate of that seen for biopsies obtained from steroid-treated or untreated patients; cell growth was also highly correlated with acute rejection. Thus, under these conditions OKT3 treatment appears beneficial with respect to inhibiting either graft infiltration and/or T cell activation. The reason for such opposite observations in heart and liver transplantation is not known.

These two studies are a further illustration of the fact that the growth (or growth failure) of T cells from allograft biopsies correlates with the incidence of rejection. Hence, the general efficacy of immunosuppression is the controlling factor in whether or not the T cell growth will occur in tissue culture. Despite the fact that different immunosuppressive protocols can be variably successful in different arenas of organ transplantation or even when applied at different transplant centers, lymphocyte growth and graft rejection always appear coincidentally.

USE OF IL-2–EXPANDED T CELLS IN ANIMAL MODELS OF TRANSPLANTATION

The method of IL-2 expansion of graft-derived T cells has proved to be a useful tool for examining rejection mechanisms outside the clinical setting. We have adapted this technique to a mouse cardiac allograft model to study the kinetics and T cell phenotypes of graft-infiltrating lymphocytes.[56, 57]

For the initial studies, we attempted to select a model that closely parallels the HLA mismatch found in clinical cardiac transplantation. We chose the C57B1/6 mouse strain as the heart donor and the C3H strain as recipient. These animals are mismatched for alleles at four loci: the K and D (class I) loci and the I-A and I-E (class II) loci). This is analogous to a human donor-recipient mismatch at the HLA A, B, DR, and DQ loci, a situation not uncommonly encountered. Graft survival for this model was determined to be 9.2 days.

To examine the graft infiltration by activated T cells, engrafted hearts were removed from recipient animals on days 2, 4, 6, 8, and 10 post-transplantation. Myocardial tissue from these grafts was placed in culture with IL-2, and the cultures were observed daily. As a control, C3H hearts were engrafted to C3H recipients, and these hearts were likewise removed. Cell growth was graded as negative, ±, or positive from 1 to 4. The results are shown in Table 2–3.

Cultures of grafts removed at days 2 and 4 post-transplantation showed little growth, indicating minimal T cell infiltration (or activation) at these times. Tissue from grafts removed at days 8 and 10 post-transplantation produced observable growth after only 2 days in culture and achieved maximal cell proliferation (3+ to 4+ growth) within 5 days of culture. Syngeneic grafts survived indefinitely and did not produce growth in culture.

Positive cultures were characterized phenotypically. The percentages of CD4+ and CD8+ cells present in cultures obtained from serially removed grafts are given in Figure 2–7. Few cells were present in cultures derived from grafts removed at days 2 and 4. Of the T cells present in these cultures, there was a predominance of the CD4+ phenotype (approximately 20 per cent of cells; CD4/CD8 ratios were 1.4 and 1.8 in each of two experiments). For day 6 cultures, large quantities, primarily of the CD8 phenotype (89 per cent and 82 per cent in each of the respective experiments), were seen. Between days 8 and 10 (the window surrounding the predicted time for graft failure), the percentage of CD8 cells remained approximately 65 per cent. The percentage of CD4+ T cells did not exceed 3 per cent in any culture initiated later than 4 days post-transplantation.

This study suggests that CD4+ T cells are of importance early in the rejection process and that the CD8+ phenotype is the principal mediator at the later stages. Despite the relatively small and transient CD4 response, one could argue that these cells are an artifact and do not play a significant role. However, in a similar study, it was shown that rejection can be prevented by treatment of recipient animals with anti-CD4 antibody.[58] In that experiment, the number of CD4+ graft-infiltrating cells was reduced (predictably) by this treatment, but also there was a significant decrease in the number of infiltrating CD8+ cells. Thus, the early (albeit minimal) CD4+ T cell response, occurring soon after transplantation in this model, is highly important for the generation of effector cells.

Table 2–3. IL-2–Stimulated Lymphocyte Growth in Cultures of Explanted Mouse Cardiac Allograft Removed Serially Following Transplantation

Day of Graft Removal (Post-transplantation)	Syngeneic*		Allogeneic	
	Experiment		*Experiment*	
	1	*2*	*1*	*2*
2	—†	—	+	+ +
4	±	±	+	+
6	+	±	+ + +	+ +
8	±	±	+ + +	+ + + +
10	±	±	+ + + +	+ + + +

*Syngeneic: C3H to C3H; allogeneic: C57B1/6 to C3H.

†Grading by microscopic assessment of cultures. Grades represent the highest degree of growth seen for triplicate cultures and employ the following scheme:

—, no growth
±, rare dividing cells
+, moderate numbers (50–100) of dividing cells

+ +, numerous dividing cells and cell clusters
+ + +, confluent growth on 25%–50% of the plate
+ + + +, 50%–100% confluency

From Carlquist JF, Shelby J, Hammond EH, Greenwood JH, Anderson JL. Recovery and phenotypic identification of in vivo-activated lymphocytes from mouse cardiac allografts. Transplantation 50:349, 1990.

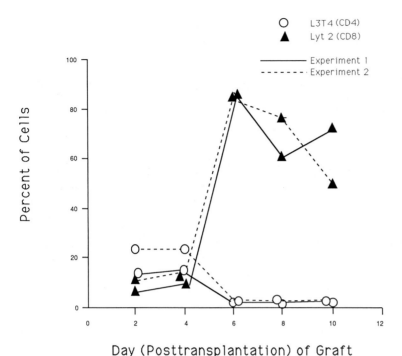

Figure 2–7. Phenotypes of lymphocytes recovered in culture from murine cardiac allografts. Cultures were generated from heart tissue removed serially post-transplantation. (From Carlquist JF, Shelby J, Hammond EH, Greenwood JH, Anderson JL. Recovery and phenotypic identification of in vivo-activated lymphocytes from mouse cardiac allografts. Transplantation 50:349, 1990.)

The phenotypic pattern of graft infiltration differs with respect to strain differences between graft donor and recipient. We further studied T cell infiltration in other donor-recipient mismatch combinations. These investigations indicated that the type of mismatch (i.e., MHC class I or class II) has a pronounced effect on the immune response mounted by the recipient. Compared with the model (class I plus class II mismatch), a donor recipient mismatch only for the H-2D class I antigen results in a reduced CD4 and increased CD8 T cell response in the early period post-transplantation. In contrast, animals mismatched only at the class II loci (I-A and I-E) but compatible at both class I loci have a strikingly pronounced and prolonged CD4+ T cell response.[59] Whereas in clinical transplantation we were unable to correlate T cell phenotypes with donor-recipient mismatch, the observations in animal models are consistent with the recognized association between CD4+ T cells and class II MHC molecules and CD8+ T cells and class I MHC molecules. Thus, in the absence of immunosuppressive therapy, the rules that govern foreign peptide presentation and recognition are similar for allorecognition.

SUMMARY

Interleukin-2 is a cytokine of primary importance in any immune response. T cells acti-

vated in response to either alloantigens or foreign peptides cannot progress beyond the G_1 phase of the cell cycle without the second signal provided by IL-2. This two-signal requirement has been exploited by investigators to expand and study T cells activated in vivo in response to allogeneic challenge (i.e., an allograft). These cultures have been shown to be specific for donor HLA antigens in both proliferative and cytolytic assays. In some cases, cytolytic activity has been found to parallel clinical outcome.

The response of T cells to IL-2 in vitro has been shown to have diagnostic and prognostic value in the case of solid organ transplantation. Numerous studies have found that lymphocyte proliferation correlates with, and often times precedes, acute rejection. The growth of T cells from graft tissue has also been shown to predict efficacy of therapy for acute rejection.

This method has also been used to obtain large quantities of alloactivated T lymphocytes for further studies of graft rejection. Although much remains to be learned about the cellular mediators of rejection and the effects of immunosuppressive therapy on these cells, this method provides a window through which the rejection process can be viewed with the potential for obtaining the answers to some of these questions.

REFERENCES

1. Medewar PB. The behaviour and fate of skin auto-grafts and skin homografts in rabbits. J Anat 78:176, 1944.

2. Billingham RE, Brent L, Medewar PB. Quantitative studies on tissue transplantation immunity. II. The origin, strength and duration of actively and adoptively acquired immunity. Proc R Soc Lond (Biol) 143:58, 1954.

3. Billingham RE, Silvers WK, Wilson DB. Further studies on adoptive transfer of sensitivity to skin homografts. J Exp Med 118:397, 1963.

4. Ertle W, Reichenspurner H, Lersch C, Hammer C, Plahl M, Lehmann M, Kemkes BM, Osterholzer G, Reble B, Reichart B, Brendel W. Cytoimmunological monitoring in acute rejection and viral, bacterial or fungal infection following transplantation. J Heart Transplant 4:390, 1985.

5. Hanson CA, Bolling SF, Stoolman LM, Schlegelmilch JA, Abrams GD, Miska P, Deeb GM. Cytoimmunologic monitoring and heart transplantation. J Heart Transplant 7:424, 1988.

6. O'Toole CM, Maher P, Spiegelhalter DJ, Walker JR, Stovin P, Wallwork J, English TAH. "Rejection or infection" predictive value of T-cell subject ratio, before and after heart transplantation. J Heart Transplant 5:518, 1985.

7. Mayer TG, Fuller AA, Lazarovits AI, Boyle LA, Kurnick JT. Characterization of in vivo–activated lymphocytes propagated from human renal allograft biopsies undergoing rejection. J Immunol 134:258, 1985.

8. Shimizu Y, Newman W, Tanaka Y, Shaw S. Lymphocyte interactions with endothelial cells. Immunol Today 13:106, 1992.

9. Hancock WW, Gee D, De Moerloose P, Rickles FR, Ewan VA, Atkins RC. Immunohistological analysis of serial biopsies taken during human renal allograft rejection. Transplantation 39:430, 1985.

10. Platt JL, LeBien TW, Michael AF. Interstitial mononuclear cell populations in renal graft rejection: Identification by monoclonal antibodies in tissue sections. J Exp Med 155:17, 1982.

11. Croker BP, Borowitz MJ. Cytotoxic T-cell allotaxis in human kidney rejection. Am J Pathol 78:707, 1982.

12. Hancock WW, Thomson NM, Atkins RC. Composition of interstitial cellular infiltrate identified by monoclonal antibodies in renal biopsies of rejecting human renal allografts. Transplantation 35:458, 1983.

13. Tufveson G, Forsum G, Claesson K, Klareskog L, Larsson E, Karlsson-Parra A, Frodin L. T lymphocyte subsets and HLA-DR bearing cells in rejected human kidney grafts. Scand J Immunol 18:37, 1983.

14. Carlquist JF, Hammond EH, Anderson JL. Propagation and characterization of lymphocytes from rejecting human cardiac allografts. J Heart Transplant 7:397, 1988.

15. Morgan DA, Ruscetti FW, Gallo R. Selective in vitro growth of T lymphocytes from normal human bone marrows. Science 193:1007, 1976.

16. Tsudo M, Kozak RW, Goldman CK, Waldman TA. Demonstration of a non-Tac peptide that binds interleukin-2: A potential participant in a multichain interleukin receptor complex. Proc Natl Acad Sci USA 83:9694, 1986.

17. Teshigawara K, Wang HM, Kato K, Smith KA. Interleukin-2 high affinity receptor expression requires two distinct binding proteins. J Exp Med 165:223, 1987.

18. Ashwell JD, Robb RJ, Malek TR. Proliferation of T lymphocytes in response to interleukin-2 varies with their state of activation. J Immunol 137:2572, 1986.

19. Smith KA. Interleukin-2: Inception, impact, and implications. Science 240:1169, 1988.

20. Cantrell DA, Smith KA. Transient expression of interleukin-2 receptors. Consequences for cell growth. J Exp Med 158:1895, 1983.

21. Smith KA. The interleukin-2 receptor. Adv Immunol 42:166, 1988.

22. Taga K, Tosato G. IL-10 inhibits human T cell proliferation and IL-2 production. J Immunol 148:1143, 1992.

23. Schwartzentruber DJ, Topalian SL, Mancini M, Rosenberg SA. Specific release of granulocyte-macrophage colony-stimulating factor, tumor necrosis factor-α and IFN-γ by human tumor infiltrating lymphocytes after autologous tumor stimulation. J Immunol 146:3674, 1991.

24. Rosenberg SA, Packard BS, Aebersold PM, Soloman D, Topalian SL, Toy ST, Simon P, Lotze MT, Yang JC, Seipp CA, Simpson C, Carter C, Bock S, Schwartzentruber D, Wei JP, White DE. Use of tumor-infiltrating lymphocytes and interleukin-2 in the immunotherapy of patients with metastatic melanoma. N Engl J Med 319:1676, 1988.

25. Karpati RM, Banks SM, Malissen B, Rosenberg SA, Sheard MA, Weber JS, Hodes RJ. Phenotypic characterization of murine tumor-infiltrating T lymphocytes. J Immunol 146:2043, 1991.

26. Binimelis J, Sutherland D, Sibley R, de Leiva A, Barbosa J. Phenotypes of in vivo–activated T lymphocytes from a pancreas allograft. Transplant Proc 19:403, 1987.

27. Pollack MS, Washington J, Matoba A. The propagation of HLA-specific T cells from failed corneal grafts. Transplant Proc 19:408, 1987.

28. Saidman SL, Demetris AJ, Zeevi A, Duquesnoy RJ. Propagation of lymphocytes infiltrating human liver allografts. Transplantation 49:107, 1990.

29. Weber T, Kaufman C, Zeevi A, Zerbe TR, Herdesty RJ, Kormos RH, Griffith BP, Duquesnoy RJ. Lymphocyte growth from cardiac allograft biopsy specimens with no or minimal cellular infiltrates: Association with subsequent rejection episode. J Heart Transplant 8:23, 1989.

30. Charpentier B, Bach MA, Lang PH, Hiesse CH, Fries D. In situ analysis of cells involved in irreversible acute rejection of human renal allografts. Transplant Proc 19:392, 1987.

31. Moreau JF, Bonneville M, Peyrat MA, Godard A, Jacques Y, Desgranges C, Soulillou JP. T lymphocyte cloning from rejected human kidney allografts. J Clin Invest 78:874, 1986.

32. Preffer FI, Colvin RB, Leary CP, Boyle LA, Tuazon TV, Lazarovits AI, Cosimi AB, Kurnick JT. Two-color flow cytometry and functional analysis of lymphocytes cultured from human renal allografts: Identification of a Leu-2 + 3 + subpopulation. J Immunol 137:2823, 1986.

33. Strom TB, Tilney NL, Paradysz JM, Bancewicz J, Carpenter CB. Cellular components of allograft rejection: Identity, specificity and cytotoxic function of cells infiltrating acutely rejecting allografts. J Immunol 118:2020, 1977.

34. von Willebrand E, Hayry P. Composition and in vitro cytotoxicity of cellular infiltrates in rejecting human allografts. Cell Immunol 41:358, 1978.

35. Zeevi A, Fung J, Zerbe TR, Kaufman C, Rabin BS, Griffith BP, Hardesty RL, Duquesnoy RJ. Allospecificity of activated T cells grown from endomyocardial

biopsies from heart transplant patients. Transplantation 41:620, 1986.

36. Chothia C, Boswell DR, Lesk AM. The outline structure of the T cell receptor. EMBO J 7:3745, 1988.

37. Davis MM, Bjorkman PJ. T cell antigen receptor genes and T cell recognition. Nature (Lond) 334:395, 1988.

38. Duquesnoy RJ, Zeevi A, Fung J J, Kaufman C, Zerbe TR, Griffith B, Trento A, Kormos R, Hardesty R. Sequential infiltration of class I and class II specific alloreactive T cells in human cardiac allografts. Transplant Proc 19:2560, 1987.

39. Carlquist JF, Hammond ME, Yowell RL, O'Connell JB, Anderson JL. Correlation between class II antigen (DR) expression and interleukin-2–induced lymphocyte proliferation during cardiac allograft rejection. Transplantation 50:582, 1990.

40. Steeg PS, Moore RN, Johnson HM, Oppenheim J J. Regulation of murine macrophage Ia antigen expression by a lymphokine with interferon activity. J Exp Med 156:792, 1982.

41. Aberer W, Stingl L, Pogantsch S, Stingl G. Effect of glucocorticosteroids on epidermal cell-induced immune responses. J Immunol 133:792, 1984.

42. Hanaumi K, Gray P, Suzuki T. Fc receptor-mediated suppression of gamma interferon-induced Ia antigen expression on a murine macrophage cell line (P38D1). J Immunol 133:2852, 1984.

43. Ina Y, Koide Y, Nezu N, Yoshida TO. Regulation of HLA class II antigen expression: Intracellular signaling molecules responsible for the regulation by IFN-gamma and cross-linking of Fc receptors in HL-60 cells. J Immunol 139:1711, 1987.

44. Howard M, O'Garra A. Biological properties of IL-10. Immunol Today 13:198, 1992.

45. Sell KW, Tadros T, Wang YC, Hertzler G, Knopf WD, Murphy DA, Ahmed-Ansari A. Studies of major histocompatibility complex class I/II expression on sequential human heart biopsy specimens after transplantation. J Heart Transplant 7:407, 1988.

46. Masuyama J, Minato N, Kano S. Mechanisms of lymphocyte adhesion to human vascular endothelial cells in culture: T lymphocyte adhesion to endothelial HLA-DR antigens induced by gamma interferon. J Clin Invest 77:1596, 1986.

47. Colson YL, Markus BH, Zeevi A, Duquesnoy RJ. Interactions between endothelial cells and alloreactive T cells involved in allograft immunity. Transplant Proc 20:273, 1988.

48. Carlquist JF, Hammond EH, O'Connell JB, Anderson JL. Increased risk of rejection associated with the

growth of lymphocytes from human cardiac allografts. Transplant Proc 23:1146, 1991.

49. Weber T, Kaufman C, Zerbe TR, Hardesty RJ, Kormos RH, Griffith BP, Duquesnoy RJ. Propagation of lymphocytes from human heart transplant biopsies: Methodologic considerations. Transplant Proc 20:176, 1988.

50. Vandekerckhove BAE, Datema G, Kining F, Goulmy E, Persijn GG, van Rood JJ, Claas FHJ, de Vries JE. Analysis of the donor-specific cytotoxic T lymphocyte repertoire in a patient with a long-term surviving allograft. J Immunol 144:1288, 1990.

51. Weber T, Zerbe T, Kaufman C, Zeevi A, Kormos R, Hardesty R, Griffith B, Duquesnoy RJ. Propagation of alloreactive lymphocytes from histologically negative endomyocardial biopsies from heart transplant patients. Transplantation 48:430, 1989.

52. Libby P, Salomon RN, Payne DD, Schoen FJ, Pober JS. Functions of vascular wall cells related to development of transplantation-associated coronary arteriosclerosis. Transplant Proc 21:3677, 1989.

53. Kaufman C, Zeevi A, Zerbe T, Keenan R, Kormos R, Griffith B, Hardesty R, Armitage J, Uretsky B, Duquesnoy RJ. In vitro culture of infiltrating lymphocytes from coronary arteries and endomyocardial biopsies: Association with graft coronary disease. Transplant Proc 23:1142, 1991.

54. Kaufman C, Zeevi A, Zerbe T, Kormos R, Griffith B, Hardesty R, Duquesnoy RJ. In vivo studies of endomyocardial biopsies from heart transplant recipients on RATG and OKT3 immunoprophylaxis protocols. Transplantation 48:621, 1989.

55. Saidman SL, Demetris AJ, Zeevi A, Duquesnoy RJ. Propagation of lymphocytes infiltrating human liver allografts. Correlation with histologic diagnosis of rejection. Transplantation 49:107, 1990.

56. Carlquist JF, Shelby J, Hammond ME, Greenwood JH, Anderson JL. Recovery and phenotypic identification of in vivo–activated lymphocytes from mouse cardiac allografts. Transplantation 50:349, 1990.

57. Shelby J, Corry RJ. The primarily vascularized mouse heart transplant as a model for the study of the immune response. Heart Transplant 2:32, 1982.

58. Bishop DK, Shelby J, Eichwald EJ. Functional analysis of donor-reactive T cells infiltrating heterotopic cardiac transplants: Effect of anti-CD4 Mab in vivo. Transplant Proc 23:287, 1991.

59. Carlquist JF, Shelby J, Hammond ME, Greenwood JH, Anderson JL. Major histocompatibility complex–regulated differences in cellular rejection mechanisms in murine cardiac allograft models. J Am Coll Cardiol 19:295A, 1992.

Chapter

3

THE ROLE OF ENDOTHELIAL CELLS IN TRANSPLANT REJECTION

Robert E. Shaddy, MD, Stephen M. Prescott, MD, Thomas M. McIntyre, PhD, and Guy A. Zimmerman, MD

The vascular endothelium is the layer of cells that lines all blood vessels and provides a cellular interface between blood and tissue. It is a highly specialized single cell layer with multiple functions. After transplantation, the endothelium provides an allogeneic barrier between the recipient's blood (including lymphocytes) and the donor transplanted organ. In this chapter, the role of the endothelium as it relates to solid organ transplant rejection is discussed.

BIOLOGIC FEATURES OF THE ENDOTHELIUM RELEVANT TO TRANSPLANT REJECTION

Morphology of the Vascular Endothelium and Endothelial Cells

The vessel wall is composed of three layers. The first of these layers is the intima, composed of endothelium, which rests upon a basement membrane composed of type IV collagen, laminin, fibronectin, von Willebrand factor, and other extracellular matrix constituents.[1] The internal elastic lamina separates the intima from the next layer, the tunica media, which is composed primarily of smooth muscle cells. Finally, the external elastic membrane separates the tunica media from the adventitia, the outermost layer of the cell wall. In muscular arteries, the tunica media consists of smooth muscle bands without bands of elastin. A typical capillary has essentially no smooth muscle cells. Veins have a very thin tunica media.

The vascular endothelium is a polarized monolayer that provides a heterogeneous, homeostatic barrier between the blood and all subendothelial tissues. It functions not only as a barrier but also as an autocrine, paracrine, and juxtacrine organ with a variety of physiologic properties, including procoagulant, antiplatelet, anticoagulant, fibrinolytic, metabolic, and immunologic functions.[2] In addition, it has a variety of other biologic features, including expression of histocompatibility antigens, binding of insulin and lipoproteins, growth factor production and regulation, cellular binding, and generation of components of the basal lamina and surrounding stroma.[3] This chapter will not review these biologic characteristics in encyclopedic fashion but will focus on certain aspects that appear at this time to be clearly relevant to transplant rejection (also, see Chapter 4, pages 53–60). After transplantation, the endothelium becomes a major component of immunologic recognition of the transplanted organ, and of its response.

Endothelial Cell Activation: Responses to Cytokines and Other Agonists

Endothelial activation is a term used to describe changes in certain phenotypic features

35

of endothelial cells in response to agonists that bind to surface receptors on endothelium, or in response to other perturbations (for example, immune or oxidant injury).[4] The concept that endothelial cells alter critical functions in a regulated fashion in response to stimulation in physiologic conditions, and in a dysregulated fashion in pathologic states, is one of the most important concepts in vascular biology. It differs from the earlier view that the endothelial cell is passive and simply serves structural and antithrombotic roles.

Activation results in changes such as major histocompatibility complex (MHC) antigen expression, increased procoagulant activity, and increased adhesiveness of the endothelium for leukocytes. Some of these changes take hours or even days to occur and involve protein synthesis.[5]

Cytokines from both T cells and endothelium mediate many of the cellular interactions seen after transplantation. Two cytokines, interleukin-1 (IL-1) and tumor necrosis factor (TNF), cause parallel but distinct effects on endothelial cells. Both cytokines induce synthesis and expression of several endothelial adhesion molecules: (1) E-selectin, a 110-kD cell-surface selectin that binds neutrophils, monocytes, and some lymphocyte subsets;[6, 7] (2) intercellular adhesion molecule-1 (ICAM-1), a 100-kD member of the immunoglobulin (Ig) gene superfamily that binds lymphocytes, PMNs, and monocytes through recognition and binding to one of two B2 integrins (the αL/B2-integrin also known as CD11a/CD18, and the αM/B2-integrin also known as CD11B/CD18);[8–10] and (3) vascular cell adhesion molecule (VCAM-1), another 100-kD Ig that binds lymphocytes and monocytes by recognizing a β1-integrin (the a4, β1-integrin, known as the very late activation antigen, VLA-4).[11, 12] These will be discussed in greater detail later. Another cytokine, interferon (IFN)-γ, enhances MHC class II expression on endothelial cells, inducing increased adhesion of T cells to endothelial cells.[13] IFN-γ also has other properties, such as the ability to increase ICAM-1 expression on endothelial cells and to activate macrophages.[9] TNF also increases expression of MHC class I molecules.[14]

An important facet of endothelial activation in transplantation is human leukocyte antigen (HLA) DR antigen expression. Normally, in humans, MHC class II antigens are only weakly expressed on some capillary endothelium.[15] Increased class I and class II MHC expression is a feature of almost all rejecting organs and is concomitant with cellular infiltration. This increased expression results from activation of the endothelium by IFN-γ and TNF. In cultured human umbilical vein endothelial cells, class II antigen expression is detectable about 6 to 8 hours after IFN-γ exposure and reaches plateau levels by 4 to 6 days.[16] TNF causes an increase in the expression of class I MHC antigens but has very little, if any, effect on MHC class II expression.[17] As with IFN-γ, the effect is gradual, and the peak effect is seen at 4 to 6 days. The significance of increased MHC induction is unclear, but it appears to be necessary, although not sufficient, for allograft rejection. Also, controversy exists as to whether the degree of HLA DR antigen expression correlates with rejection.[18–21]

Activation responses, such as the increase in intracellular calcium, arachidonate release, and transient synthesis and expression of platelet-activating factor (PAF) by endothelial cells stimulated with thrombin, can also occur in endothelium in a manner of minutes.[22] Although controversial,[23] some investigators believe that IL-1 and TNF induce the synthesis of PAF, which enhances lymphocyte binding to and penetration through endothelium.[24] These rapid activation events may be important in immediate or short-term responses of endothelium in transplanted organs.

Endothelial Molecules That Regulate Adhesion and Activation of Leukocytes

The regulation of leukocyte adhesion at the intimal surface is one of the most intensely studied aspects of endothelial biology in recent years, and it is particularly germane to transplantation. Several recent reviews of endothelial-leukocyte interactions are included in the bibliography.[7, 10, 25–27] The mechanisms involved are complex and vary with the different classes of leukocytes (granulocytes, monocytes, and lymphocytes). However, certain general principles apply.[7] First, activation of endothelial cells alters the number and type of adhesion molecules, compared with those found in the resting state. Second, different patterns of adhesion molecules are expressed by endothelial cells in a time-dependent fashion and can cause different patterns of leukocyte adhesion and activation. Third, alterations in adhesive phenotype of both endothelial cells and leukocytes can be induced by inflammatory or immune mediators, such as cytokines.

The adhesion of T lymphocytes to endothelium is an important component of several mechanisms of rejection (see later sections) and will be used as an example to illustrate the spectrum of endothelial adhesion molecules that can be called into play. Certain of the adhesion molecules are constitutively expressed on high endothelial cells of the lymph node venules, or on postcapillary venules in systemic tissues, and they are used by naive and memory T cells for normal homing and recirculation. However, pathologic inflammation, of the sort that occurs in transplant rejection, dramatically alters adhesive interactions, principally by inducing increased numbers of certain ligands for T cells on the endothelial cell surface, expression of new ligands for T cells on the endothelial cell surface, or both. The pattern of ligands for T cells depends, in part, on the specific cytokines or other agonists that activate the endothelial cells, the time after initiation of the inflammatory response, and the local milieu.[26] The proadhesive molecules for the T lymphocytes that are expressed by activated endothelial cells fall into one of two major groups: the selectins, or the members of the immunoglobulin gene superfamily (Table 3–1).

The selectins are a family of membrane glycoproteins that are expressed on endothelial cells, platelets, and leukocytes, which mediate cell-cell interactions at vascular surfaces. The three members of the family are described in Table 3–2. Two of these, P-selectin and E-selectin, are expressed by activated endothelial cells; however, they have different mechanisms of expression and temporal patterns and are induced in response to different agonists.[reviewed in 7] Both mediate adhesion of memory T cells and other lymphocyte subsets.[reviewed in 27] Both these selectins also mediate adhesion of granulocytes and monocytes (Table 3–2).[7] P- and E-selectin each bind to one or more ligands on target cells that contain complex carbohydrates; the precise structures of these ligands are not yet known. L-selectin, the third member of the selectin family, is not found on endothelial cells but instead is expressed on the surface of T lymphocyte subsets, other lymphocyte subsets, and all myeloid cells.[7, 27] L-selectin binds to one or more ligands induced on the surfaces of cultured umbilical vein endothelial cells, which are informative models of postcapillary venous endothelium, when they are activated with cytokines.[28] This suggests that structures recognized by L-selectin may be induced on endothelium lining vessels of transplanted organs. The ligand recognized by L-selectin on cultured umbilical vein endothelium is induced to a variable degree by TNFα, IL-1b, lipopolysaccharide, IFN-γ, and IL-4, and it is sensitive to cleavage with neuraminidase.[28] A candidate ligand for L-selectin, which appears to present complex carbohydrate structures to it, has been purified and the cDNA cloned from mouse lymph nodes.[29] It remains to be determined whether the structure recognized by L-selectin on cultured human endothelium

Table 3–1. Proadhesive Molecules for T Lymphocytes Expressed by Human Endothelial Cells

Proadhesive Molecule	Expressed on Resting EC	Increased by Activation	Agonists for Increased Expression	T Cell Ligand
Selectin Family				
E-selectin	no	yes	IL-1, TNFα, LPS	Unknown; probably sialated glycoprotein or glycolipid
P-selectin	no	yes	Thrombin, LTC4, histamine, C5b-9, peroxides	Unknown; probably sialated glycoprotein
Immunoglobulin Gene Superfamily				
ICAM-1	low	yes	IL-1, TNFα, LPS, IFN-γ	CD11a/CD18, CD11b/CD18
ICAM-2	high	no	—	CD11a/CD18
VCAM-1	none or low	yes	IL-1, TNFα, LPS	α_4/β_1-integrin
PECAM-1	moderate (junctional localization)	?	?	PECAM-1

Adhesive interactions of T lymphocytes with endothelium mediated by proadhesive molecules shown in this table, binding of the purified molecule to T cells, or both, have been demonstrated in vitro. In some cases, interactions mediated by the molecules have been demonstrated in vivo as well. The adhesive mechanisms involved differ between molecules; see text and references for details.

(Note: E-selectin and P-selectin were previously known as ELAM-1 and GMP-140 or PADGEM protein, respectively. CD11a/CD18 is also known as αL/B2-integrin. CD11b/CD18 is also known as αM/B2-integrin.)

Table 3–2. The Selectin Family of Adhesion Molecules

Selectin	Earlier Names	Expressed by	Target Cell
L-selectin	MEL-14 LAM-1 LEU-8 TQ1 LEC.AM-1 LEC.CAM-1 DREG.56	PMNs, monocytes, lymphocyte subsets	High EC venules of lymph nodes; activated systemic ECs
E-selectin	ELAM-1	Cytokine-activated ECs	PMNs, monocytes, lymphocyte subsets
P-selectin	GMP-140 PADGEM	Rapidly activated ECs, platelets	PMNs, monocytes, lymphocyte subsets

activated with IL-1 is the same, or a similar, ligand.

Each of the second group of adhesion molecules that is expressed by resting or activated endothelial cells and that influence T cell adhesion is structurally related to immunoglobulins. Therefore, each is classified as a member of the immunoglobulin (Ig) gene superfamily (see Table 3–1). Two Ig-like molecules expressed on endothelial cells, ICAM-1 and ICAM-2, are ligands for leukocyte function-associated antigen-1 (LFA-1), which is constitutively expressed on the plasma membranes of T cells and other leukocytes.[30, 31] LFA-1 is a member of the class of adhesion molecules termed integrins[32] and is also known as CD11a/CD18 or α_1/β_2-integrin. ICAM-1 was shown to be a counterreceptor, or ligand, for CD11a/CD18 in both purified systems and experiments with cells expressing these molecules.[reviewed in 24] ICAM-1 is expressed at low levels on resting endothelial cells, and its expression is increased by inflammatory mediators such as IL-1 and TNF. In contrast, ICAM-2 is expressed at relatively high levels on unactivated endothelial cells, and surface expression of the protein is not increased by inflammatory mediators. Because they are expressed at variable levels in the basal state, ICAM-1 and ICAM-2 appear to be involved in binding of lymphocytes to unstimulated endothelial cells and lymphocyte homing.[33] They are also part of the system that mediates adhesion and transmigration of T lymphocytes across inflamed endothelium.[26]

Vascular cell adhesion molecule-1 (VCAM-1), a third member of the immunoglobulin family, is absent or expressed at low levels on resting endothelial cells, but it is strongly induced on TNFα- or IL-1–activated endothelial cells. Both VCAM-1 and ICAM-1 are increased on endothelium in cardiac and renal biopsy specimens during cellular rejection.[34, 35]

VCAM-1 mediates binding of lymphocytes and monocytes by ligating an integrin of the β_1 class, α_4,β_1-integrin, also known as VLA-4.[25] Thus, in two key interactions, a member of the immunoglobulin family on the endothelial cell pairs with an integrin on the lymphocyte: VCAM-1 with a β_1-integrin, VLA-4, and ICAM-1 or ICAM-2 with a β_2-integrin, CD11a/CD18. CD11a/CD18-dependent adhesion requires activation of the lymphocyte, resulting in a functional change in the CD11a/CD18 heterodimer that enhances its avidity for ICAM-1 and ICAM-2.[24, 36] Activation of the lymphocyte, resulting in "triggering" of CD11a/CD18-dependent adhesive interactions, appears to mediate both tight binding of T lymphocytes to endothelium and transmigration.[26] Other molecular events may trigger or signal activation of CD11a/CD18; for example, interactions of lymphocytes mediated by the T cell receptor may activate integrin function in inflamed vessels of transplanted organs.[37] VLA-4 also undergoes functional activation under some conditions.[26]

A fourth member of the immunoglobulin gene superfamily, PECAM-1, may also be involved in T cell binding to endothelium. PECAM-1 is the acronym for platelet endothelial cell adhesion molecule-1, a name given to it because it was originally identified on platelets as well as on endothelial cells. PECAM-1, which is also designated CD31, is constitutively expressed on endothelial cells and is enriched at intercellular junctions. It is proposed that it binds in a homotypic fashion to other PECAM-1 molecules expressed on T cell subsets.[38] Engagement of PECAM-1 on T cells induces the adhesive functions of VLA-4 and CD11a/CD18 under some conditions, providing a potential mechanism for recruiting the participation of these integrins in adhesive interactions (see earlier). VLA-4 appears to be preferentially activated when PECAM-1 on T cells is engaged.[38]

The diversity of proadhesive molecules for T cells that are expressed by endothelial cells implies that multiple adhesive interactions are involved in targeting and transmigration of these lymphocytes. One advantage of the use of multiple ligands in physiologic inflammatory interactions is that this strengthens the avidity of adhesion, over and above the relatively weak adhesion provided by a single ligand pair. Certain molecular interactions may play particular roles in initiation of adhesion or in adhesion strengthening; for example, adhesion mediated by molecules of the selectin class is relatively resistant to shear forces and may initially capture the T lymphocyte, allowing the interaction mediated by binding of CD11a/CD18 on the leukocyte to ICAM-1 and ICAM-2 on the endothelial cell to amplify adhesion. The latter molecular interaction is relatively sensitive to disruption by shear forces.[26] Certain interactions not mentioned earlier, such as binding of CD44 T lymphocytes to glycosaminoglycans on endothelial cells, and the CD-2–LFA-3 interactions, may be involved in adhesion strengthening, although the exact significance of these interactions is unclear.[33, 39, 40] A second advantage of multiple ligand interactions is that one or more of them may induce critical functional alterations in the lymphocyte. For example, the putative mechanism involving binding of PECAM-1 on endothelium to PECAM-1 on T lymphocytes, mentioned earlier, may trigger the adhesive function of VLA-4. Such an "adhesion and activation cascade"[38] may facilitate transmigration, in addition to strengthening binding, of T lymphocytes.[26]

Multiple molecular events that mediate both adhesion and activation of the leukocyte are also involved in interactions of neutrophils and other myeloid leukocytes with activated endothelium. Proadhesive molecules for myeloid leukocytes that are expressed by endothelial cells have "tethering" or "signaling" functions.[7] Coordinated expression of combinations of tethering and signaling molecules leads to both adhesion and juxtacrine activation of the neutrophil. This was first shown for P-selectin and platelet-activating factor, which are temporally expressed by endothelial cells activated by thrombin or histamine and which, respectively, mediate tethering and juxtacrine

activation.[41] Juxtacrine activation in this fashion, which is both spatially and temporally regulated, may initiate neutrophil polarization, priming, and other requisite functions in physiologic inflammatory responses.[7] However, dysregulated expression of one or more of these molecules may be involved in the pathogenesis of diverse forms of vascular injury.[42] Such dysregulated molecular interactions may mediate components of hyperacute rejection (see following) or neutrophil accumulation in other forms of injury to transplanted organs.

Growth Factor Production

Growth factors produced by endothelial cells that are implicated in the chronic transplant rejection response include IL-1, basic fibroblast growth factor (bFGF), platelet-derived growth factor (PDGF)-like protein, and connective tissue growth factor.[43] The mitogenic properties of IL-1 for fibroblasts and smooth muscle cells appear to be mediated through its ability to stimulate the production of PDGF A chain.[44] PDGF is a cationic polypeptide stored in the α-granules of platelets and released locally after platelet activation. The main function of PDGF in vivo is thought to be stimulation of mesenchymal proliferation at sites of tissue injury.[45] Endothelial cells have been shown to synthesize and secrete a protein similar to PDGF. This activity can be stimulated by a variety of agents, including thrombin, IL-1, and TNF.[44, 46, 47] A recent study described a new mitogen called connective tissue growth factor, which is a 38-kD monomeric molecule that appears to be antigenically and functionally related to PDGF but is not a product of the PDGF A or B chain genes.[43] This molecule appears to be secreted in much higher concentrations than the PDGF A or B chain molecules. This new connective tissue growth factor may account for the majority of growth factor activity secreted by endothelial cells that has been attributed to the "PDGF-like protein" by many investigators.

Ross and colleagues, using immunohistochemical techniques, have shown PDGF-like protein to be localized within atheromatous lesions.[48] Moreover, an increased expression of PDGF B receptors on vascular smooth muscle has been seen in kidney transplant biopsy specimens from patients undergoing rejection.[49] This suggests that increased local production of PDGF, or possibly connective tissue growth factor, potentially results from allograft rejection. This could contribute to the development of accelerated graft vasculopathy.

Work from our laboratory has shown that T cells are capable of inducing secretion of PDGF-like protein from endothelial cells.[50] Furthermore, secretion of mitogens in response to T cells may be primarily, or exclusively, a property of arterial endothelial cells, since human umbilical vein endothelial cells demonstrated a very blunted response to T cells in comparison with arterial endothelial cells (Fig. 3–1). It is possible that a similar interaction with T cells induces endothelial cells to produce and secrete PDGF-like protein during cellular rejection (see following), resulting in excessive myointimal proliferation and subsequent accelerated graft vasculopathy. Preliminary work by others has shown that binding of natural killer cells to endothelium itself induces signal transduction in endothelial cells, suggesting that endothelial membrane structures engaged by lymphocyte adhesion are capable of transducing activation signals.[51] However, the adhesion pathways (see last section) involved in this T cell–stimulated signaling are unknown.

Endothelial cells also synthesize bFGF. bFGF is a potent mitogen for fibroblasts and smooth muscle cells, as well as a potent autocrine growth factor for endothelial cells.[52, 53] In contrast to PDGF-like protein, after bFGF is synthesized by endothelial cells it either remains cell-associated or is deposited into the subendothelial matrix.[54] bFGF does not contain a signal peptide and thus is not able to be secreted from endothelial cells by the usual mechanisms. The only known factors to modulate bFGF release by endothelial cells are lytic cell injury[55, 56] and phorbol esters.[57] Although bFGF has been implicated as a potential contributor to accelerated graft vasculopathy, it is not known whether its synthesis or its secretion is immunologically regulated.

PATTERNS OF ENDOTHELIAL INJURY AND RESPONSE IN REJECTION OF TRANSPLANTED ORGANS

Hyperacute Rejection

Hyperacute rejection occurs when the recipient has preformed antibodies (from previous transplantation, pregnancy, or blood transfusions) or when transplantation occurs across an ABO blood group barrier, especially in xenotransplantation. Histologic features described in hyperacute rejection include platelet aggregation, endothelial cell damage, fibrin deposition, capillary rupture, interstitial edema, neutrophil emigration, and thrombosis; in transplanted hearts undergoing hyperacute rejection, myocardial necrosis has been described.[58] A unique antigen system expressed on the surface of both vascular endothelial cells and monocytes has been implicated in hyperacute rejection in renal[59] and cardiac[60, 61] transplantation. This molecular system may be involved in the mechanism of hyperacute rejection reported in individuals without ABO or HLA incompatibility and with a negative lymphocyte cross-match, indicating no HLA incompatibility.[60, 62]

The initiating event in hyperacute rejection is an antibody-mediated injury caused by recognition of antigens on the vascular endothelium of the transplanted organ by the antibody. The type and extent of antibody-mediated injury depends upon the quantity and localization of the antigen as well as the type of antibody response (e.g., anti-T cell, anti-B cell, warm and cold, autoimmune, and ABO blood group antibodies).[63] Since the antibody response is usually quite profound, hyperacute rejection usually results in graft loss.

This process causes recruitment and activation of inflammatory cells, resulting in increased vascular permeability, arteriolar vasoconstriction, and diffuse cellular damage.

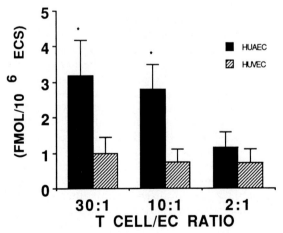

Figure 3–1. Secretion of PDGF-like protein above background levels from human umbilical artery endothelial cells (HUAECs) and human umbilical vein endothelial cells (HUVECs) after coincubation with T cells at T cell/endothelial cell ratios of 30:1, 10:1, and 2:1. *$p < 0.05$ when compared with respective 2:1 ratio.

Experimentally, IgM from human sera induces the release of heparan sulfate from xenogeneic porcine endothelial cells, suggesting a direct effect of natural antibodies on induction of mediator synthesis by endothelium in hyperacute rejection.[64] Hyperacute rejection can be blunted in xenografts by removal of the endothelium.[65]

It has been proposed that one mechanism by which the endothelium participates in hyperacute rejection is through induction or expression of adhesion molecules, such as P-selectin and E-selectin, for inflammatory cells on its surface.[66] Complement may also participate in the pathogenesis of hyperacute rejection by mediating the activation of endothelial cells and adhesion of leukocytes to endothelium.[64, 67] The complement C5b-9 complex induces surface expression of P-selectin.[68] Support for the importance of complement in hyperacute rejection comes from the fact that endothelial cytotoxicity after xenotransplantation can be blocked by decay-accelerating factor, a membrane-associated inhibitor of complement.[69] PAF could also be a potential mediator of the thrombosis as well as the neutrophil binding and emigration seen in hyperacute rejection.[70]

Acute Cellular Rejection

Acute cellular rejection is seen as perivascular or interstitial infiltrates of leukocytes, primarily T cells, into the allograft. Eosinophils and neutrophils can also be present, particularly as the extent and degree of the rejection worsens. In the transplanted heart, myocyte necrosis and hemorrhage are hallmarks of more severe rejection.

A standardized histologic grading system has been adopted for cellular rejection in heart transplantation that classifies rejection as mild to severe.[71] A more severe form of this type of rejection is a vasculitis consisting of transmural and intramural collections of inflammatory cells with plump or destroyed endothelial cells.[72] The effector T cells infiltrating the graft consist of both CD4+ and CD8+ cells.[73] Although not universal, areas of endothelial cell necrosis and proliferation have been described in acute cellular rejection.[74] The mechanism of endothelial cell injury during rejection is unclear but may be secondary to direct cellular effects. Work from our laboratory has shown that sera from heart transplant patients undergoing moderate-severe rejection contains a component that induces peripheral blood mononuclear cells to injure endothelial cells.[75]

Cellular rejection is a complex process initiated by the interaction of antigen-presenting cells (e.g., endothelial cells) within the allograft with recipient CD4+ T cells via the MHC class II antigen and T cell receptor[76] (Fig. 3–2). IL-2 stimulates CD4+ and CD8+, as well as other lymphocytes, to proliferate and differentiate into cytotoxic effector cells that have the capacity to adhere to and lyse endothelial cells. CD4+ cells also secrete IL-4, which increases antibody production from B cells.[76] CD4+ and CD8+ lymphocytes bind primarily to the endothelial MHC class II and MHC class I molecules, respectively, both members of the Ig gene superfamily. This binding increases overall interactions between T lymphocytes and endothelium and may contribute to signal transduction.[76] It is thought that increased expression and subsequent recognition of MHC class I and class II antigens on the allograft is one of the early events in acute cellular rejection[77, 78] (Fig. 3–2). Experimentally, IFN-γ increases HLA DR antigen expression on endothelial cells and thus has been implicated as a potential initiator of this process in transplant rejection. A cascade of events then takes place, including release of IL-1 from antigen-presenting cells, such as endothelial cells themselves, or macrophages.[77] In this capacity, endothelial cells function quite well as antigen-presenting cells for T cell–mediated acute cellular rejection.[79] In turn, activated T cells secrete IL-2, which, in vitro, causes T cell proliferation, adherence to endothelial cells, and migration below the endothelium.[80] Infiltrating monocytes and macrophages are capable of secreting cytokines such as IL-1 and TNF, which increase expression of MHC class I and II antigens on fibroblasts and endothelial cells and increase endothelial cell metabolic activity.[81] These cytokines also induce expression of E-selectin and synthesis of other proinflammatory mediators.[82] MHC class II antigen expression on endothelial cells, potentially mediated through IFN-γ, is a common finding after heart transplantation, particularly during episodes of rejection.[78, 83]

Effector mechanisms for acute cellular allograft rejection and graft destruction are less well understood than the afferent arc of the rejection process. The majority of CD4+ lymphocytes recognize MHC class II antigens, and CD8+ lymphocytes recognize primarily MHC class I antigens. Furthermore, two classes of

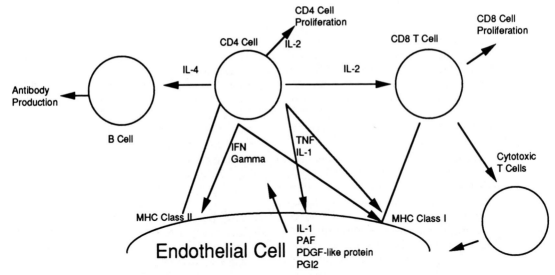

Figure 3–2. CD4 cells bind to MHC class II antigens on endothelial cells and regulate rejection through secretion of mediators that affect T cells, B cells, and endothelial cells. IFN-γ and TNF induce expression of MHC class I and II antigens and increase production and/or secretion of IL-1, PAF, PDGF-like protein, and PG12. IL-2 secretion causes proliferation of CD4 and CD8 cells. IL-4 increases antibody production from B cells. CD8 cells bind to MHC class I antigens and can differentiate into cytotoxic T cells.

CD4+ T cell clones have been described in the mouse: (1) Th1, which produce IL-2, TNFβ and IFN-γ but not IL-4, IL-5, or IL-10; and (2) Th2, which produce the latter but not the former cytokines.[84] The precise role of each of these classes of CD4+ cells in allograft rejection is unclear. However, the interaction between CD4+ and CD8+ cells as it relates to allograft rejection is much more complex than initially realized. In this setting, CD4+ cells function as helper cells for both CD4+ and CD8+ effector cells. Effector T cells can then either release cytokines to attract and activate macrophages to mediate tissue destruction or can cause direct cell-mediated cytotoxicity. In the latter mechanism, T cells recognize a target cell and lyse it.[73] The role of natural killer cells is not well defined. These cells are present in the rejecting graft either as CD3+ cells or as CD16+ cells and are probably capable of cytolytic activity.[77] There is also evidence that upregulation of class I, class II, and ICAM-1 expression by cytokines released from T cells may increase the vulnerability of endothelial cells and other cells to lysis.[85]

Vascular Rejection

This form of rejection was initially described in kidney transplant patients. The presence of immunoglobulin deposition on peritubular capillaries, and/or endothelial swelling and proliferation, is considered evidence of vascular rejection.[86, 87] Vascular rejection in heart transplant patients has now been well described. The histologic findings consist of immunofluorescent staining of immunoglobulin (IgG or IgM), complement (C3 and/or C1q), and fibrin in a vascular pattern.[88] This mechanism of rejection is believed to require an antibody-mediated event distinct from that implicated in hyperacute rejection and to involve immune complex deposition on or under endothelial cells. Endothelial cells are often prominently swollen and project into the lumen of vessels (Fig. 3–3). In one study, heart transplant patients with generalized endothelial cell swelling, coupled with immunofluorescent evidence of vascular immunoglobulin and complement in the vessels, were at higher risk for allograft loss.[88] These patients were younger and tended to have a higher frequency of preformed antibodies against a panel of HLA antigens (positive panel-reactive antibody) in serum samples collected before transplantation, or of antibodies against the donor HLA antigens in post-transplant sera (positive donor-specific cross-match).

The mechanism of vascular rejection is unclear. It has been hypothesized that it may represent either inadequate immunosuppression, a serum sickness type of response to therapy, or an allergic response to OKT3 (a mouse

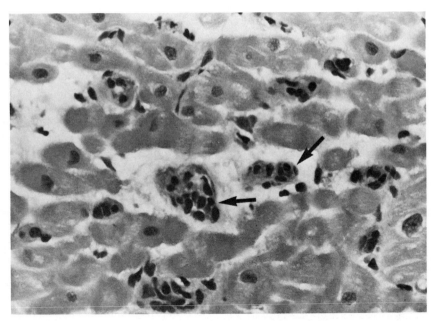

Figure 3–3. Photomicrograph of cross-section of myocardium from a patient undergoing vascular rejection, demonstrating endothelial activation (arrows) involving capillaries. Note occlusion of the lumen by swollen endothelial cells.

monoclonal antibody against CD3 cells).[89] In kidney transplantation, it has been hypothesized that cyclosporine may modify the endothelium of recipient vessels and thus make them more susceptible to rejection of this vascular type.[72] In one study, vascular rejection was associated with elevated plasma endothelin levels as well as endovasculitis, characterized by intimal thickening, infiltration of the intima by mononuclear cells, and fibrinoid necrosis of the vessel wall.[90]

Chronic Rejection

Chronic rejection after solid organ transplantation is often difficult to identify. It is usually diagnosed by a combination of clinical, histopathologic, and angiographic findings, and it is responsible primarily for late loss of allografted organs. Manifestations of this disease include the development of obliterative fibrosis of hollow structures within the graft, regardless of whether they are blood vessels, bronchioles, or bile ducts.[91] This is seen as glomerulosclerosis, nephrosclerosis, and vasculopathy in kidney transplant patients; coronary vasculopathy in heart transplant patients; biliary sclerosis and vasculopathy in liver transplant patients; and bronchiolitis obliterans or vasculopathy in lung transplant patients. The term *chronic rejection* has been used synony-

mously with accelerated graft vasculopathy after heart transplantation.[92, 93] (see next section).

The etiology of chronic rejection is almost certainly multifactorial and may involve factors distinct to the individual organs. Endothelial cells appear to play a very important role. T cells, particularly CD4+ and CD8+ T cells, are found in these lesions in histologic samples, suggesting a chronic cellular cytotoxic rejection.[91, 94] Indeed, a marked lymphocytic vasculitis has been described in human heart allografts with chronic rejection.[95] It has been hypothesized that ongoing stimulation of recipient T lymphocytes by HLA-DR+ endothelium of donor vessels may contribute to the sustained immune response of chronic rejection.[94] However, cellular mechanisms are not solely responsible since, in experimental renal allograft rejection, an antibody response to glomelular endothelial non-MHC antigens may also bring about chronic vascular rejection.[95]

Graft Vasculopathy

As noted, accelerated graft vasculopathy after heart transplantation is felt to represent a type of chronic rejection and is currently the major limiting factor to long-term survival after human heart transplantation.[96] This form of arteriosclerosis is termed *accelerated* because it can occur within a few months or years after heart transplantation rather than over many years with more usual forms. It affects 33 per cent to 50 per cent of all heart transplant recipients within 5 years after transplantation. Although graft vasculopathy has been most widely recognized after heart transplantation, it is in no way unique to the transplanted heart. In fact, accelerated vasculopathy has been described in all transplanted solid organs, including heart, kidney, liver, and lung.[97] Although "immunologic injury" secondary to rejection or infection has been widely implicated as a contributing factor to the pathogenesis of accelerated graft vasculopathy, the mechanisms of this process remain unknown.

The histologic features of the vasculopathy seen after heart transplantation are quite variable, ranging from diffuse to segmental, and from atheromatous to entirely composed of myointimal proliferation.[98] After heart transplantation, rats and rabbits fed low cholesterol diets show significant intimal proliferative lesions of the coronary arteries with little or no lipid deposition, whereas those fed high cholesterol diets show fatty-proliferative lesions, more resembling ordinary (nontransplant) human coronary arteriosclerosis.[99, 100] In the absence of hypercholesterolemia or other risk factors for atheromatous lesions, graft vasculopathy usually consists of myointimal proliferation without atheromatous plaques. In general, the endothelium remains intact, suggesting that this process does not involve a severe, destructive vasculitis or necrosis.

In the usual form of arteriosclerosis not associated with transplantation, the "response to injury" hypothesis states that endothelial cell damage leads to the synthesis and/or secretion of paracrine and autocrine factors that promote myointimal and smooth muscle cell proliferation.[101] Vascular cells implicated in graft arteriosclerosis include endothelial cells, smooth muscle cells, and the so-called myofibroblasts, which are internal to the internal elastic lamina.[102] In the earlier stages of intimal proliferation, clusters of subendothelial lymphocytes may be seen, although their numbers may be sparse.[103] For these reasons, it has been hypothesized that graft vasculopathy represents a type of chronic rejection with subsequent development of chronic vascular changes.[93] Other hypotheses of its etiology include a delayed-type hypersensitivity reaction mediated through leukocyte–endothelial cell

interactions and subsequent cytokine release.[104] As described earlier, during rejection, a complex series of interactions involving leukocyte–endothelial cell adhesion (cellular rejection) or antibody-induced endothelial activation (vascular rejection) cause cytokine release and endothelial activation. It is not yet clear how (or even whether) these interactions result in accelerated graft vasculopathy. However, it is speculated that immune-mediated events result in excessive growth factor production and subsequent myointimal cell migration and proliferation. As stated earlier, the primary growth factors implicated in this process include bFGF and PDGF-like proteins such as connective tissue growth factor. The stimulus for this excessive secretion is unknown, but it could be a result of either the direct contact of lymphocytes with endothelial cells or as a result of antibody production or inflammatory cytokine production (Fig. 3–4).

THERAPEUTIC STRATEGIES

Therapeutic strategies to prevent or treat rejection traditionally have been directed toward global immunosuppression with medications such as corticosteroids, azathioprine, and cyclosporine (see Chapter 11, page 227). Glucocorticoids and cyclosporine inhibit early gene activation events in T cells.[105] Corticosteroids inhibit release of IL-1, cyclosporine inhibits release of IL-2 and IFN-γ, and azathioprine inhibits DNA replication.[106] More recently, therapeutic strategies based on cellular and molecular events thought to be critical in the pathogenesis of rejection have been proposed. Antibodies against specific cytokines have met with some success in experimental studies. Anti-TNF antibodies have prolonged survival in rat cardiac allografts.[107, 108] Similarly, anti-IL-2 antibodies have been shown to prolong survival in cardiac allografts in rats[109] and primates[110] without significant side effects.

Monoclonal antibodies directed at specific molecules or receptors involving leukocyte-endothelial interactions have also been investigated. The first therapeutic monoclonal antibody approved by the Food and Drug Administration for therapeutic human use was the anti-CD3 murine monoclonal antibody (OKT3), which has now been used extensively in heart and renal transplantation for both prevention and treatment of rejection.[106, 111] OKT3 causes an immediate reduction in circulating T cells and interferes with T cell anti-

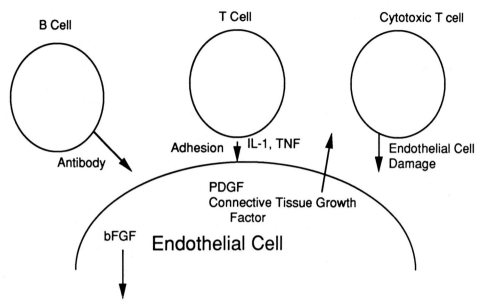

Figure 3–4. Possible interactions between lymphocytes and endothelial cells that could promote growth factor production and thus accelerated graft vasculopathy. B cells (through antibody production) and T cells (through cytokine production or direct cytotoxic effects) could induce increased production of bFGF, PDGF, and connective tissue growth factor. In vitro, bFGF is secreted into the extracellular matrix, whereas PDGF and connective tissue growth factor are secreted into the supernatant medium.

gen recognition through binding of the antibody to the CD3 receptor.[106] Antibodies to CD4 (OKT4-A) have also been shown to prevent allograft rejection in renal and cardiac transplantation but have not been as widely used.[112, 113] Monoclonal antibodies directed against ICAM-1 and LFA-1 (CD11a/CD18) prolong skin and renal allograft survival in monkeys,[114, 115] although anti-LFA-1 (CD11a/CD18) has not been effective in the treatment of acute rejection in human kidney transplantation.[116] More recently, antibodies to ICAM-1 and LFA-1 have been shown to provide indefinite survival for incompatible mice strains synergistically when administered for 6 days after transplantation.[117] Further investigation into antibody therapies and other novel treatment strategies may provide more specific and effective approaches to prevention and treatment of allograft rejection.

SUMMARY AND CONCLUSION

Endothelial cells are the first line of defense of the allografted solid organ against the rejection response from the recipient white blood cells and circulating antibodies. The endothelium is not a passive structure, but rather it is an active organ with the potential for pleio-

tropic biologic responses. In vitro and in vivo studies have demonstrated the importance of the endothelium for amplifying or decreasing the rejection response. Future strategies for prevention and treatment of transplant rejection will undoubtedly include therapies directed at the vascular endothelium.

REFERENCES

1. Libby P. The active roles of cells of the blood vessel wall in health and disease. Molec Aspects Med 9:499, 1987.
2. Jaffe EA. Cell biology of endothelial cells. Hum Pathol 18:234, 1987.
3. Fajardo LF. The complexity of endothelial cells. Am J Clin Pathol 92:241, 1989.
4. Cotran RS, Pober JS. Recent insights into the mechanisms of vascular injury. *In* Simionescu N, Simionescu M (eds). *Endothelial Cell Dysfunctions.* New York, Plenum Press, 1992, p 183.
5. Pober JS, Cotran RS. The role of endothelial cells in inflammation. Transplantation 50:537, 1990.
6. Bevilacqua MP, Pober JS, Mendrick DL, et al. Identification of an inducible endothelial-leukocyte adhesion molecule. Proc Natl Acad Sci USA 84:9238, 1987.
7. Zimmerman GA, Prescott SM, McIntyre TM. Endothelial cell interactions with granulocytes: Tethering and signaling molecules. Immunol Today 13:93, 1992.
8. Rothlein R, Dustin ML, Marlin SD, et al. A human intercellular adhesion molecule (ICAM-1) distinct from LFA-1. J Immunol 137:1270, 1986.

9. Pober JS, Gimbrone MA, Lapierre LA, et al. Overlapping patterns of activation of human endothelial cells by interleukin 1, tumor necrosis factor and immune interferon. J Immunol 137:1893, 1986.

10. Springer TA. Adhesion receptors of the immune system. Nature 346:425, 1990.

11. Osborn L, Hession R, Tizard R, et al. Direct expression cloning of vascular cell adhesion molecule-1, a cytokine-induced endothelial protein that binds lymphocytes. Cell 59:1203, 1989.

12. Shimizu Y, Newman W, Gopal TV, et al. Four molecular pathways of T cell adhesion to endothelial cells: Roles of LFA-1, VCAM-1, and ELAM-1 and changes in pathway hierarchy under different activation conditions. J Cell Biol 113:1203, 1991.

13. Masuyama J, Minato N, Kano S. Mechanisms of lymphocyte adhesion to human vascular endothelial cells in culture. J Clin Invest 77:1596, 1986.

14. Collins T, Lapierre LA, Fiers W, et al. Recombinant human tumor necrosis factor increases RNA levels and surface expression of HLA-A, B antigens in vascular endothelial cells and dermal fibroblasts in vitro. Proc Natl Acad Sci USA 83:446, 1986.

15. Daar AS, Fuggle SV, Fabre JW, et al. The detailed distribution of MHC Class II antigens in normal human organs. Transplantation 38:293, 1984.

16. Collins T, Korman AJ, Wake CT, et al. Immune interferon cultivates multiple class II major histocompatibility complex genes and the associated invariant chain gene in vascular endothelial cells and dermal fibroblasts in vitro. Proc Natl Acad Sci USA 83:446, 1984.

17. Lapierre LA, Fiers W, Pober JS. Three distinct classes of regulatory cytokines control endothelial cell MHC antigen expression: Interactions with immune interferon differentiate the effects of tumor necrosis factor and lymphotoxin from those of leukocyte and fibroblast interferon. J Exp Med 167:794, 1988.

18. Ahmed-Ansari A, Tadros TS, Knopf WD. Major histocompatibility complex class I and class II expression by myocytes in cardiac biopsies post-transplantation. Transplantation 45:972, 1988.

19. Carlquist JF, Hammond ME, Yowell RL, et al. Correlation between class II antigen (DR) expression and interleukin-2-induced lymphocyte proliferation in acute cardiac allograft rejection. Transplantation 50:582, 1990.

20. Rose ML, Coles MI, Griffin RJ, et al. Expression of class I and class II major histocompatibility antigens in the normal and transplanted heart. Transplantation 41:776, 1986.

21. Belitsky P, Miller SM, Gupta R, et al. Induction of MHC class II expression in recipient tissues caused by allograft rejection. Transplantation 49:472, 1990.

22. Prescott SM, Zimmerman GA, McIntyre TM. Human endothelial cells in culture produce platelet-activating factor (1-alkyl-2-acteyl-sn-glycero-3-phosphocholine) when stimulated with thrombin. Proc Natl Acad Sci USA 81:3534, 1984.

23. Pober JS, Cotran RS. Cytokines and endothelial cell biology. Physiol Rev 70:427, 1990.

24. Renkonnen R, Mattila P, Turunen JP, et al. Lymphocyte binding to and penetration through endothelium is enhanced by platelet-activating factor. Scand J Immunol 30:673, 1989.

25. Osborn L. Leukocyte adhesion to endothelium in inflammation. Cell 62:3, 1990.

26. Shimizu S, Newman W, Tanaka Y, et al. Lymphocyte interactions with endothelial cells. Immunol Today 13:106, 1992.

27. McEver RP. Leukocyte–endothelial cell interactions. Curr Opin Cell Biol 4:840, 1992.

28. Spertini O, Luscuskas FW, Kansas GS, et al. Leukocyte adhesion molecule (LAM-1, L-selectin) interacts with an inducible endothelial cell ligand to support leukocyte adhesion. J Immunol 147:2565, 1991.

29. Lasky LA, Singer MS, Dowbenko D, et al. An endothelial ligand for L-selectin is a novel mucin-like molecule. Cell 69:927, 1992.

30. Mentzer SJ, Burakoff SJ, Faller DV. Adhesion of T lymphocytes to human endothelial cells is regulated by the LFA-1 membrane molecule. J Cell Physiol 126:285, 1986.

31. Staunton DE, Dustin ML, Springer TA. Functional cloning of ICAM-2, a cell adhesion ligand for LFA-1 homologous to ICAM-1. Nature 339:61, 1989.

32. Hynes RO. Integrins: Versatility, modulation, and signaling in cell adhesion. Cell 69:11, 1992.

33. Makgoba MW, Saunders ME, Shaw S. The CD-2-LFA-3 and LFA-1-ICAM-1 pathways: Relevance to T cell recognition. Immunol Today 10:417, 1989.

34. Briscoe DM, Schoen FJ, Rice GE, et al. Induced expression of endothelial-leukocyte adhesion molecules in human cardiac allografts. Transplantation 51:537, 1991.

35. Faull RJ, Russ GR. Tubular expression of intracellular adhesion molecule-1 during renal allograft rejection. Transplantation 48:226, 1989.

36. Figdor CG, van Kooyk Y, Keizer GD. On the mode of action of LFA-1. Immunol Today 11:277, 1990.

37. Colson YL, Markus BH, Zeevi A, et al. Increased lymphocyte adherence to human arterial endothelial cell monolayers in the context of allorecognition. J Immunol 144:2975, 1990.

38. Tanaka Y, Albelda SM, Horgan KJ, et al. CD31 expressed on distinctive T cell subsets is a preferential amplifier of beta 1 integrin-mediated adhesion. J Exp Med 176:245, 1992.

39. Oppenheimer-Marks N, Davis LS, Lipsky PE. Human T lymphocyte adhesion to endothelial cells and transendothelial migration. J Immunol 145:140, 1990.

40. Aruffo A, Stamenkovic I, Melnick M, et al. CD44 is the principal cell surface receptor for hyaluronate. Cell 61:1303, 1990.

41. Lorant DE, Patel KD, McIntyre TM, et al. Coexpression of GMP-140 and PAF by endothelium stimulated by histamine or thrombin: A juxtacrine system for adhesion and activation of neutrophils. J Cell Biol 115:223, 1991.

42. Gill EA, McIntyre TM, Prescott SM, et al. Mechanisms of vascular injury in the pathogenesis of infectious disease. Curr Opin Infect Dis 5:381, 1992.

43. Bradham DM, Igarashi A, Potter RL, et al. Connective tissue growth factor: A cysteine-rich mitogen secreted by human vascular endothelial cells is related to the SRC-induced immediate early gene product CEF-10. J Cell Biol 114:1285, 1991.

44. Raines EW, Dower SK, Ross R. Interleukin-1 mitogenic activity for fibroblasts and smooth muscle cells is due to PDGF-AA. Science 134:393, 1989.

45. Ross RR, Raines EW, Bowen-Pope DF. The biology of platelet-derived growth factor. Cell 46:155, 1986.

46. Harlan JM, Thompson J, Ross RR, et al. Alpha-thrombin induces release of platelet-derived growth factor-like molecules by cultured endothelial cells. J Cell Biol 103:1129, 1986.

47. Hajjar KA, Hajjar DP, Silverstein RL, et al. Tumor

necrosis-mediated release of platelet-derived growth factor from cultured endothelial cells. J Exp Med 166:235, 1987.

48. Ross RR, Masuda J, Raines E, et al. Localization of PDGF-B protein in macrophages in all phases of atherogenesis. Science 248:1009, 1990.

49. Rubin K, Hansson GK, Ronnstrand L, et al. Induction of B-type receptors for platelet-derived growth factor in vascular inflammation: Possible implications for development of vascular proliferative lesions. Lancet 1:1353, 1988.

50. Shaddy RE, Hansen JC, Cowley CG. Effects of T cells on platelet-derived growth factor-like protein from endothelial cells. J Heart Lung Transplant 11:48, 1992.

51. Pardi R, Bender JR. Signal transduction in cultured endothelial cells induced by lymphocyte adhesion. Clin Res 38:466A, 1990.

52. Gospodarowicz D, Neufeld G, Schweigerer L. Fibroblast growth factor: Structural and biological properties. J Cell Physiol (Suppl) 5:15, 1987.

53. Schweigerer L, Neufeld G, Friedman J, et al. Capillary endothelial cells express basic fibroblast growth factor, a mitogen that promotes their own growth. Nature 325:257, 1987.

54. Vlodavsky I, Folkman J, Sullivan R, et al. Endothelial cell-derived basic fibroblast growth factor: Synthesis and deposition into the subendothelial extracellular matrix. Proc Natl Acad Sci USA 84:2292, 1987.

55. Gajdusek CM, Carbon S. Injury-induced release of basic fibroblast growth factor from bovine aortic endothelium. J Cell Physiol 139:570, 1989.

56. McNeil PL, Muthukrishnare L, Warder E, et al. Growth factors are released by mechanically wounded endothelial cells. J Cell Biol 109:811, 1989.

57. Bikfalvi A, Inyang AL, Dupuy E, et al. Basic fibroblast growth factor expression in human omental microvascular endothelial cells and the effect of phorbol ester. J Cell Physiol 144:144, 1990.

58. Cooper DKC, Lanza RP. Pathology of acute rejection. In: Heart Transplantation. Lancaster, United Kingdom, MTP Press Ltd, 1984, p 175.

59. Cerilli J, Brasile L, Galouzis T, et al. The vascular endothelial cell antigen system. Transplantation 39:286, 1985.

60. Trento A, Hardesty RL, Griffith BP, et al. Role of antibody to vascular endothelial cells in hyperacute rejection in patients undergoing cardiac transplantation. J Thorac Cardiovasc Surg 95:37, 1988.

61. Brasile L, Zerbe T, Rabin B, et al. Identification of the antibody to vascular endothelial cells in patients undergoing cardiac transplantation. Transplantation 40:672, 1985.

62. Jordan SC, Yap HK, Sakai RS, et al. Hyperacute allograft rejection mediated by anti-vascular endothelial cell antibodies with a negative monocyte crossmatch. Transplantation 46:585, 1988.

63. Dubernard JM, Flye MW. Xenografts. In Flye MW (ed). Principles of Organ Transplantation. Philadelphia; WB Saunders, 1989, pp 612–633.

64. Platt JL, Vercellotti GM, Lindman BJ, et al. Release of heparan sulfate from endothelial cells: Implication for pathogenesis of hyperacute rejection. J Exp Med 171:1363, 1990.

65. Galumbeck MA, Sanfilippo FP, Hagen PO, et al. Inhibition of vessel allograft rejection by allograft removal: Morphologic and ultrastructural changes. Ann Surg 206:757, 1987.

66. Sedmak DD, Orosz CG. The role of vascular endothelial cells in transplantation. Arch Pathol Lab Med 115:260, 1991.

67. Marks RM, Todd RF III, Ward PA. Rapid induction of neutrophil-endothelial adhesion by endothelial complement fixation. Nature 339:314, 1989.

68. Hattori R, Hamilton KK, Fugate RD, et al. Complement proteins C5b-9 induce secretion of high molecular weight multimers of endothelial von Willebrand factor and translocation of granule membrane protein GMP-140 to the cell surface. J Biol Chem 264:768, 1989.

69. Dalmasso AP, Vercellotti GM, Platt JL, et al. Inhibition of complement-mediated endothelial cell cytotoxicity by decay-accelerating factor. Transplantation 52:530, 1991.

70. Carveth HJ, Shaddy RE, Whatley RE, et al. Regulation of platelet-activating factor (PAF) synthesis and PAF-mediated neutrophil adhesion to endothelial cells activated by thrombin. Semin Thromb Hemost 18:126, 1992.

71. Billingham ME, Cary NRB, Hammond ME, et al. A working formulation for the standardization of nomenclature in the diagnosis of heart and lung rejection: Heart rejection study group. J Heart Transplant 9:587, 1990.

72. Herskowitz A, Soule LM, Ueda K, et al. Arteriolar vasculitis on endomyocardial biopsy: A histologic predictor of poor outcome in cyclosporine-treated heart transplant recipients. J Heart Transplant 6:127, 1987.

73. Hall BM. Cells mediating allograft rejection. Transplantation 51:1141, 1991.

74. Colvin RB. Cellular and molecular mechanisms of allograft rejection. Annu Rev Med 41:361, 1990.

75. Shaddy RE, Mak C, Zimmerman GA. Evidence that the serum of moderate-to-severely rejecting heart transplant patients induces peripheral blood mononuclear cells to injure endothelial cells. Transplantation 49:1013, 1990.

76. Denning SM. T-lymphocyte interactions in cardiac transplant rejection. Trends Cardiovasc Med 1:75, 1991.

77. Marboe CC, Buffaloe A, Fenoglio JJ. Immunologic aspects of rejection. Prog Cardiovasc Dis 32:419, 1990.

78. Milton AD, Fabre JW. Massive induction of donor class I and class II major histocompatibility complex antigens in rejecting cardiac allografts in the rat. J Exp Med 161:98, 1985.

79. Rose ML, Page C, Hengstenberg C, et al. Identification of antigen presenting cells in normal and transplanted human heart: Importance of endothelial cells. Hum Immunol 28:179, 1990.

80. Robbins RA, Klassen L, Rasmussen J, et al. Interleukin-2-induced chemotaxis of human T-lymphocytes. J Lab Clin Med 108:340, 1986.

81. Cavender DE, Edelbaum D, Ziff M. Endothelial cell activation induced by tumor necrosis factor and lymphotoxin. Am J Pathol 134:551, 1989.

82. Bevilacqua MP, Stengelin S, Gimbrone MA, et al. Endothelial leukocyte adhesion molecule 1: An inducible receptor for neutrophils related to complement regulatory proteins. Science 243:1160, 1989.

83. Bouwman E, Ijzermans JNM, Heineman E, et al. Class II antigen expression on vascular endothelium of the graft in rat heart transplantation. Transplant Proc 19:198, 1987.

84. Mossman TR, Cherwinski H, Bond MW, et al. Two types of murine helper T cell clones: I. Definition

according to profiles of lymphokine activities and secreted proteins. J Immunol 136:2348, 1986.

85. Suranyi MS, Bishop GA, Clayburger C, et al. Lymphocyte adhesion molecules in T cell mediated lysis of human kidney cells. Kidney Int 39:312, 1991.

86. Paul LC, van Es LA, van Rood JJ, et al. Antibodies directed against antigens on the endothelium of peritubular capillaries in patients with rejecting renal allografts. Transplantation 27:175, 1979.

87. Mihatsch MJ, Thiel G, Basler V, et al. Morphologic patterns in cyclosporine treated renal transplant recipients. Transplant Proc 17:101, 1985.

88. Hammond EH, Yowell RL, Nunoda S, et al. Vascular (humoral) rejection in heart transplantation: Pathologic observations and clinical implications. J Heart Transplant 8:430, 1989.

89. Hammond EH, Ensley RD, Yowell RL, et al. Vascular rejection of human cardiac allografts and the role of humoral immunity in chronic allograft rejection. Transplant Proc 23:26, 1991.

90. Watschinger B, Vychytil A, Schuller M, et al. The pathophysiologic role of endothelin in acute vascular rejection after renal transplantation. Transplantation 52:743, 1991.

91. Tilney NL, Whitley D, Diamond JR, et al. Chronic rejection—an undefined conundrum. Transplantation 52:389, 1991.

92. Chomette G, Auriol M, Cabrol C. Chronic rejection in human heart transplantation. J Heart Transplant 7:292, 1988.

93. Paul LC, Fellstrom B. Chronic vascular rejection of the heart and the kidney: Have rational treatment options emerged? Transplantation 53:1169, 1992.

94. Salomon RN, Hughes CCW, Schoen FJ, et al. Human coronary transplant-associated arteriosclerosis. Am J Pathol 138:791, 1991.

95. Duijvestijn AM, van Breda R, Vriesman PJC. Chronic renal allograft rejection. Transplantation 52:195, 1991.

96. O'Neill BJ, Pflugfelder PW, Singh NR, et al. Frequency of angiographic detection and quantitative assessment of coronary arterial disease one and three years after cardiac transplantation. Am J Cardiol 63:1221, 1989.

97. Miller LW. Allograft vascular disease: A disease not limited to hearts. J Heart Lung Transplant 11:S32, 1992.

98. Johnson DE, Gao SZ, Schroeder JS, et al. The spectrum of coronary artery pathologic findings in human cardiac allografts. J Heart Transplant 8:349, 1989.

99. Laden AMK. Experimental atherosclerosis in rat and rabbit cardiac allografts. Arch Pathol 93:240, 1972.

100. Alonso DR, Starek PK, Minick CR. Studies on the pathogenesis of atheroarteriosclerosis induced in rabbit cardiac allografts by the synergy of graft rejection and hypercholesterolemia. Am J Pathol 87:415, 1977.

101. Ross R, Faggiotto A, Bowen-Pope D, et al. The role of endothelial injury and platelet and macrophage interactions in atherosclerosis. Circulation 70(Suppl III):77, 1984.

102. Williams SK. Regulation of intimal hyperplasia: Do endothelial cells participate? Lab Invest 64:721, 1991.

103. Billingham ME. Histopathology of graft coronary disease. J Heart Lung Transplant 11:S38, 1992.

104. Libby P, Payne DD, Schoen FJ. Functions of the vascular wall cells related to development of transplantation-associated coronary arteriosclerosis. Transplant Proc 21:3677, 1989.

105. Krensky AM, Weiss A, Crabtree G, et al. T-lymphocyte-antigen interactions in transplant rejection. N Engl J Med 322:510, 1990.

106. Bristow MR, Gilbert EM, Renlund DG, et al. Use of OKT3 monoclonal antibody in heart transplantation: Review of the initial experience. J Heart Transplant 7:1, 1988.

107. Lin H, Chensue SW, Strieter RM, et al. Antibodies against tumor necrosis factor prolong cardiac allograft survival in the rat. J Heart Lung Transplant 11:330, 1992.

108. Bolling SF, Kunkel SL, Lin H. Prolongation of cardiac allograft survival in rats by anti-TNF and cyclosporine combination therapy. Transplantation 53:283, 1992.

109. Sakagami K, Ohsaki T, Ohnishi T, et al. The effect of anti-interleukin 2 monoclonal antibody treatment on the survival of rat cardiac allografts. J Surg Res 46:262, 1988.

110. Brown PS, Parenteau GL, Dirbas FM, et al. Anti-Tac-H, a humanized antibody to the interleukin 2 receptor, prolongs primate allograft survival. Proc Natl Acad Sci USA 88:2663, 1991.

111. Cosimi AB, Burton RC, Colvin RB. Treatment of acute renal allograft rejection with OKT3 monoclonal antibody. Transplantation 32:535, 1981.

112. Cosimi AB, Burton RC, Kung PC, et al. Evaluation in primate renal allograft recipients of monoclonal antibody to human T-cell subclasses. Transplant Proc 13:499, 1981.

113. Herbert J, Roser B. Strategies of monoclonal antibody therapy that induce permanent tolerance of organ transplants. Transplantation 46(Suppl):128S, 1988.

114. Cosimi AB, Geoffrian C, Anderson T, et al. Immunosuppression of Cynomolgus recipients with renal allografts by R6.5, a monoclonal antibody to ICAM-1. *In* Springer TA, Anderson DC, Rothlein R, Rosenthal AS (eds). *Leukocyte Adhesion Molecules*. Berlin, Springer-Verlag, 1989, pp 274–281.

115. Berlin PJ, Bacher JD, Sharrow SO, et al. Monoclonal antibodies directed against human T cell adhesion molecules—Modulation of immune function in nonhuman primates. Transplantation 53:840, 1992.

116. Le Mauff B, Hourmant M, Rougier J, et al. Effect of anti-LFA-1 (CD11a) monoclonal antibodies in acute rejection in human kidney transplantation. Transplantation 52:291, 1991.

117. Isobe M, Yagita H, Okumura K, et al. Specific acceptance of cardiac allograft after treatment with antibodies to ICAM-1 and LFA-1. Science 255:1125, 1992.

4

FIBRINOLYTIC AND ANTICOAGULANT CONTROL OF HEMOSTASIS IN HUMAN CARDIAC AND RENAL ALLOGRAFTS

W. PAGE FAULK, MD, FRC PATH, and CARLOS A. LABARRERE, MD

The thrust of immunologic research in transplantation has focused on cells, cytokines, antibodies, and amplification systems such as complement. These aspects of immunity are recognized as key elements in the success or failure of grafts, but also it is recognized that grafts in invertebrates that lack immunologic systems manifest similar degrees of success or failure.[1] It thus appears that fundamental pieces are missing in the puzzle of recipient responses to grafted tissues. This is supported by the clinical awareness that allografts do not last forever, and by the statistical reality that the survival of solid organ allografts is an inverse function of time.[2]

Survival of any tissue depends upon the maintenance of a circulatory route that delivers oxygen and nutrients and carries away metabolic debris. Defects in either the afferent or efferent arms of the circulation result in diminished function. Such functional failures usually are not characterized by morphologic changes, but the tissue consequences of such failures can be identified. These are classified by pathologists according to a nosology that relates structure to function. Using this approach, pathologists realized many years ago that vascular obstruction was a premier defect in renal allografts.[3, 4]

This chapter discusses vascular changes in allografts. We have structured our discussion to deal with the systems that normally function to prevent fibrin deposits (Fig. 4–1). The presence of fibrin can be viewed as representing either an upstream defect (i.e., failure in natural anticoagulant pathways), or a downstream defect (i.e., inadequate function of the fibrinolytic pathways). For the most part, we have pursued these discussions unencumbered by considerations of cellular infiltrates, antibodies, and so on, but this was done with fore-

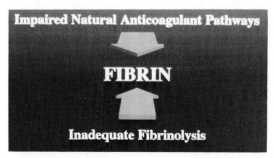

Figure 4–1. Physiology of fibrin deposition. Note that fibrin can result from either upstream (i.e., natural anticoagulant pathways) or downstream (i.e., fibrinolytic pathways) defects.

knowledge that such immunologic aspects are discussed in other chapters.

TECHNICAL CONSIDERATIONS

Patients

The material discussed in this chapter is drawn primarily from our experience since 1987 with heart and kidney recipients at Methodist Hospital of Indiana. These populations represent 150 cardiac and 250 renal allografts. The patients are followed by surgeons, physicians, and transplant coordinators. Patients are evaluated by clinical status, functional tests, angiography, and biopsies, and results of these evaluations are used to classify individual patients as being either stable or unstable. For cardiac allograft recipients, criteria for being unstable are coronary artery disease, falling ejection fractions, and/or three or more classifications of 2 or higher for functional status or histologic biopsy grading.[5] For renal allograft recipients, criteria for being unstable are clinical evaluation, creatinine of more than 2 mg per dl, and/or evidence of cellular infiltrates in the biopsy.

Biopsies

All hearts and many kidneys are biopsied before being perfused with recipients' blood. These tissues provide information about the donor organs at time-zero, and data from these biopsies have been used to build a picture of the hemostatic, fibrinolytic, and natural anticoagulant pathways in normal hearts and kidneys. It might be argued that time-zero hearts are not normal, for they are obtained from donors who technically are dead. However, when we compared time-zero findings with autopsy and surgically obtained tissues from normal nontransplanted hearts, only trivial differences were found. Nonetheless, there do appear to be differences in the hemostatic pathway for tissue factor between time-zero biopsies obtained from cadaver and living-related donors.[6]

Processing and Evaluation of Biopsies

Technical publications should be consulted for these details,[7–9] but it is a matter of both policy and philosophy that prior decisions are made regarding whether biopsies are going to be evaluated by immunocytochemical techniques. This is essential because (a) the hemostatic, fibrinolytic, and natural anticoagulant pathways cannot be evaluated without using immunocytochemical techniques, and (b) many fixation procedures used to prepare tissues for histologic evaluations cannot be used to prepare tissues for immunocytochemical evaluations. If in doubt, it is prudent to snap-freeze tissues in liquid nitrogen, for this is a generic first step in preservation for most immunocytochemical procedures. If properly frozen, wrapped in aluminum foil, and kept at least at minus 20°C, such tissues can be studied years later.

Immunocytochemical preparations made by using enzyme-labeled antibodies (e.g., immunoperoxidase) can be evaluated with any competent microscope, but preparations made by using antibodies labeled with fluorochromes (e.g., fluorescein isothiocyanate) must be evaluated with microscopes equipped for immunofluorescence. Such microscopes are expensive and somewhat intimidating. The same complaints were voiced about electron microscopy, but discovery of the immunocolloidal gold technique[10] has helped immunoelectron microscopy evolve into a powerful diagnostic technique.[11]

Immunoperoxidase preparations are stable and can be stored for future study; immunofluorescence preparations are unstable, tend to fade upon examination, and cannot be stored for future study. It is not surprising that most pathology laboratories tend to favor the use of immunoperoxidase. However, these economic and logistic advantages should not obscure the precision and flexibility of immunofluorescence. For example, as many as three antibodies can be studied simultaneously on the same tissue section by using fluorochrome labels that emit characteristic colors, thus allowing investigations of the interaction of different systems at specific sites within biopsy specimens. Regardless of the advantages of immunocytochemistry, none of these techniques will yield satisfactory results if the tissues are not obtained rapidly and processed properly.

HEMOSTASIS

Coagulation describes clotting in a liquid phase (e.g., in a test tube), and hemostasis describes an interruption of blood flow (e.g.,

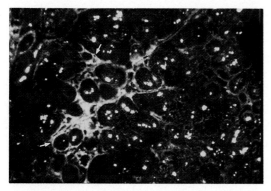

Color Figure 4–1. Heart biopsy from an unstable allograft reacted with monoclonal antibody to the amino terminal neotope of the fibrin β-chain. This antibody recognizes fibrin and not fibrinogen. Note the fibrin in microcirculation, the interstitium, and around myocardial cells (arrows). (× 400)

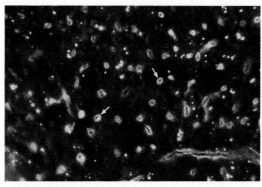

Color Figure 4–2. Heart biopsy from a stable allograft reacted with antibody to thrombomodulin. Note endothelial reactivity (arrows). (× 400)

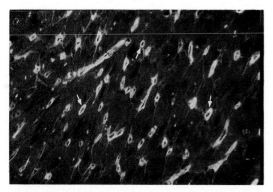

Color Figure 4–3. Localization of antithrombin III in biopsy of cardiac allograft with a history of serious signs of failure, but the patient survived. Note AT III reactivity of capillaries (arrows). (× 400)

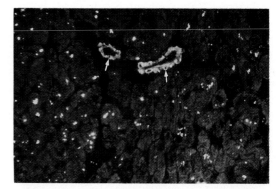

Color Figure 4–4. Heart biopsy from a stable allograft incubated with antibody to tissue plasminogen activator. Note that arterial smooth muscle cells are reactive (arrows). (× 400)

within a blood vessel). The process that occurs in vessels of allografted organs is described more precisely as hemostasis. Both processes result in the thrombin-mediated conversion of fibrinogen to fibrin. Fibrinogen is a ubiquitously distributed plasma protein present in normally functioning organs, and fibrin is not present in normally functioning organs.[12] Thus, fibrin is a marker of hemostasis and as such it can be used as an index of vascular damage.

Fibrin Versus Fibrinogen

Most textbooks are singularly unhelpful about how fibrin should be identified. There are many histochemical techniques to identify fibrin/fibrinogen, but none identify fibrin and not fibrinogen. This problem is aggravated by cavalier use of the noun fibrin when discussing fibrinogen, and vice versa. Indeed, the recent edition of an otherwise useful book on histochemistry states that fibrin can be identified by using fluorescein-labeled antibody to fibrinogen!

In our experience, fibrin deposits within vessels of allografted organs is the earliest and most reliable index of graft failure.[12] Inasmuch as fibrinogen always is present, it is essential to identify fibrin independent of the presence of fibrinogen. This can be done reliably by using a monoclonal antibody that recognizes fibrin but not fibrinogen.[12-14] Such antibody reacts with an epitope exposed at the amino terminus of the beta-chain of human fibrin.

Generation of Fibrin Deposits

Fibrin deposits can be generated by discrete and indiscrete mechanisms. The indiscrete mechanism involves hemostasis triggered by platelets subsequent to their activation by vascular basement membrane collagen, endothelially derived platelet-activating factor,[15] or exposure to epinephrine, adenosine diphosphate (ADP), thrombin, or prostaglandin endoperoxides.[16]

We have not been able to identify immunocytochemically a consistent role for platelets in graft rejection, but radiolabeled platelets have been identified within renal allografts during rejection,[17] suggesting an as yet undefined role for platelets in rejection. In addition, many investigators in the field of atherosclerosis research are of the opinion that products of activated platelets play a role in the pathogenesis of atherosclerosis.[18] In this chapter, we will not present data on platelets, but this should not imply that we think they are unimportant.

The discrete mechanism for generation of fibrin deposits involves the intrinsic and extrinsic coagulation pathways. Detailed information on these pathways can be obtained from any hematology textbook, but readers should be aware of changing ideas about the roles of these pathways in biology and disease. Briefly, it used to be taught that the intrinsic pathway was paramount, and that the extrinsic pathway was somewhat of an academic side show. Much has been learned from studies of the intrinsic pathway, and today there is a prevailing opinion (and masses of data) that endothelial control of hemostasis is expressed almost exclusively through the so-called extrinsic pathway.[19, 20] In light of this, it perhaps is less confusing simply to refer to the extrinsic pathway as the tissue factor pathway, for the availability of tissue factor modulates the role and extent of hemostasis at the level of plasma membranes.[21]

Tissue Factor Pathway

The substance in tissues considered to be responsible for coagulation used to be referred to as tissue thromboplastin. This has been isolated and characterized as a 37-kD glycoprotein and now is referred to as tissue factor.[21-23] The molecule normally is not available on endothelial plasma membranes but is upregulated and made available on endothelium following exposure to certain cytokines (e.g., tumor necrosis factor, interleukin-1), endotoxin,[24] or hypoxia and metabolic acidosis.[25] In its upregulated position, tissue factor binds and activates factor VII. Activated factor VII activates factor X (and factor IX), causing the assembly of prothrombin convertase (i.e., activated factors X and V, calcium, and phospholipid), which generates thrombin that converts fibrinogen to fibrin. In addition, significant concentrations of tissue factor are present in the brain and amniotic fluid,[26] and the exposure of either of these substances to blood (e.g., following head trauma or amniotic fluid embolism) results in life-threatening disseminated intravascular coagulation.

Although the exposure of tissue factor in brain or amniotic fluid to blood results in disseminated intravascular coagulation, a type of localized intravascular coagulation can result from the upregulation of endothelial tissue factor in a circumscribed area of vessels. For example, this occurs in human placentas in areas of chronic villitis[27] and in the peritubular venous capillary plexus of dysfunctional transplanted kidneys.[6] This thrombogenic process is augmented by complement activation at cell surfaces, which increases tissue factor expression.[28] The availability of tissue factor in these vascular beds converts endothelium from a thromboresistant to a thrombogenic surface. This results in fibrin deposition and the development of microthrombi that obstruct blood flow and promote hypoxia and metabolic acidosis, further aggravating the thrombogenic state and resulting in localized intravascular coagulation.

Diagnosis of Hemostasis

Antibodies to most clotting factors are commercially available, but the specificities of many of these antibodies have not been established by rigid immunochemical criteria. In an effort to identify the most useful antibodies to diagnose intravascular hemostasis, we have studied the immunocytochemical reactivities of antibodies to all clotting factors in normal and transplanted hearts and kidneys. In our experience, monoclonal antibody to the fibrin neotope is the most sensitive, specific, and reproducible marker of hemostasis, and results obtained from antibodies to other hemostatic factors do not extend the information obtained from antifibrin.

Normal human hearts and kidneys do not contain fibrin, and fibrin is not identified in biopsies of stable and well-functioning heart and kidney allografts. However, allograft failure, regardless of the time since transplantation, is associated with the identification of fibrin deposits, and the degree of failure is associated with the amount of fibrin deposited.[12] The amount of fibrin deposited can be quantified by using double-antibody techniques that simultaneously identify fibrin and von Willebrand factor (as a marker of endothelium). This allows a calculation of the percentage of vessels containing fibrin.

Since vessels of normal hearts and stable allografts contain no fibrin, we assign this a grade of 1.0. Fibrin in 10 per cent or less of the vessels is graded as 2.0, and a grade of 3.0 is assigned to biopsy specimens that contain fibrin in more than 10 per cent of the vessels.

Grade 3.0 hearts do not contain fibrin-reactive vessels in all four quadrants of a high-power ($\times$ 400) microscopic field, but they do contain interstitial fibrin that often extends around cardiomyocytes (Color Fig. 4–1). Intracardiomyocytic reactivity usually is not observed in grade 3.0 biopsy material. In contrast, grade 4.0 hearts contain fibrin-reactive vessels in all quadrants of a high-power field, as well as fibrin deposits in interstitial, perimyocardiocytic, and intramyocardiocytic locations. The functional significance of grading fibrin deposits in cardiac biopsies is that the grade often corresponds to the New York Heart Association's functional criteria, yet we have been impressed by the lack of concordance between fibrin scores and cellular infiltrates.[12]

Systemic Manifestation of Hemostasis in Allograft Recipients

In light of the preceding evidence of hemostasis in allografts, we have asked whether allograft recipients manifest measurable coagulation changes in their peripheral blood. Results of immunocytochemical studies suggest that failure of natural anticoagulant pathways is central to hemostasis.[29, 30] These pathways are designed primarily to regulate thrombin.[31] Since thrombin times are a measure of the ability of exogenously added thrombin to exceed the several thrombin control mechanisms of plasma and convert fibrinogen to fibrin, we have determined the thrombin times in samples of citrated plasma from renal and cardiac allograft recipients.

Results of these studies have revealed three hitherto unrecognized coagulational characteristics of peripheral blood from allograft recipients. First, we have observed that prolongation of thrombin times is a pathophysiologic response to allografting (Table 4–1). Second, there is an inverse relationship between plasma creatinine concentrations and thrombin times in renal allograft recipients. Third, cardiac allograft recipients with immunocytochemical evidence of vascular damage in their endomyocardial biopsies (e.g., fibrin deposits, impaired fibrinolysis, and/or diminished natural anticoagulant pathways) have shorter thrombin times than recipients without evidence of vascular damage in their biopsies.[12]

Several possible reasons for a relationship between thrombin times and graft function are possible, yet no single reason has been

Table 4–1. Average Thrombin Times for Groups of Stable Allograft Recipients*

Allografts	Thrombin Times†	NYHA Class‡	Creatinine *(mg/dl)*
Heart	14.4/11.9	1	—
Kidney	13.3/11.9	—	1.16

*Hearts: 50 samples from 33 recipients; kidneys: 50 samples from 46 recipients.
†Test value/control value.
‡New York Heart Association's functional classification.

established. Possible explanations for a prolonged thrombin time are endogenous heparan and in vivo fibrinogenolysis.[32] We presently do not know why this relationship exists, but it appears to be a systemic manifestation of damage within the vascular bed of allografted organs. In our experience, patients with shortened thrombin times have a high probability of decreased graft function and increased vascular damage, although more research needs to be done to define these associations more precisely.

NATURAL ANTICOAGULANT PATHWAYS

De Motu Cordis, written by William Harvey in 1628, described circulation of the blood. Harvey had studied in Padua with Fabricius (1537–1619), who described venous valves as well as a lymphoid organ in the terminal gut of birds. This organ, subsequently named the bursa of Fabricius, 400 years later provided the critical clue to understanding that the immunologic system was composed of T (i.e., thymus-derived) and B (i.e., bursa-derived) lymphocytes. It is prophetic that these men, separated by great distance during turbulent times, were able to work together on problems that profoundly touch our lives today.

Although it has been known for several centuries that blood circulates, it has not been known how circulating blood normally avoids hemostasis. Recently, light has been cast into this dark corner by the emerging concept of natural anticoagulant pathways. There presently are five natural anticoagulant pathways

Table 4–2. Natural Anticoagulant Pathways

- Thrombomodulin–protein C
- Heparan sulfate proteoglycan–antithrombin III
- Dermatan sulfate proteoglycan–heparin cofactor II
- Secretion of endogenous heparan sulfate
- Tissue factor pathway inhibitor

(Table 4–2). Each of these will be discussed regarding their known or speculative role in the success and/or failure of allografts.

Thrombomodulin–Protein C Pathway

Thrombomodulin is an intrinsic glycoprotein of endothelial plasma membranes that serves as a receptor for thrombin (Fig. 4–2). Subsequent to formation of the thrombomodulin-thrombin complex, the specificity of thrombin undergoes a macromolecular shift from being a procoagulant to an anticoagulant molecule.[31] This transition in the biologic activity of thrombin is represented by a diminished ability to activate platelets and convert fibrinogen to fibrin, and a newly acquired ability to convert a plasma protein called protein C to activated protein C.[33] Activated protein C, in collaboration with its cofactor (protein S),

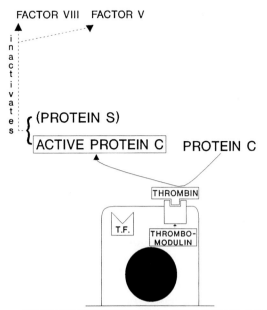

Figure 4–2. Thrombomodulin—protein C natural anticoagulant pathway.

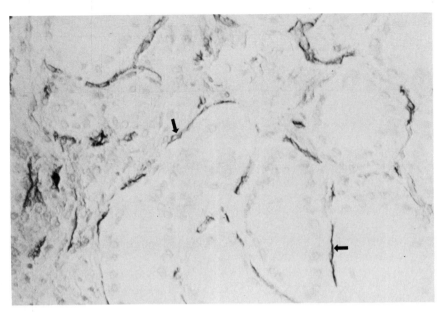

Figure 4–3. Thrombomodulin—protein C natural anticoagulant pathway. Biopsy of stable renal allograft reacted with antibody to thrombomodulin. Note reactivity of peritubular venous capillary plexus (arrows). (Antibody peroxidase technique, × 250)

exerts an anticoagulant effect by attacking activated factors V and VIII, which are the principal cofactors in the coagulation cascade.

The thrombomodulin–protein C natural anticoagulant pathway functions at the level of endothelial plasma membranes only when thrombomodulin is in an upregulated position (i.e., positioned in the membrane to allow access to blood). The molecule normally is upregulated, but certain chemical or physical changes in the microenvironment of endothelial cells cause thrombomodulin to be downregulated (i.e., no longer positioned in plasma membranes to allow access to blood). Although not established as an invariable consequence of downregulation, loss of thrombomodulin positions tissue factor to contact blood, thereby converting endothelial plasma membranes from thromboresistant to thrombogenic surfaces.

In light of the ability of thrombomodulin to maintain a state of endothelial thromboresistance, much research has focused on characterizing conditions that downregulate the molecule. Results indicate that downregulation is mediated by endotoxin, certain cytokines (especially interleukin-1 and tumor necrosis factor), and pH values below the physiologic range.[34] Unfortunately, no substance of possible therapeutic use has been identified to upregulate thrombomodulin.

The finding that thrombomodulin is down-regulated by interleukin-1 and tumor necrosis factor, both of which are produced by activated macrophages, helps explain the frequent observation of fibrin in vessels surrounded by activated macrophages; that is, cytokines released by macrophages cause endothelial downregulation of thrombomodulin and concomitant positioning of endothelial tissue factor to activate the enzymatic chain that leads to fibrin deposition. Alternatively, activated macrophages themselves produce a tissue factor-like procoagulant that can precipitate fibrin deposition independent of endothelial cells.[35]

The practical aspect of these observations is that stable allografts contain the endothelial thrombomodulin natural anticoagulant pathway in characteristic locations, and infiltration of these grafts by activated macrophages often is accompanied by a loss of endothelial thrombomodulin.[29, 36] For example, antibodies to thrombomodulin react in biopsies of normal kidneys and stable renal allografts with endothelium of the peritubular venous capillary plexus (Fig. 4–3). When this reactivity is lost, cellular infiltrates usually are found. Alternatively, we have observed a loss of thrombomodulin in what are assumed to be antibody-mediated episodes of acute rejections that sometimes are associated with deposits of complement components (usually products of activated C3 or C9).

Renal glomeruli normally do not react with antibody to thrombomodulin, but we often observe glomerular reactivity in biopsies of failing allografts. The reason for this is not clear, but glomerular structures in dysfunctional grafts undergo several other changes. For instance, they become reactive for urokinase (see section on fibrinolysis), and they lose reactivity for both tissue factor[6] and alpha smooth muscle cell actin.[37] We also have found that arteriolar endothelium of glomeruli in failing renal allografts, regardless of the presence of cellular infiltrates, reacts with a monoclonal antibody called PAL-E that ordinarily reacts only with venous endothelium. These data indicate that vessels in failing allografts undergo fundamental changes.[6, 12, 18, 29, 30, 37–41]

Like renal allografts, the endothelium of cardiac allografts reacts with antibody to thrombomodulin (Color Fig. 4–2), and this reactivity often is lost in biopsy specimens that contain cellular infiltrates. However, it is relevant that vessels have more than one anticoagulant pathway, so the absence of thrombomodulin is not necessarily accompanied by the deposition of fibrin.[29, 41] Indeed, there is no direct evidence that any of the other natural anticoagulant pathways are downregulated by cytokines released by activated macrophages.

Heparan Sulfate Proteoglycan–Antithrombin III Pathway

This pathway is composed of heparan sulfate anchored to endothelial plasma membranes by a core protein. The core protein contains extended sequences of alternating residues of serine and glycine. Serines are coupled through a connecting sequence (Xyl-Gal-Gal-Glu) to glucuronic acid and N-acetylglucosamine. This simple disaccharide structure is extended by a series of postsynthetic modifications to form heparan sulfate proteoglycan. Depending upon the amount and location of its sulfation, heparan sulfate binds antithrombin III from blood by reacting with particular lysine groups.[42]

Antithrombin III thus is captured by heparan sulfate, which is anchored to endothelial plasma membranes through its core protein.[43] In this position, a critical arginine residue of antithrombin III is conformationally armed to bind thrombin. This binding neutralizes thrombin and alters the conformation of antithrombin III in such a way that it is released from heparan sulfate and circulates as a

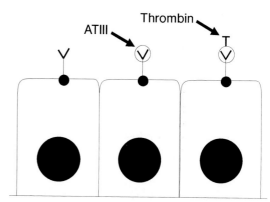

Figure 4–4. The heparan sulfate proteoglycan-antithrombin III natural anticoagulant pathway.

thrombin-antithrombin complex until being removed from the blood by specialized receptors in the liver. Meanwhile, the endothelial heparan sulfate binds and conformationally arms another molecule of antithrombin III, in preparation for neutralization of more thrombin (Fig. 4–4).

Since heparan sulfate proteoglycan is produced by endothelium and binds antithrombin III produced by liver cells, we have asked whether antithrombin III can be identified on endothelium of normal hearts and stable cardiac allografts. Results of experiments designed to answer this question have shown that antithrombin III can be identified in characteristic locations in blood vessels of transplanted hearts.[29] In fact, the distribution varies between veins, arteries, and capillaries (Table 4–3), and we have found that the localization is an index of the success or failure of cardiac allografts.[44]

Normal hearts and stable cardiac allografts contain antithrombin III on venous endothelium and on the smooth muscle cells and in the intima of small arteries and arterioles; we call this a type I distribution.[44] Cardiac allografts in early failure (independent of cellular infiltrates) contain antithrombin III only on smooth muscle cells and in the intima of small arteries and arterioles; we call this a type II

Table 4–3. Vascular Localization of Antithrombin III in Normal Hearts

Vessels	Locations
Veins	Endothelium
Small arteries	Smooth muscle cells
	Intima
Capillaries	Negative

Table 4–4. Vascular Localization of Antithrombin III in Cardiac Allografts

Type	Localization
Type I	Arterial smooth muscle cells and intima
	Venous endothelium
Type II	Arterial smooth muscle cells and intima
Type III	No antithrombin III reactivity
Type IV	Arterial smooth muscle cells and intima
	Venous endothelium
	Capillary endothelium

distribution. If type II is associated with fibrin deposits, the prognosis is not good. Unstable allografts that contain no vascular antithrombin III are associated with fibrin deposits and denote a poor prognosis; we call this a type III distribution.[44] Allografts with type III distribution usually pursue one of three possible courses: some of them die, some of them revert to a type II distribution, and approximately one third of them develop a striking pattern of capillary endothelial reactivity that includes venous endothelium and arteriolar intima and smooth muscle cells (Table 4–4); we call this a type IV distribution (Color Fig. 4–3).

The biochemical explanation for changes in the microanatomic distribution of antithrombin III probably relates to the ability of the Golgi apparatus in endothelial and smooth muscle cells to sulfate heparan at positions within the molecule to allow binding of antithrombin III.[42] These findings relate for the first time an immunocytochemically defined biochemical defect to graft failure. The therapeutic implication is that treatment with heparin appears to promote the synthesis of a species of heparan sulfate that binds anti-

thrombin III, thereby shifting the poor prognosis type III distribution backward to a type II distribution (i.e., arteriolar reactivity only) or forward to a type IV distribution (i.e., arteriolar, venous, and capillary reactivities), as shown in Figure 4–5. In our experience, patients with a type IV distribution (n = 18) had a 25 per cent survival advantage over control patients (n = 72) who did not have a type IV distribution of their vascular antithrombin III.[44]

Dermatan Sulfate Proteoglycan–Heparin Cofactor II Pathway

This natural anticoagulant pathway is analogous to the heparan sulfate proteoglycan–antithrombin III pathway, inasmuch as dermatan sulfate rather than heparan sulfate is the glucosaminoglycan, and heparin cofactor II rather than antithrombin III is the glycoprotein. There presently is evidence that the heparin cofactor II pathway is involved in the transplantation analogy of human pregnancy,[45] but a deficiency of this pathway does not appear to be involved in the development of thrombosis in renal allograft recipients.[46] In light of limited data, this pathway will not be discussed further.

Secretion of Endogenous Heparan Sulfate

It has been known for many years that human newborns have significantly prolonged coagulation times compared with adults, and this has been shown to be due to a circulating, heparin-like molecule.[47] Subsequent studies have shown that cancer patients with different types of tumors have prolonged coagulation times, also due to a circulating, heparin-like molecule.[48] This indicates that the gene responsible for secretion of this anticoagulant in fetuses/newborns can be reactivated/derepressed in adults with certain cancers.

The relevance of prolonged coagulation times in fetuses and some cancer patients to transplantation can be appreciated from our finding that recipients with stable renal or cardiac allografts have prolonged thrombin times compared with control values (see Table 4–1). Cardiac recipients with unstable allografts have thrombin times equal to or less than control values.[12] However, it is not clear that the

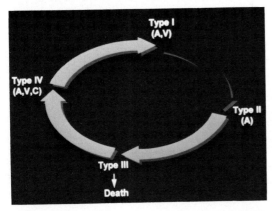

Figure 4–5. Modulation of vascular antithrombin III in cardiac allografts.

prolonged thrombin times are due to the secretion of endogenous heparan sulfate, because the prolonged times frequently are not corrected by addition of protamine (a positively charged molecule that neutralizes the anticoagulation effects of heparin), yet the prolonged thrombin times usually are corrected by the addition of fresh plasma.

The finding that recipients with successful allografts have prolonged thrombin times is compatible with a growing body of evidence that success is favored by treatment of allograft recipients with heparin,[49] which also prolongs the thrombin time. Our medical center presently is involved in a long-term study of the effects of low-molecular-weight heparin on the outcome of cardiac allograft recipients. As a part of this investigation, we have developed a sensitive radiometric assay to measure heparin in samples of peripheral blood, so it should be possible to determine whether the prolonged thrombin times of recipients with functionally successful allografts are due to the secretion of endogenous heparan sulfate. If their success is due to the secretion of endogenous heparan, new therapeutic strategies will have to be developed to maximize the beneficial effects of this largely ignored natural anticoagulant pathway.

Tissue Factor Pathway Inhibitor

Almost 50 years ago, Professor Lewis Thomas reported that the lethal disseminated intravascular coagulation that occurs following infusion of thromboplastin (i.e., tissue factor) is inhibited if the thromboplastin is preincubated with serum.[50] This seminal observation pointed a direction for the long held idea that there was something in serum that inhibited thromboplastin-triggered coagulation. We know today that the protecting factor in serum is a 32-kD glycoprotein containing three Kunitz-type protease inhibitors.[22] A Kunitz-type inhibitor is a serine protease inhibitor. The most characterized member of this inhibitor family is bovine basic pancreatic trypsin inhibitor, or aprotinin (Trasylol). Tissue factor pathway inhibitor (TFPI) normally circulates associated with lipoproteins.[51]

Readers will recall that the tissue factor pathway (i.e., the so-called extrinsic pathway of coagulation) consists of extravascular, subendothelial, or endothelial tissue factor that activates factor VII, and the activated factor VII activates factor X (and factor IX). The second

Kunitz group of TFPI binds activated factor X, and then the first Kunitz group of the TFPI–factor Xa complex binds factor VII of the tissue factor–factor VIIa complex, thus specifically binding and inactivating all components of the extrinsic pathway. Platelets also contain TFPI, so when they become involved in an ongoing hemostatic reaction, they release TFPI that is capable of shutting down upstream mediators of hemostasis.[22]

The intravenous injection of heparin causes blood concentrations of TFPI to increase quickly and significantly,[52] suggesting a competitive displacement of the molecule bound to endothelial heparan sulfate proteoglycan.[22] Thus, baseline values of plasma TFPI can be augmented both from platelets and what is thought to be a loosely bound TFPI reservoir on endothelium. In light of the concept that hemostasis is a central cause of allograft failure, it can be anticipated that the TFPI natural anticoagulant pathway will assume a prominent role in transplantation. However, there presently are no data on this emerging possibility.

FIBRINOLYSIS

A certain amount of hemostasis occurs in life (e.g., hemorrhoids, menstruation, tooth brushing), and it generally is assumed that the resulting fibrin deposits are resolved by fibrinolysis.[13] The fibrinolytic system is composed of plasminogen, two plasminogen activators (i.e., tissue plasminogen activator, or tPA, and urokinase) and two inhibitors of the plasminogen activators. Uninhibited plasminogen activators have the specific ability to convert plasminogen to plasmin, and, in the absence of plasmin inhibitors such as alpha-2-plasmin inhibitor, plasmin enzymatically removes fibrin (Fig. 4–6).

Plasminogen Activators in Cardiac Allografts

The vascular smooth muscle cells (SMC) in biopsies of normal hearts and stable cardiac allografts react with monoclonal antibody to tPA.[53] The reactive tissue has been identified morphologically as arterial SMC, and the tPA-reactive cells have been shown to react with antibody to alpha smooth muscle actin,[12] which is characteristic of SMC.[54, 55] Biopsies of

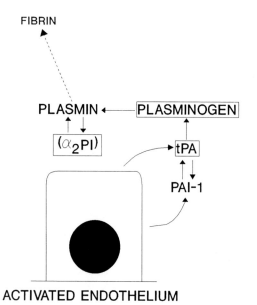

Figure 4–6. The fibrinolytic pathway.

hearts and stable allografts do not react with antibodies to urokinase, although vascular SMC have been shown to have receptors for urokinase. In spite of a vast number of publications that document the presence of both tPA and the mRNA for tPA in cultured endothelial cells, the endothelium of normal hearts and stable allografts (during the first 3 years of allografting) does not react with monoclonal antibody to tPA.[53]

We have reported that the loss of tPA from vascular SMC is a reliable index of allograft rejection, regardless of the presence or absence of cellular infiltrates.[12, 53] The degree of depletion of tPA from SMC of small arteries and arterioles appears to be proportional to the amount of fibrin deposited in and around vessels in cardiac biopsies. This has led us to the impression that depleted SMC tPA indicates a poor prognosis. Similarly, the reappearance of tPA-reactive SMC in subsequent biopsies indicates a good prognosis.

The quantification of vascular SMC is based on small arteries and arterioles that do not exceed the size of adjacent cardiomyocytes. Reactivity of all SMC is graded as 1.0 (Color Fig. 4–4). Reactivity of most of the cells (with interspersed negative SMC) is graded as 2.0; reactivity of only a minority of cells at the periphery of vessels is graded as 3.0, and no reactivity is graded as 4.0.[12] As with fibrin scores, tPA scores generally are associated with clinically defined functional criteria.[12, 18, 53, 56]

Native hearts removed from recipients at the time of transplantation usually have diminished tPA-reactive SMC, and endothelial cells of the same hearts frequently contain tPA-reactive endothelium. This finding in end-stage hearts, coupled with our finding that endothelium in normal hearts and stable allografts does not react with antibody to tPA, suggests that tPA-reactive endothelium is indicative of compromised vascular function (e.g., impaired oxygenation) with existing or impending compromised myocardial function (e.g., infarction). This impression is supported by the observation that tPA grade 4.0 hearts sometime contain tPA-reactive endothelium. In contrast, we have observed tPA-reactive endothelium in biopsies of some long-term allografts (i.e., more than 3 years) that are functioning normally and do not contain deposits of fibrin.

Plasminogen Activators in Renal Allografts

The vascular SMC of normal kidneys and stable renal allografts react with antibody to tPA in a manner similar if not identical to that observed in normal hearts and stable cardiac allografts, and the depletion of tPA from failing renal allografts can be scored according to the grading system used for cardiac allografts. However, any quantification scheme for tPA should be limited to small arteries and arterioles, for depletion of the molecule from large vessels does not correlate reliably with either function or clinical status.

Urokinase is a second plasminogen activator found in kidneys, and it is not associated with vascular SMC. The proximal tubular epithelial cells of normal kidneys and stable renal allografts react with antibody to urokinase, and all other cell types are nonreactive.[57] However, as graft function begins to deteriorate (as measured by blood creatinine concentrations), the distribution of urokinase changes (Fig. 4–7). The first change is an increase in the reactivity of proximal tubular epithelial cells and the identification of urokinase in glomeruli. Progressive loss of function is associated with diminished tubular and increased glomerular reactivity,[37] and biopsies from advanced dysfunctional allografts show glomerular but not tubular reactivity with antibody to urokinase (Fig. 4–7).

Since tPA is located in the same vascular compartment in kidneys and hearts, and since vascular aspects of rejection are associated with similar patterns of SMC tPA depletion, it ap-

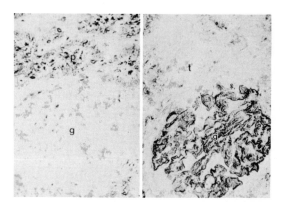

Figure 4–7. Urokinase in biopsies of stable (left) and failing (right) renal allografts. Note reactivity of proximal renal tubular epithelial cells (p) and negative glomerulus (g) in stable graft, and loss of tubular epithelial reactivity (t) and positive glomerulus (g) in unstable graft. (Antibody peroxidase technique × 250)

pears that the structure-function aspects of tPA are analogous in renal and cardiac allografts. However, the transition of urokinase from proximal tubular epithelial cells in normal kidneys to glomeruli in failing renal allografts suggests that the structure-function aspects of this molecule depend upon the microanatomy of its location. In its tubular location, urokinase is positioned to resolve fibrin clots in urine, and, in its glomerular location, urokinase is positioned to resolve fibrin deposits in glomeruli. Depletion of urokinase helps explain the presence of fibrin in both of these locations in dysfunctional renal allografts.

Identification of Plasmin

Plasminogen circulates in blood as a zymogen (i.e., an inactive enzyme) that can be converted to plasmin by plasminogen activators such as tPA and urokinase. Both plasminogen and tPA have high-affinity binding sites for fibrin. When they both bind fibrin, tPA cleaves plasminogen to plasmin. Since plasmin is a powerful proteolytic enzyme, both tPA and plasmin are inhibited by inhibitors; these are plasminogen activator inhibitor-1 (PAI-1) and alpha-2-plasmin inhibitor (α_2PI), respectively. Thus, under physiologic conditions, fibrinolysis is a balanced interaction between fibrin, plasminogen, tPA or urokinase, PAI-1, plasmin, and α_2PI.

Information about fibrinolysis can be obtained from biopsies by using immunocytochemical techniques to evaluate the reactivities of antibodies to defined components of the fibrinolytic system. Examples of this approach are given in the foregoing sections on plasminogen activators. In contrast to the situation with plasminogen activators, information gained from the use of antibodies to plasminogen is not useful in evaluating fibrinolysis, because plasminogen is a ubiquitous plasma protein. The logic flow in this objection is the same as that used in the preceding discussion of fibrinogen versus fibrin (see first section of Hemostasis).

The unavailability of antibodies to plasmin is not an impediment to its immunocytochemical identification, for activation of plasminogen results in the production of plasmin that is bound by α_2PI, and formation of this complex opens two possibilities for the identification of plasmin. First, the complex itself forms new antigens, and antibodies are available that identify these neoantigens.[58] Second, antibody to α_2PI also reliably identifies plasmin (Fig. 4–8). Indeed, identical results are obtained from double-antibody experiments done with polyclonal antibody to either α_2PI or plasmin neoantigen and monoclonal antibody to fibrin, indicating the presence of a fibrinolytic triad consisting of substrate (fibrin), enzyme (plasmin), and enzyme inhibitor (α_2PI).

Though presently limited to research interest only, we have observed that fibrin deposits in biopsies unaccompanied by α_2PI suggest a poorer prognosis than such deposits accompanied by α_2PI. We interpret this as indicating that fibrinolysis is not keeping pace with hemostasis, and our present efforts are to calculate a fibrin-α_2PI index that reflects the adequacy of fibrinolysis.

Identification of Plasminogen Activator Inhibitors

Both tPA and urokinase are inhibited by PAI-1 and another inhibitor (PAI-2) that is produced primarily during pregnancy.[59] The biochemical isolation of PAI-1 is complicated by technical factors, but present data indicate that the tPA-PAI-1 complex does not effectively activate plasminogen. Indeed, in some conditions, such as human pregnancy, plasma concentrations of tPA are increased, but this is associated with increased tPA-PAI-1 complexes giving a net effect of no increased plasminogen activation.[59] Thus, a complete picture of fibrinolytic potential cannot be obtained without considering the role of plasminogen activator inhibitors.

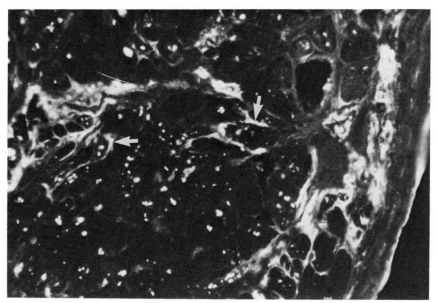

Figure 4–8. Heart biopsy from an unstable allograft reacted with antibody to human α_2–antiplasmin-plasmin complex. Note bright reactivity within the microcirculation (arrows). ($\times$ 400)

Assessment of fibrinolytic potential has been assisted by the availability of a monoclonal antibody that reacts with a PAI-1 epitope available only on PAI-1 complexed with tPA.[60] We have used this antibody in an effort to determine the functional status of endothelial tPA. As discussed earlier (first section of Fibrinolysis), the reactivity of anti-tPA in stable allografts is limited to vascular SMC, but failing allografts have tPA-reactive endothelium. However, it is problematic that this tPA can convert plasminogen to plasmin, for the same endothelial cells react with monoclonal antibody to the PAI-1 epitope of tPA-PAI-1 complexes.

The role of plasminogen activator inhibitors in control of tPA-mediated plasminogen activation on endothelial plasma membranes is not entirely clear. Our data show that tPA and complexed PAI-1 on endothelium of biopsy specimens with fibrin deposits and depleted SMC tPA indicate a poor prognosis. However, tPA on endothelium of biopsy specimens with tPA-reactive vascular SMC and no fibrin deposits do not indicate a poor prognosis for stable allografts of long duration (i.e., greater than 3 years after transplantation). These findings suggest that the significance of endothelial tPA cannot be evaluated without knowing the status of other hemostatic and fibrinolytic components.

Diagnosis of Fibrinolysis

We do not use immunocytochemical techniques to diagnose fibrinolysis. Our interest is to identify and quantify components of the fibrinolytic system in allograft biopsies.[12] Findings from these experiments have been evaluated with biochemical, functional, radiologic, and clinical assessments to build a data base that allows the extraction of prognostic information from biopsies. On balance, this has been successful. For example, we have found that depletion of SMC tPA from arterioles in heart biopsies and depletion of urokinase from proximal tubular epithelium in kidney biopsies indicate a poor prognosis.[12, 37, 53, 57] The value of such observations is enhanced greatly when considered together with information about the hemostatic and natural anticoagulant pathways.

We have found that immunocytochemical evaluations of the fibrinolytic potential yield more useful data about the capabilities of allografts to sustain and mobilize products of hemostasis than the identification of fibrin degradation products, which are more direct markers of fibrinolysis. However, if the aim is to diagnose fibrinolysis, there are several reliable and commercially available antibodies to fibrin degradation products, such as D-dimer, and these have been used commonly to identify products of fibrinolysis in well-defined situations, as in the lesions of spontaneous atherosclerosis.[61]

IMMUNOPATHOLOGY

It has been our intention in this chapter to discuss vascular changes in allografts as they relate to the hemostatic, fibrinolytic, and natural anticoagulant pathways. We have focused on these pathways because of two groups of compelling observations. The first group of observations is drawn from recipient hearts removed at the time of transplantation. Vessels in these hearts consistently are found to have abnormalities in hemostasis, fibrinolysis, and anticoagulation, suggesting that these pathways are involved in the pathophysiology if not the pathogenesis of chronic heart disease. We also rarely find immunopathologic evidence to support a role for immunologic mechanisms in recipient hearts.

The second group of observations that has focused our attention on the hemostatic, fibrinolytic, and natural anticoagulant pathways is the large number of allograft biopsy specimens we examine that present no evidence of cellular infiltrates or complement activation. Indeed, we have studied many cases of cardiac and renal allograft failure that manifested no evidence of immunopathology, yet the same organs contained clear evidence of accelerated hemostasis, depressed fibrinolysis, and impaired natural anticoagulant pathways.[12]

These observations say nothing about either the role or importance of cellular infiltrates in allograft biopsies. In our experience, vascular changes can occur in the absence of cellular infiltrates,[12] cellular infiltrates can occur in the absence of vascular changes, and they can occur together. The same is true for deposits of immunoglobulins/complement and vascular changes.[62] Taken together, these observations have spawned the putative classification of rejection as being either cellular or vascular in origin. There are many reasons to pursue this idea, not the least of which is its possible impact on the use of immunosuppressive therapies.

It clearly is important to define the causes of vascular compromise that may result in graft failure. Several years ago it would have been axiomatic that vascular damage in allografts is part of the immunopathology of transplantation, but today it still is not clear what immunopathologic reactions are involved, although many mechanisms have been proposed. Attractive candidates include antibodies to endothelial cells,[63] T lymphocyte–endothelium interactions,[64] cytokine-mediated endothelial activation,[65] and the cytokine network as a regulator of immune responses to allografts.[66] None of these has been shown consistently to account for objective parameters of vascular damage observed in biopsy material from allografts of established functional status.

We receive many biopsy specimens from failing allografts that contain no macrophages or lymphocytes, yet the vessels contain fibrin and manifest objective findings of impaired natural anticoagulant pathways and depleted fibrinolysis.[6, 12, 18, 29, 30, 37, 41, 44, 53, 56, 57] However, an immunocytochemical finding that does link immunologic with endothelial changes is the absence of IgM on endothelium of failing allografts.[67] Results of double antibody experiments have shown a negative correlation between the presence of IgM and fibrin on endothelial cells in allografts. These data suggest that recipient IgM antibody disallows fibrin deposition, perhaps by inhibiting one of the serine proteases in the hemostatic pathway. This finding stands in stark contrast to the role of naturally existing IgM in xenograft recipients, in whom the antibody is associated with massive hemostasis.[17, 68] It is possible, of course, that this IgM is of another specificity. We propose that it could have the same specificity as that described for human cardiac allografts,[67] but it reacts with xenogeneic epitopes that are appropriately spaced to fix complement, which alters endothelial plasma membranes and allows tissue factor to initiate uncompensated hemostasis.

VASCULOPATHY

Transplant-induced vasculopathy develops in several months,[69] thus providing a model for the spontaneous development of atherosclerosis.[70] Other models are found in venous graft bypass procedures and percutaneous transluminal coronary angioplasty.[69] It is reasonable to propose that transplant-induced vasculopathy results from immune-mediated damage, but it is difficult to accept that immune-mediated damage causes the atheromatous changes found in autologous vein grafts or coronary angioplasty.

In an effort to define vascular components that might be instructive in defining the pathophysiology of transplant-induced vasculopathy, we have used immunocytochemical markers to study the vessels themselves. The vessels were identified in thin sections of snap-frozen biopsy material from human cardiac and renal allografts, and the results indicated that graft function can be assessed by evaluating thrombogenic and thromboresistant properties of vessels.[18] Biopsy material with cellular infiltrates often contained damaged vessels, but damaged vessels also were identified in specimens that were devoid of cellular infiltrates.

Aspects of the development of atheroma are endothelial damage, SMC proliferation, cellular invasion and expansion of intima, and thrombosis.[71, 72] The metabolic changes that result from these lesions are ischemia, hypoxia, and eventual infarction. Such ischemic changes can result from perturbations in the hemostatic, fibrinolytic, and anticoagulant pathways, and examples of these have been the subject of this chapter. However, the factors that initiate perturbations in these pathways are not precisely known. Metabolic changes in cultured endothelial cells can affect the heparan sulfate proteoglycan-antithrombin III anticoagulant pathway, and the biochemical basis of some of these changes has been reported for cultured and transformed endothelial cells.[43] This may account for some of the changes in endothelium that lead to the syndrome of transplant-induced vasculopathy.

Proliferation of SMC is key in the pathophysiology of atherosclerosis.[73] It is not clear whether such proliferation is initiated by endothelial damage,[74] for proliferation within the media and invasion of the intima in cardiac allografts can occur in coronary arteries with ultrastructurally intact endothelium.[75] We have reported that arterial SMC in rejecting cardiac allografts and in hearts with transplant-induced vasculopathy lose their tPA reactivity,[18, 53] indicating that rejecting and vasculopathic grafts have similar deficiencies in their fibrinolytic pathways. In both these conditions tPA-reactive SMC can be identified within the intima of affected vessels. This suggests that intimal SMC have the ability to activate plasminogen to remodel fibrin, for the intima of vasculopathic vessels contains characteristic degradation products of cross-linked fibrin.[61] Thus, the vascular SMC in transplant-induced vasculopathy have the same type of changes in their fibrinolytic pathways as are found in the vessels of failing allografts, regardless of the presence or absence of cellular infiltrates.

CONCLUSIONS

The information presented in this chapter has been weighted in favor of vascular changes as being more informative than cellular infiltrates in allograft biopsies. This has been done to bring forward the emerging reality that the immunocytochemical assessment of vascular changes in biopsies offers telling insights into the pathophysiology of allogeneic recognition and rejection reactions. It would be incorrect to conclude from the foregoing discussion of vascular changes that cellular infiltrates are not important.

Investigators who examine allograft biopsy material commonly are presented with situations in which both the allograft recipient and the allograft itself are clinically and functionally compromised, but examination of the specimen provides no findings that help explain the compromise. If this chapter has accomplished anything, we hope that it has been to demonstrate that biopsy specimens that are devoid of cellular infiltrates can contain unambiguous immunocytochemical evidence of vascular damage that correlates with clinical findings.

Evolving technology in vascular biology has laid a scientific foundation for an explanation of the age-old question of why blood in the circulation does not clot. The reason for the maintenance of a fluid state in blood appears to relate to newly described antithrombogenic systems called natural anticoagulant pathways.[12, 22, 29–31, 38, 42, 44] Some of these (e.g., the thrombomodulin–protein C pathway) are sensitive to cytokines released by immune cells,[64, 65] but for the most part it is not known what regulates these anticoagulant pathways. Nonetheless, it is clear that abnormalities in the pathways are associated with fibrin deposits, and that fibrin deposits are associated with rejection.

Communication is essential between pathologists and physicians, and the meaning and implication of critical words used in communication are centrally important in patient management. In this case, the meaning of "rejection" conveys different implications to different people, depending upon their background, experience, and position in the chain of responsibility for patients. For example, some people equate rejection with cellular infiltrates; others think of the word in terms of vascular phenomena; yet others accept the word as implying loss of function; and many interpret rejection as an indicator for immunosuppression. Since rejection means different things to different people, it would appear to be rather more than academic to establish clearly the meaning(s) and implications(s) of this important word in the transplantation vocabulary.

SUMMARY

This chapter discusses the role of vascular changes in allograft function. This is done by first considering the pathways by which fibrin deposits arrive in the vessels of transplanted organs. It is stressed that the tissue factor (i.e., extrinsic) pathway initiates hemostasis in vivo, and that this usually occurs as a result of failures in upstream or downstream pathways. Upstream failures are in the natural anticoagulant pathways, and each of the five anticoagulant pathways is discussed. Downstream failures are in the fibrinolytic pathways, and the role of tissue plasminogen activator in fibrinolysis is discussed. The chapter ends with a discussion of the relationship of these pathways to cellular infiltrates and the development of transplant vasculopathy. It is concluded that there are many mechanisms of graft failure, and that it is misleading, inaccurate and perhaps dangerous to describe them all as rejection.

REFERENCES

 1. Chorney MJ, Cheng TC. Discrimination of self and non-self invertebrates. Contemp Top Immunobiol 9:37, 1980.
 2. Cecka JM, Terasaki PI. The UNOS scientific renal transplant registry. *In* Terasaki PI, Cecka JM (eds). *Clinical Transplants 1991*. Los Angeles, UCLA Tissue Typing Laboratory, 1991, pp 1–11.
 3. Porter KA, Thomson WB, Owen K, Keagon JR, Mowbray JF, Peart WS. Obliterative vascular changes in four human kidney homotransplants. Br Med J 2:639, 1963.
 4. Kincaid-Smith P. Vascular changes in homotransplants. Br Med J 1:178, 1964.
 5. Billingham ME, Cary NRB, Hammond ME, Kemnitz J, Marboe C, McCallister HA, Snovar DC, Winters GL, Zerbe A. A working formulation for the standardization of nomenclature in the diagnosis of heart and lung rejection: Heart Rejection Study Group. J Heart Transplant 9:587, 1990.
 6. Bukovsky A, Labarrere, CA, Haag B, Carter C, Faulk WP. Tissue factor in normal and transplanted human kidneys. Transplantation 54:644, 1992.
 7. Faulk WP, Hijmans W. Recent developments in immunofluorescence. Prog Allergy 16:9, 1972.
 8. Faulk WP, Labarrere CA, Carson SD. Tissue factor: Identification and characterization of cell types in human placentae. Blood 76:86, 1990.
 9. Labarrere CA, Esmon CT, Carson SD, Faulk WP. Concordant expression of tissue factor and class II MHC antigens in human placental endothelium. Placenta 11:309, 1990.
10. Faulk WP, Taylor GM. An immunocolloid method for the electron microscope. Immunochemistry 8:1081, 1971.
11. Verkleij AJ, Leunissen JLM. *Immuno-Gold Labeling in Cell Biology*. Boca Raton, Florida, CRC Press, 1990.
12. Faulk WP, Labarrere CA, Pitts D, Halbrook H. Vascular lesions in biopsies devoid of cellular infiltrates: Qualitative and quantitative immunocytochemical studies of human cardiac allografts. J Heart Lung Transplant 12:219, 1993.
13. Faulk WP. Placental fibrin. Am J Reprod Immunol 19:132, 1989.
14. Faulk WP, Labarrere CA, Pitts D, Strate R. Immunopathology of unexplained graft failure. J Heart Transplant 9:68, 1990.
15. Camussi G, Niesen N, Tetta C, Saunders RN, Milgrom F. Release of platelet-activating factor from rabbit heart perfused in vitro by sera with transplantation alloantibodies. Transplantation 44:113, 1987.
16. Weksler BB. Platelet interactions with the blood vessel wall. *In* Colman RW, Hirsh J, Marder VJ, Salzman EW (eds). *Hemostasis and Thrombosis*, 2nd ed. Philadelphia, JB Lippincott, 1987, pp 804–815.
17. Faulk WP, Gargiulo P, McIntyre JA, Bang NU. Hemostasis and fibrinolysis in renal transplantation. Semin Thromb Hemost 15:88, 1989.
18. Faulk WP, Labarrere CA. Vascular immunopathology and atheroma development in human allografted organs. Arch Pathol Lab Med 116:1337, 1992.
19. Repke D, Gemmell CH, Gruha A, Turitto VT, Broze GJ, Nemerson Y. Hemophilia as a defect of the tissue factor pathway of blood coagulation: Effect of factors VIII and IX on factor X activation in a continuous-flow reactor. Proc Natl Acad Sci USA 87:7623, 1990.
20. Hassan HJ, Leonardi A, Chelucci C, Mattia G, Macioce G, Gruerriero R, Russo G, Mannucci PM, Peschle C. Blood coagulation factors in human embryonic-fetal development: Preferential expression of the FV11/tissue factor pathway. Blood 76:1158, 1990.
21. Rapaport SI. The extrinsic pathway inhibitor: A regulator of tissue factor-dependent blood coagulation. Thromb Haemost 66:6, 1991.
22. Broze GJ, Girard TJ, Novotny WF. Regulation of coagulation by a Kunitz-type inhibitor. Biochemistry 29:7539, 1990.
23. Nemerson Y. Tissue factor and hemostasis. Blood 71:1, 1988.
24. Moore KL, Andreoli SP, Esmon NL, Esmon CT, Bang NU. Endotoxin enhances tissue factor and suppresses thrombomodulin expression of human vascular endothelium in vitro. J Clin Invest 79:124, 1987.
25. Almus FE, Rad LVM, Rapaport SI. Decreased inducibility of tissue factor activity on human umbilical vein endothelial cells cultured with endothelial cell growth factor and heparin. Thromb Res 50:339, 1988.
26. Lockwood CJ, Bach R, Guha A, Zhou X, Miller WA, Nemerson Y. Amniotic fluid contains tissue factor, a potent initiator of coagulation. Am J Obstet Gynecol 165:1335, 1991.
27. Labarrere CA, Carson SD, Faulk WP. Tissue factor in chronic villitis of unestablished etiology. J Reprod Immunol 19:225, 1991.
28. Carson SD, Johnson DR. Consecutive enzyme cascades: Complement activation at the cell surface triggers increased tissue factor expression. Blood 76:361, 1990.
29. Labarrere CA, Pitts D, Halbrook H, Faulk WP. Natural anticoagulant pathways in normal and transplanted human hearts. J Heart Lung Transplant 11:342, 1992.
30. Absher E, Labarrere CA, Carter C, Haag B, Faulk WP. The endothelial heparan sulfate-antithrombin III natural anticoagulant pathway in normal and transplanted human kidneys. Transplantation 53:828, 1992.
31. Esmon CT. The regulation of natural anticoagulant pathways. Science 235:1348, 1987.
32. Sherry S. The thrombolytic agents. *In* Sherry S (ed). *Fibrinolysis, Thrombosis and Hemostasis*. Philadelphia, Lea & Febiger, 1992, p 123.

33. Dittman WA, Majerus PW. Structure and function of thrombomodulin: A natural anticoagulant. Blood 75:329, 1990.

34. Esmon CT. The roles of protein C and thrombomodulin in the regulation of blood coagulation. J Biol Chem 264:4743, 1989.

35. Carson SD, Faulk WP. Blood clotting and immunity. *In* Coulam CB, Faulk WP, McIntyre JA (eds). *Immunological Obstetrics.* New York, WW Norton, 1992, pp 61–72.

36. Tsuchida A, Salem H, Thomson N, Hancock WW. Tumor necrosis factor production during human renal allograft rejection is associated with depression of plasma protein C and free protein S levels and decreased intragraft thrombomodulin expression. J Exp Med 175:81, 1992.

37. Bukovsky A, Labarrere CA, Carter C, Haag B, Faulk WP. Novel immunohistochemical markers of human renal allograft dysfunction: Antithrombin III, Thy-1, urokinase and α-smooth muscle actin. Transplantation 54:1064, 1992.

38. Hunt BJ, Segal H, Yacoub M. Endothelial cell hemostatic function after heart transplantation. Transplant Proc 23:1182, 1991.

39. Hengstenberg C, Rose ML, Page C, Taylor PM, Yacoub MH. Immunocytochemical changes suggestive of damage to endothelial cells during rejection of human cardiac allografts. Transplantation 49:895, 1990.

40. Cherry R, Nielsen H, Reed E, Reemtsma K, Suciu-Foca N, Marboe CC. Vascular (humoral) rejection in human cardiac allograft biopsies: Relation to circulating anti-HLA antibodies. J Heart Lung Transplant 11:24, 1992.

41. Labarrere CA, Faulk WP. Microvascular perturbations in human allografts: Analogies in pre-eclamptic placentae. Am J Reprod Immunol 27:109, 1992.

42. Rosenberg RD. Regulation of the hemostatic mechanism. *In* Stamatoyaunnopoulos G, Nienhuis AW, Leder P, Majerus PW (eds). *The Molecular Basis of Blood Diseases.* Philadelphia, WB Saunders, 1987, pp 534–574.

43. Wight TN. Cell biology of arterial proteoglycans. Arteriosclerosis 9:1, 1989.

44. Faulk WP, Labarrere CA. Modulation of endothelial antithrombin III in human cardiac allografts. Haemostasis 23:194, 1993.

45. Andrew M, Mitchell L, Berry L, Paes B, Delorme M, Ofosu F, Burrows R, Khambolia B. An anticoagulant dermatan sulfate proteoglycan circulates in the pregnant woman and her fetus. J Clin Invest 89:321, 1992.

46. Toulon P, Moulonguet-Doleris L, Costa JM, Aich M. Heparin cofactor II deficiency in renal allograft recipients: No correlation with the development of thrombosis. Thromb Haemost 65:20, 1991.

47. Muller AD, van Doorm JM, Hemker HC. Heparin-like inhibitor of blood coagulation in the normal newborn. Nature 267:616, 1977.

48. Khoory MS, Nesheim ME, Bowie EJW, Mann KG. Circulating heparan sulfate proteoglycan anticoagulant from a patient with a plasma cell disorder. J Clin Invest 65:660, 1980.

49. Ubhi CS, Lam FT, Mavor AI, Giles GR. Subcutaneous heparin therapy for cyclosporin-immunosuppressed renal allograft recipients. Transplantation 48:886, 1989.

50. Thomas L. Studies on the intravascular thromboplastic effect of tissue suspensions in mice. II. A factor in normal rabbit serum which inhibits the thromboplas-tic effect of the sedimentable tissue component. Bull Johns Hopkins Hosp 81:26, 1947.

51. Novotny WF, Girard TJ, Miletich JP, Broze GJ. Purification and characterization of the lipoprotein-associated coagulation inhibitor from human plasma. J Biol Chem 64:18832, 1989.

52. Lindahl AK, Abildgaard U, Larsen ML, Aamodt LM, Nordfang O, Beck TC. Extrinsic pathway inhibitor (EPI) and the post-heparin anticoagulant effect in tissue thromboplastin induced coagulation. Thromb Res Suppl XIV:39, 1991.

53. Labarrere CA, Pitts D, Halbrook H, Faulk WP. Tissue plasminogen activator in human cardiac allografts. Transplantation 55:1056, 1993.

54. Desmouliere A, Rubbia-Brandt L, Gabbiani G. Modulation of actin isoform expression in cultured arterial smooth muscle cells by heparin and culture conditions. Arterioscler Thromb 11:244, 1991.

55. Clowes AW, Clowes MM, Kocher O, Ropraz P, Chaponnier C, Gabbiani G. Arterial smooth muscle cells in vivo: Relationship between actin isoform expression and mitogenesis and their modulation by heparin. J Cell Biol 107:1939, 1988.

56. Faulk WP, Labarrere CA. Vascular events in human placentae and organ allografts. Am J Reprod Immunol 28:176, 1992.

57. Bukovsky A, Labarrere CA, Bang NU, Faulk WP. Renal fibrinolysis and transplantation. Fibrinolyse 4:3, 1991.

58. Holvoet P, Boer ADE, Verstreken M, Collen D. An enzyme-linked immunosorbent assay (ELISA) for the measurement of plasmin-α_2-antiplasmin complex in human plasma. Thromb Haemost 56:124, 1986.

59. Kruithof EKO, Tran-Thang C, Gudinchet A, Hauert J, Nicoloso G, Genton C, Welti H, Bachmann F. Fibrinolysis in pregnancy: A study of plasminogen activator inhibitors. Blood 69:460, 1987.

60. MacGregor IR. Characterization of epitopes on human tissue plasminogen activator recognised by a group of monoclonal antibodies. Thromb Haemost 53:45, 1985.

61. Smith EB, Keen GA, Graut A, Stirk C. Fate of fibrinogen in human arterial intima. Arteriosclerosis 12:263, 1990.

62. Hammond EH, Yowell RL, Nunoda S, Menlove RL, Renlund DG, Bristow MR, Gay WA Jr, Jones KW, O'Connell JB. Vascular (humoral) rejection in heart transplantation: Pathologic observations and clinical implications. J Heart Transplant 8:430, 1989.

63. Dunn MJ, Crisp SJ, Rose ML, Taylor PM, Yacoub MH. Anti-endothelial antibodies and coronary artery disease after cardiac transplantation. Lancet 339:1566, 1992.

64. Pober JS, Cotran RS. Immunologic interactions of T lymphocytes with vascular endothelium. Adv Immunol 50:261, 1992.

65. Pober JA. Cytokine-mediated activation of vascular endothelium: Physiology and pathology. Am J Pathol 133:426, 1988.

66. Dallman MJ. The cytokine network and regulation of the immune response to organ transplants. Transplant Rev 6:209, 1992.

67. Labarrere CA, Pitts D, Halbrook H, Faulk WP. Immunoglobulin M antibodies in transplanted human hearts. J Heart Lung Transplant 12:394, 1993.

68. Bach FH, Dalmasso AP, Platt JL. Xenotransplantation: A current perspective. Transplant Rev 6:163, 1992.

69. Ip JH, Fuster V, Badimon L, Badimon J, Taubman MB,

Chesebro JH. Syndromes of accelerated atherosclerosis: Role of vascular injury and smooth muscle cell proliferation. J Am Coll Cardiol 15:1667, 1990.

70. Fyfe AI. Transplant atherosclerosis: The clinical syndrome, pathogenesis and possible model of spontaneous atherosclerosis. Can J Cardiol 8:509, 1992.

71. Wilcox JN, Smith KM, Schwartz SM, Gordon D. Localization of tissue factor in the normal vessel wall and in the atherosclerotic plaque. Proc Natl Acad Sci USA 86:2839, 1989.

72. Fuster V, Badimon L, Badimon JJ, Chesebro JH. The pathogenesis of coronary artery disease and the acute coronary syndromes. N Engl J Med 326:310, 1992.

73. Ross R. The pathogenesis of atherosclerosis: An update. N Engl J Med 314:488, 1986.

74. Jamal A, Bendeck M, Langille BL. Structural changes and recovery of function after arterial injury. Arterioscler Thromb 12:307, 1992.

75. Kuwahara M, Jacobsson J, Kuwahara M, Kagan E, Ramwell P, Foegh ML. Coronary artery ultrastructural changes in cardiac transplant atherosclerosis in the rabbit. Transplantation 52:759, 1991.

II

Pathology of Rejection of Solid Organ Allografts

In this section are chapters dealing with the specific pathologic features of rejection in different solid organ allografts. Although many of us have directly and specifically observed rejection processes in individual organs, we have little collective experience in evaluation of the similarities and differences among them. In some organs, like the kidney and heart, cellular rejection is considered to be more common and less severe than rejection involving the microvasculature. In the lung and liver, the microvascular alterations are considered part of the usual rejection picture, since they are commonly both present. Because our understanding of the precise mechanisms of rejection that operate in these organs in vivo is limited, we must await further studies to elucidate the similarities and differences in the rejection process.

These chapters provide specific information about how to diagnose rejection in the various sites. Each chapter also includes references that will amplify the information presented. Three chapters deal with cardiac allograft rejection: one discusses cellular rejection, the most common form; one discusses microvascular rejection; and a third deals with coronary allograft vasculopathy, an entity that is similar to vasculopathic processes occurring in other solid organ allografts. The pathology of rejection involving other allografts is considered in single chapters, accompanied by liberal illustrations and references.

5

CARDIAC TRANSPLANT PATHOLOGY

Margaret E. Billingham, MB, BS, FRC Path

Since 1967, when the first human cardiac transplantation was performed by Barnard in Capetown, South Africa,[1] followed a few weeks later by the first successful adult cardiac transplantation in the United States by Shumway, cardiac transplantation has evolved from an experimental procedure to an accepted therapeutic option for patients with end-stage cardiac disease. In 1981, the first successful human heart-lung transplantation was performed by Reitz and associates at Stanford University.[2] Heart-lung transplantation has also become fairly routine now and is beyond the experimental stage. The Registry of the International Society for Heart and Lung Transplantation in 1993 shows that now over 130 medical centers worldwide perform heart and heart-lung transplantation.[3] The Registry for 1993 also shows 22,516 orthotopic heart transplants worldwide, of which 1347 are combined heart-lung transplants. The overall 1-year survival rate for cardiac transplantation worldwide is now 78.4 per cent, and 67.0 per cent for 5-year survival worldwide. The longest surviving cardiac transplant patient recently died at 22 years postcardiac transplantation at Stanford. Stanford University, where the first combined heart-lung transplantation was performed, now has a 64 per cent 5-year survival rate and a 35 per cent survival rate at 10 years for heart-lung transplantation (compared with rates of 30 per cent

for 5-year survival and 45 per cent for 10-year survival prior to the introduction of cyclosporine in 1980). Pediatric heart transplants (0 to 18 years of age) now number 1577 worldwide, with a 1-year survival rate of 75 per cent and a 5-year survival rate of 66.3 per cent. Pediatric combined heart-lung (first time) transplants number 184, with a 1-year survival rate of 61 per cent.[3]

Recipient diagnosis for heart transplantation is mainly for end-stage idiopathic dilated cardiomyopathy and end-stage coronary atherosclerotic disease in adults. The next largest group of cardiac recipients are those who have failed valvular repairs; nowadays, congenital heart disease is becoming the fourth largest group. A small, heterogeneous group of cardiac recipients includes those with diseases such as amyloidosis, sarcoidosis, cardiac tumor, Marfan's disease, and myocarditis; however, these are relatively rare. Stanford, which has the longest ongoing cardiac transplant program in the United States, has performed 694 cardiac transplants (482 1-year survivors) as of January, 1993. Of these cardiac recipients, 86 per cent have been fully rehabilitated, and currently living are 318 patients who have survived from 1 month to 19 years as of January, 1993.

Over the years, different immunosuppressive regimens have been used in different transplantation centers, and these in turn have affected not only the survival but also the pathology of the transplanted heart. At this time, most centers are using variations of triple or quadruple therapy (azathioprine, steroids, and

Supported by the Clinical Heart and Heart-Lung Transplantation Grant HL-13108-23, National Heart, Lung and Blood Institute, Bethesda, Maryland.

cyclosporine with or without OKT3 or antithymocyte globulin), with and without induction.

Cardiac transplantation has been performed mainly in adults and adolescents; it was not until 1982 that patients as young as 10 years became cardiac recipients and not until 1984 that the first neonates were transplanted for complex congenital heart disease. The age range for cardiac transplantation has now been extended from birth to 70 years. It is clear that those most likely to benefit from cardiac transplantation tend to be patients with end-stage heart disease who have a very poor prognosis for survival (less than 6 to 9 months) and who have potentially reversible organ damage in spite of their long-standing heart disease. It must be remembered that treatment with steroids, which is used in many centers as an immunosuppressive agent, may also exacerbate long-standing generalized atherosclerotic disease in those patients transplanted for coronary artery disease.

The main cause of death in transplant recipients still remains acute cardiac rejection or infection from over-immunosuppression in the early stages and graft vascular disease in the later stages (Table 5–1). Although cardiac transplantation is in its 25th year in this country, the prevention of acute rejection is still elusive despite the many different therapeutic protocols being tried. Also, although noninvasive methods have been tried, particularly in the younger age groups, at the time of writing this chapter the definitive diagnosis of acute rejection still requires a morphologic confirmation. It is surprising that although endomyocardial biopsy was first used for the diagnosis of acute rejection in 1973,[4] it is still being used in most cardiac transplant centers to this day. This chapter outlines the temporal and sequential changes occurring in the morphology of cardiac tissue obtained by endomyocardial biopsy and at autopsy in failed cardiac recipients.

THE DIAGNOSIS OF ACUTE REJECTION

Since the onset of cardiac transplantation in 1967,[1] many noninvasive methods have been tried and others are being developed in an attempt to monitor acute cardiac rejection. Recently, with the transplantation of neonates and very young infants, there is a further impetus to develop a noninvasive technique. So far, despite some methods that are used to follow patients, most of them are guidelines to reduce the number of endomyocardial biopsies, which to this day still remain the most accurate way to diagnose acute cellular rejection. The many noninvasive methods tried and used to monitor rejection are clinical, radiologic, electrocardiographic, hemodynamic, echocardiographic, serologic, and immunologic. These noninvasive methods will be mentioned only briefly as they will be expanded in other chapters in this book.

The clinical symptoms of acute rejection include fever, gallop rhythm, cardiomegaly, and other signs of heart failure. In the early days, a reduced summated electrocardiographic (ECG) voltage was used as an indication of acute rejection. It is now known that clinical

Table 5–1. Causes of Death in 694 Cardiac Recipients (Stanford Cardiac Transplantation)

	First Postop Year		>1 Year Postop	
	CSA*	AZA†	CSA*	AZA†
Rejection	17	7	9	4
Infection	36	28	36	18
Graft coronary	1	—	26	7
Graft failure	9	—	—	—
Lymphoproliferative	2	—	5	3
Nonlymphoid Malignancy	1	—	9	3
Embolus (pulmonary)	3	—	—	—
Pulmonary Hypertension	2	2	—	—
CVA	3	—	2	—
Other	10	—	18	8
Total Deaths	84	37	105	43

*Cyclosporine.
†Azathioprine.

and ECG changes do not appear until there is at least widespread moderate acute rejection, which may be difficult to reverse. A number of different immunologic markers have been used for acute rejection monitoring. Interleukin-2 receptors, together with T helper cell and T cytotoxic cell ratios, have been described but have also been found to be unreliable. Monitoring the excretion of neopterin and lymphocyte transferrin receptor levels has been tried. Plasma prolactin and β2-microglobulin secretion, as well as spontaneous lymphocyte blastogenesis counts, has also been used for this purpose. The sensitivity and specificity of many of these techniques have not revealed sufficient accuracy or consistency.

M-mode echocardiography and two-dimensional echocardiography have probably been the most successful techniques in picking up septal and left ventricular wall thickness and wall motion in a developing acute rejection.[5] The presentation of fractional shortening has been found useful as a marker, particularly in children when used in serial monitoring; however, these markers are also known to give false results. The isovolumic relaxation time (IVRT) has also been shown to be a useful method for evaluating acute rejection, although its accuracy is questionable until the patient reaches at least moderate acute rejection.[6] Magnetic resonance imaging (MRI) promises to provide an increased characterization of the tissue components in acute myocardial rejection; however, this technique has not yet been fully developed for this purpose.[7] Radionucleotide imaging with perfusion scans of thallium-201, gallium-67, and technetium[8] and indium-labeled lymphocytes and antimyosin antibody fragments has also been used in an attempt to discover an inflammatory infiltrate as well as damage to the myocardium. There is, however, much variability in the way this technique is performed, and therefore there is no consensus as to its use in ascertaining acute cardiac rejection. In some institutions, some of these noninvasive techniques are used as guidelines or auxiliary methods to diagnose acute cardiac rejection and to guide the timing of endomyocardial biopsies. Other immunologic aspects of heart transplantation are well reviewed in a recent book by Wijngaard.[9, 10]

It has also been claimed that a diagnostic potential exists for the assessment of cytokines or cytokine receptor levels in the diagnosis of rejection.[11] Elevated levels of cytokine, interleukin-6 (IL-6), soluble IL-2 receptors, and tumor necrosis factor (TNF) have been shown to increase during acute rejection in some solid organ transplants.[12] In our own laboratory, and corroborated by work in Wijngaard's laboratory, these findings have no diagnostic usefulness and could not be relied upon. We found particularly in the case of heart transplantation that cytokines were not always elevated during acute allograft rejection, using the endomyocardial biopsy histopathology as a correlation. We observed, as did Wijngaard,[11] that there were increased levels of cytokines after cardiac transplantation regardless of acute rejection. Furthermore, increased levels of cytokines could not discriminate among rejection, infection, and other inflammatory disorders. Work should be continued with noninvasive studies, as this technique obviously has tremendous advantages, but at this time I believe it is correct to say that the diagnostic and clinical usefulness of these techniques is limited.

Invasive Methods for the Diagnosis of Acute Cellular Rejection

The endomyocardial biopsy is the procedure by which tissue samples are obtained from the right and left ventricles of the donor heart. The endomyocardial biopsy was first described by the Japanese team of Konno and Sakakibara, who introduced the intravenous approach to the heart.[13, 14] Although the Japanese instrument is still used, especially in Japan, several new modifications of the transvenous catheter have emerged: the Caves-Schulz Stanford bioptome,[15] the modified Olympus or King bioptome,[16] the Kawai bioptome,[17] and the disposable Cordis bioptome. New bioptomes are being developed all the time. Philip Caves deserves the credit for the development of the new and shorter transjugular catheter biopsy forceps that can be used on an outpatient and does not require the femoral approach.[15] The clinical experience of Stanford and many other institutions with these modified bioptomes has been well reviewed in many articles and previous reports. At present, in most cardiac transplant programs, this method is performed safely on an outpatient basis in adults and children. The technique for endomyocardial biopsy has also been well described in the literature.[18, 19]

Serial biopsies over time have not presented any particular problem, and many cardiac transplant recipients have had more than 42 consecutive biopsy procedures in which 4 to 6 pieces of tissue have been removed at any one procedure. Both left and right ventricular biopsies can be performed with the bioptome, including transseptal (atrial) techniques, although most biopsies are confined to the right side. To date, more than 20,000 endomyocardial biopsies have been performed at the Stanford University Medical Center in all age groups, with only one biopsy-related death, in a 3 month old infant. The morbidity is less than that for liver or renal biopsies.

The more serious complications of endomyocardial biopsy are those of ventricular perforation with tamponade, severed chordae tendineae causing tricuspid incompetence, and coronary artery–right ventricular fistulas. The indications for endomyocardial biopsy are outlined in Table 5–2.

It is considered advisable to perform routine pretransplant biopsies of the recipient's heart to confirm the suspected diagnosis. This has become more necessary since it has been shown that amyloidosis and giant cell myocarditis, both of which can simulate end-stage idiopathic cardiomyopathy, can recur in the donor heart following transplantation.[20–22] Sarcoidosis and acute myocarditis also simulate idiopathic cardiomyopathy hemodynamically, and these should be ruled out since they are potentially curable diseases. For these reasons, pretransplant endomyocardial biopsy evaluation is important in our judgment. The least controversial use of the biopsy is in the diagnosis of acute rejection, which will be described later.

In cardiac transplantation, endomyocardial biopsies are usually performed at 1-week intervals until the patient leaves the hospital and then at 3-month intervals, although these time frames vary with different transplant centers. The endomyocardial biopsy is used not only to diagnose acute rejection but also to rule out infectious myocarditis in cardiac recipients. It is also useful for monitoring changes in therapy. Since cyclosporine and steroids have to be reduced for infection or lymphomas, the biopsy can monitor the potential development

Table 5–2. Indications for Endomyocardial Biopsy in Cardiac Recipients

Pretransplant evaluation
Diagnosis of acute rejection
Diagnosis of infectious myocarditis
To monitor changes in therapy
Long-term survivor follow-up
Removal of foreign fragments

of acute rejection. Patients may be taken off steroids for the usual complications, but particularly for osteoporosis. Although not necessary, it has been useful to monitor long-term survivors of acute rejection at least annually to rule out ischemia, which can sometimes be picked up on cardiac biopsy, but at this stage it is more useful for research than for clinical monitoring. We have also found that acute rejection may occur many years post-transplantation after infection with cytomegalovirus (CMV) or a marked increase in the patient's weight, which effectively "dilutes" the effect of the immunosuppression. More recently, in the case of rebellious teenagers no longer under parental control, noncompliance may result in reduction of immunosuppression. Endomyocardial biopsy, therefore, plays a useful part in the follow-up of all these patients.

Endomyocardial Biopsy Tissue Collection

The greatest criticism of the endomyocardial biopsy is the problem of sampling error.[23, 24] This was recognized early, and to reduce this problem it has always been the policy of major centers to obtain a minimum of four and up to six pieces of tissue at any one biopsy procedure. The size of the biopsy pieces is also important; different bioptomes vary in size from 6F (for children) up to 9F. Obviously, if smaller bioptomes are used, then it is better to obtain more tissue pieces to avoid sampling error. It is probably better to have more tissue with smaller pieces than to have fewer pieces with larger samples.

The biopsy tissue should be handled carefully and should be fixed immediately in 10 per cent buffered formalin, preferably at room temperature to avoid increased contraction of the myocardium. One piece of tissue is often frozen in liquid nitrogen or other freezing mixtures for immunofluorescence, immunohistochemistry, and, in some cases, in situ hybridization or polymerase chain reaction (PCR) studies for cytomegalovirus and other organisms. After being fixed and processed in the usual manner, the tissue is paraffin- or plastic-embedded and sections cut at not more than 4- to 6-micron thickness. It is recommended that the block be sampled with at least three deeper levels and preferably through the entire block. Staining with hematoxylin and eosin, as well as Masson's trichrome or a similar connective tissue stain, is recommended. The trichrome stain is particularly useful for highlighting myocyte damage in early ischemia (Fig. 5–1), and it is also helpful to delineate vessels and to ascertain whether or not lymphocytic infiltrates are within patches of fibrosis or healed areas. Additional histochemical stains should be ordered as required, so it is useful to keep blank slides for this purpose or in case special stains should be required to rule out acidfast bacilli or other organisms.

Most centers agree that electron microscopy is impractical for the routine surveillance of acute rejection, but it may be required for research or other diagnostic purposes.[25] For electron microscopy, the tissue should also be placed immediately into glutaraldehyde at room temperature and processed accordingly. Many centers used the plastic Beem capsules filled with Tissue Tech freezing mixture to keep small biopsy pieces safely frozen and to prevent them from drying out. Once labeled, the frozen specimens can be stored at −70°C for many years and still retain their immunogenicity for studies.

Morphology of Cardiac Rejection

Gross Changes. The gross changes of acute cardiac rejection are included here for completeness. Knowledge of these changes is use-ful at the time of retransplantation or for autopsy diagnosis. Grossly, the acutely rejected heart is a heavy, stiff heart with a darker plum color, in contrast to the light tan color of the recipient's native heart, when compared along the suture line. The darker color is due to subendocardial and intramyocardial hemorrhages. The heart is edematous, with turgid papillary muscles (rather like an amyloid heart), and the heart valves also may be edematous. In the case of a long-term survivor of 2 or 3 years or more, graft coronary disease may have ensued, and the coronary arteries may be felt as firm "tubes" and have concentric yellow material within their walls on cross-section. In some cases, the pericardium may be thickened and adhering to the epicardial surface of the heart. In other cases, cystic spaces or loculated effusions may be found between the epicardium and the pericardium. In almost all cases, evidence of acute or chronic pericarditis can be found. The atrial suture lines are often endothelialized, although this is not so common in the suture lines of the aorta and pulmonary artery.

Histopathology of Cardiac Transplantation

Cardiac transplantation histopathology can best be described by dividing the subject into

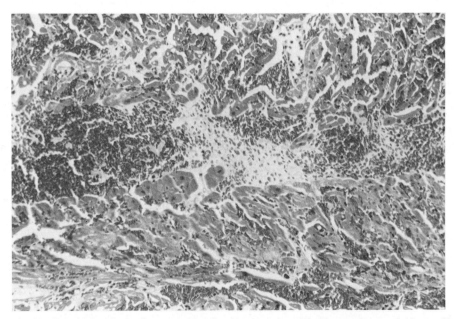

Figure 5–1. Section from heart of a cardiac transplant showing extensive, global hemorrhage and edema of hyperacute rejection. (Hematoxylin & eosin, × 200)

the sequential changes occurring in the first 24 hours following transplantation, in the first few weeks, and then in the intermediate period up to 1 year, as well as the late changes occurring after 1 year as outlined in Table 5–3.

Immediate Graft Pathology. This occurs within 24 hours of transplantation and includes sudden graft failure, which may occur in the operating room. The most common reason for this in the past has been right ventricular failure due to high pulmonary vascular resistance because of many years of heart failure or other reasons. In this event the right ventricle fails and becomes edematous and dilated. It is obvious that a normal right ventricle without hypertrophy will be unable to contract against a high pulmonary vascular pressure. This is the reason that patients who have high vascular pressure are either rejected as recipients for cardiac transplantation or have combined heart-lung transplants. In some cases, called "domino heart transplants," a previously hypertrophied right ventricle may be used as a donor heart for a patient with moderately high pulmonary vascular resistance. Other reasons for graft failure have been found to be unsuspected contusions of the myocardium from automobile or crushing accidents or prolonged hypotensive ischemia damaging the myocardium in the resuscitated donor hearts.

Hyperacute rejection is a rare complication resulting in failure of the donor heart within the first 24 hours. In one study of a total of 524 heart transplants, only 2 cases of hyperacute rejection occurred. Histopathologically, this entity is composed of pronounced interstitial edema and global interstitial hemorrhage. If the heart is kept in situ during the retrieval of a new donor heart, neutrophilic infiltration may also occur. The reasons for hyperacute rejection have been described as (1) the previous formation of antibodies to the HLA system in the transplanted graft, particularly antibodies to class 1 antigens (HLA, B, or C); (2) the existence of preformed ABO antibodies in the graft recipient at the time of transplantation; and finally, (3) in the case of xenotransplantation, transplantation between phylogenetically distinct species. Patients more likely to develop hyperacute rejection have often had exposure to previous blood transfusions, repeated pregnancies, multiple cardiac operations, or previous transplantation. Hyperacute rejection may also result from inaccurate cross-matching of the blood.[26] Hyperacute rejection usually occurs immediately, and therefore cardiac biopsies are not obtained; however, for the sake of completeness, the morphologic changes are described:

The Histopathology of Hyperacute Rejection. This consists of marked interstitial edema and hemorrhage, with a global distribution of hemorrhage throughout the entire myocardium as opposed to focal hemorrhages (see Figure 5–1). In addition, small vessels, particularly capillaries, may contain "sludging" of red cells and fibrin. Neutrophils may be seen if the donor heart is kept in situ for long.

Early Histopathologic Changes of Acute Rejection (1 to 3 Weeks). The first routine biopsy following cardiac transplantation may show evidence of reperfusion injury[27] or ischemia. Myocardial ischemia seen in endomyocardial biopsies is usually focal and sometimes subendocardial. These changes result from prolonged ischemic time of the donor heart or prolonged surgery if complications develop. The changes typical of ischemia are microinfarcts, which are best highlighted by a connective tissue stain such as Masson's trichrome that shows the myocardium as light red or gray rather than the deep red normal color. The ischemic myocardium is often shrunken, and the surrounding infiltrate, which often includes neutrophils, is scanty, unlike the pattern seen in acute rejection (Fig. 5–2). Contraction bands may be seen within the myocytes, and pyknotic myocyte nuclei are often present. In slides stained with hematoxylin and eosin, the myocytes may show hyper-

Table 5–3. Summary of Sequential Cardiac Allograft Pathology

Immediate	0–24 hours	Graft failure (Contusions, prolonged ischemia, high pulmonary vascular resistance) Hyperacute rejection
Early	1–3 weeks	Myocardial ischemia Reperfusion damage Pressor agent effect Accelerated rejection
Intermediate	1–52 weeks	Acute cellular rejection Infectious myocarditis Lymphomas (EBV-related*) Humoral rejection
Late	1–22 years	Graft coronary disease Hypertrophy and fibrosis Graft denervation

*Epstein-Barr virus.

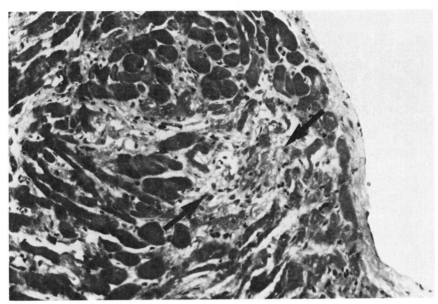

Figure 5–2. Endomyocardial biopsy from a cardiac recipient 1 week after transplantation, showing paler ischemic myocardium (arrows). Note minimal inflammatory infiltrate. (Masson's trichrome, × 360)

eosinophilia and pyknotic nuclei, thus helping separate them from the biopsy artifacts of contraction bands, which do not include pyknotic nuclei. Microinfarcts, thought to be due to trapped air bubbles within the coronary circulation at the time of reperfusion, may appear as focal myocyte damage without a lymphocytic infiltrate (see Fig. 5–1). In later biopsies, these areas of myocyte damage due to microinfarcts or reperfusion injury convert to granulation tissue, which should be easily distinguished from the monomorphous lymphocytic infiltrate seen in acute rejection. In ischemia there is always more myocyte damage than surrounding infiltrate, whereas in rejection the opposite is true.

Myocardial Damage Due to Pressor Agents. Pressor amines, used to support the donor prior to cardiac transplantation and the recipient following cardiac transplantation, may also show an effect in the donor heart. These focal areas of myocyte damage are much smaller and more discrete than in the ischemia described earlier (Fig. 5–3). These foci also have a few mixed inflammatory cells and should not be confused with acute rejection. Of course, it is possible to have accelerated acute rejection in the first few weeks following transplantation; however, this is most often seen in later weeks and will be described under the intermediate changes.

Intermediate Pathology of Transplantation (1 to 52 Weeks). During the first year following

cardiac transplantation and particularly during the first 3 months, depending on the immunosuppression protocol, acute rejection of the myocardium is present in most patients. The histopathologic changes of acute rejection have been described.[28–30] Following treatment with an increase in immunosuppression, the rejection usually resolves. In a few cases, a low-grade acute rejection may persist for the first 2 or 3 months, and further immunosuppressive treatment may be required, such as methotrexate, retransplantation, or total lymphoid irradiation.

Over the years, several different grading systems for acute rejection have been developed. Table 5–4 shows several of the grading systems in use. The need for a standardized grading system became apparent from the difficulty of trying to compare results of different institutions and also in an effort to establish competent clinical trials among different institutions.[31] In 1990, the Society for Heart and Lung Transplantation convened an international group of cardiac transplant pathologists in an attempt to develop a standardized grading system. The goal of the standardized system was to provide a grading that was simple, easily taught, and reproducible, as well as one that could be extrapolated to other grading systems. It was deemed desirable to have a numerical grading system that was statistically manipulable rather than the older descriptive one. This new standardized grading system[32] is

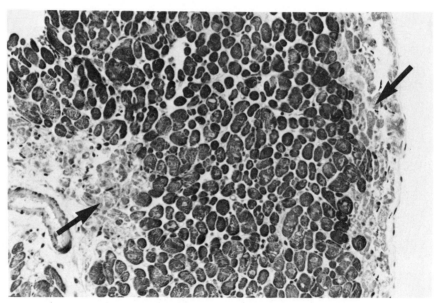

Figure 5–3. Endomyocardial biopsy showing a focal pale area in a typical "catecholamine effect" (arrows) following high dose pressor amines. (Masson's trichrome, × 500)

now used by many centers, and in some journals it is a requirement for the acceptance of papers on transplantation pathology. The outline of the new grading system is seen in Table 5–5, and it is described in more detail next. This new grading system has already been the impetus of multicenter research trials.

International Society for Heart and Lung Transplantation (ISHLT) Standardized Grading System

Grade 0. No evidence of acute rejection. If ischemia is present, for example, then this fact is listed under the additional required information.

Grade I (Mild Acute Rejection). *Grade IA* (focal mild acute rejection) represents a sparse, but distinctive, perivascular infiltrate of large, activated lymphocytes in one or two locations within a single biopsy fragment or in several biopsy pieces. Myocyte damage is not seen. The perivascular infiltrate should be distinguished from activated endothelial cells (Fig. 5–4). *Grade IB* (diffuse mild acute rejection) also presents a sparse, but more diffuse, infiltrate of large, activated lymphocytes extending into the interstitium between the myocytes and sometimes surrounding the myocytes but without causing obvious myocyte damage (Fig. 5–4). This sparse infiltrate may also be seen in one or several pieces of the biopsy tissue. It is not yet clear whether separation of IA and IB grades is clinically useful. Since 1980, with the use of cyclosporine, only 28 per cent of grade IA or IB follow-up biopsies are of a higher ISHLT grade in the first postoperative year. After the first postoperative

Table 5–4. Grading Systems for Acute Rejection

Stanford[28] (Billingham)	Standardized[32] (ISHLT)	Texas* (McAllister)	Hannover[38] (Kemnitz)
No rejection	0	0–1	A0
Mild acute	1A, 1B	1–4	A1, A2
Focal moderate	2	4	—
Moderate	3A, 3B	4–9	A3, A4
Severe	4	10	A4, A5
Resolving	(lower grade)	—	R1
Resolved	0	—	R2

*McAllister HA: A system for grading allograft rejection. Texas Heart Inst J 13:123, 1986.

Table 5–5. Standardized Cardiac Biopsy Grading*
(International Society for Heart and Lung Transplantation)

"Old" Nomenclature	"New" Nomenclature	Grade
No rejection	No rejection	0
Mild rejection	A = Focal (perivascular or interstitial infiltrate) B = Diffuse but sparse infiltrate	I
"Focal" moderate rejection	One focus only with aggressive infiltration and/or focal myocyte damage	II
"Low" moderate rejection "Borderline/severe"	A = Multifocal aggressive infiltrates B = Diffuse inflammatory process	III
Diffuse, aggressive, polymorphous, ± edema, ± hemorrhage, ± vasculitis	"Severe acute" rejection	IV
Denoted by a lesser grade:		"Resolving" rejection
Denoted by grade 0		"Resolved" rejection

Additional Required Information

*Biopsy less than four pieces
*Humoral rejection (positive immunofluorescence, vasculitis, or severe edema in absence of cellular infiltrate)
*"Quilty" effect   A = No myocyte encroachment
                      B = With myocyte encroachment
*Ischemia   A = Up to 3 weeks post-transplant
                      B = Late ischemia
*Infection present—biopsy therefore uninterpretable
*Lymphoproliferative disorder
*Other

*Modified and reproduced with permission from Billingham ME, Cary NRB, Hammond ME, et al. A working formulation for the standardization of nomenclature in the diagnosis of heart and lung rejection: Heart Rejection Study Group. J Heart Lung Transplant 9:587, 1990.

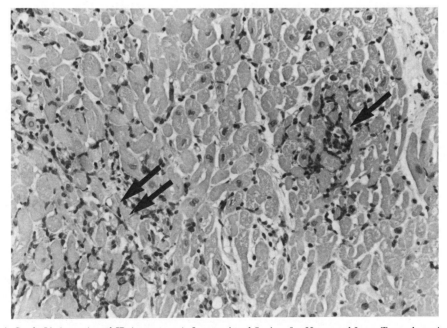

Figure 5–4. Grade IA (arrow) and IB (two arrows), International Society for Heart and Lung Transplantation (ISHLT) Standardized Grading System. (Hematoxylin & eosin, × 360)

year, only 4 per cent of follow-up biopsies are of a higher grade (personal unpublished data).

Grade II (Focal Moderate Acute Rejection). This grade represents a single circumscribed infiltrate of activated lymphocytes with or without eosinophils and with focal myocyte damage (Fig. 5–5). This grade was introduced simply because it was not known clinically whether it was necessary to treat a single focus, and it was hoped that the introduction of this grade would lead to randomized trials so the question could be answered. However, this grade does represent a "moderate" acute rejection. It is sometimes the case that there is one grade II focus, but there may be other foci of IA or IB among the biopsy pieces, and it is conventional in that case to assign the highest grade, which is grade II. Early studies suggest that there is no difference in the outcome of grade II whether treated or not. Like grade I, it is less likely to be followed with a higher grade 1 year or more post-transplantation.

Grade III (Moderate Acute Rejection). Grade IIIA represents multifocal lymphocytic infiltrates with or without eosinophils and with two or more foci causing obvious myocyte damage or obvious myocyte replacement (Fig. 5–6). Often the lymphocytes are lined up along the myocytes, indenting and overlapping them. Sometimes a single "naked" myocyte nucleus is seen within the lymphocytic infiltrate, indicating that a myocyte has been damaged. Grade IIIB indicates a more diffusely aggressive inflammatory infiltrate within several pieces of the biopsy tissue. Myocyte damage should be obvious, as well as definite myocyte replacement by the inflammatory cells. Occasional neutrophils may be found and even hemorrhage, although this is not usually present at this stage. Grade IIIB simply indicates a more aggressive and prominent infiltrate and is sometimes designated "borderline severe" (Fig. 5–7). The clinical usefulness of splitting biopsies into grade IIIA or IIIB has yet to be determined.

Grade IV (Severe Acute Rejection). In this grade, the inflammatory infiltrate is quite obvious, and it may become polymorphous with the inclusion of neutrophils as well as eosinophils (Fig. 5–8). In some cases an endothelialitis or a vasculitis is seen (Fig. 5–9); in these cases, interstitial hemorrhage is also present. Grade IV should be so extensive as to affect more than just one of the pieces of the biopsy. Edema may also be present, although this may be difficult to evaluate on a cardiac biopsy. Myocyte necrosis should be present.

Resolving or Resolved Acute Rejection. Under the new nomenclature, it was decided that the diagnosis of resolving or resolved acute rejection should not be made unless there had been a previous biopsy, in which case the numerical grade is reduced from IIIA or IV down to I, or whatever grade is appropriate, rather than using the term "resolved." It is useful,

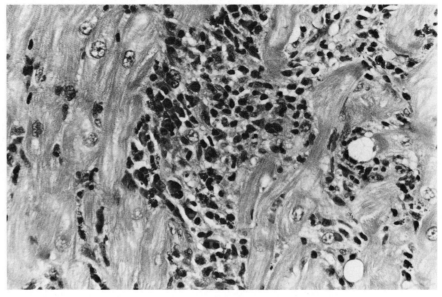

Figure 5–5. Grade II (ISHLT grade), showing a single focus of infiltrate with obvious myocyte replacement. (Hematoxylin & eosin, × 400)

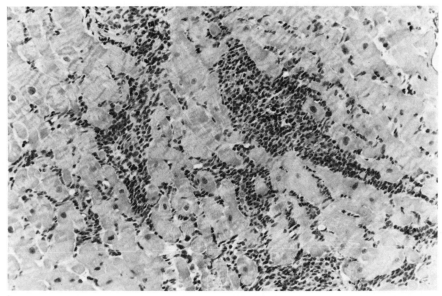

Figure 5–6. Grade IIIA (ISHLT grade), showing multifocal areas of lymphocytic infiltrate with myocyte replacement. (Hematoxylin & eosin, × 360)

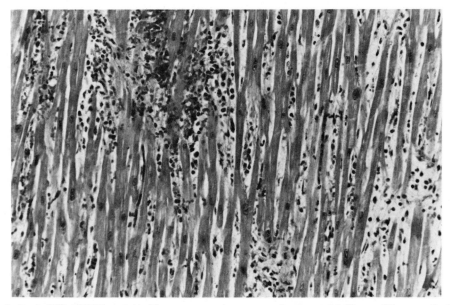

Figure 5–7. Grade IIIB (ISHLT grade), with more extensive myocyte damage and infiltrate. (Hematoxylin & eosin, × 360)

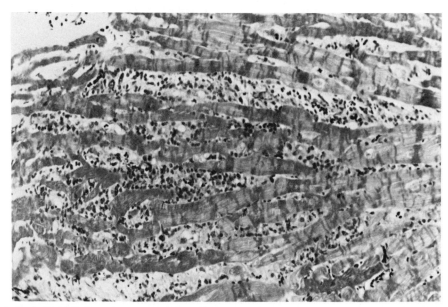

Figure 5–8. Grade IV (ISHLT grade), showing an extensive, mixed inflammatory infiltrate (neutrophils and eosinophils) with damaged myocardium. (Hematoxylin & eosin, × 360)

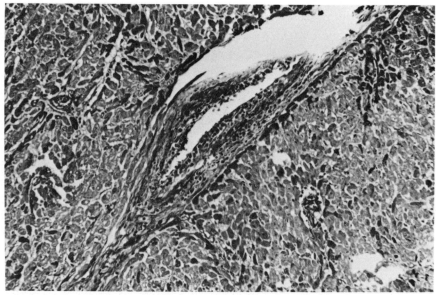

Figure 5–9. Section of myocardium at autopsy showing vasculitis from a patient who died of acute cardiac rejection. (Masson's trichrome, × 250)

however, to put down those terms as well (so that it is quite clear to the clinician that the rejection is receding rather than beginning).

Additional Required Information. As can be seen in Table 5–5, for the purpose of understanding rejection better, the ISHLT standardized grading system also requires the reporting of certain other characteristics to help multicenter trials and the understanding of published data. It is required that an inadequate or borderline adequate biopsy be reported; also whether there is any evidence of humoral rejection, denoted by positive immunofluorescence for immunoglobulins, vasculitis, or severe edema in the absence of a cellular infiltrate. Humoral or vascular acute rejection will be dealt with in detail in another chapter in this book. The presence of the "Quilty" effect should be noted; the Quilty effect is an infiltrate of lymphocytes confined predominantly to the endocardium. The ISHLT grading system has suggested the reporting of the Quilty effect as Quilty A if there is no myocyte encroachment and Quilty B if there is "spillover" of the lymphocytes into the subadjacent myocardium, causing myocyte damage. The purpose of this, again, is to see the significance of a Quilty B and whether or not myocyte encroachment should require treatment. If an infectious myocarditis is present, then this should be reported, as it is very difficult in some cases to tell the difference between acute rejection and infection. Likewise, if seen, lymphoproliferative disorders should be reported on the biopsy specimen. This detailed information will be useful in evaluating the results from different institutions. It has been suggested, for example, that there are more Quilty effects in children than there are in adults, and this type of information needs not only to be corroborated by other centers but also studied for its effect.

The Quilty Effect

The Quilty effect is characterized by a predominantly endocardial infiltrate of predominantly T lymphocytes and a mixture of B lymphocytes and accompanying small vascular spaces (Fig. 5–10). This type of infiltrate was not seen prior to the use of cyclosporine in 1981. More recently, these infiltrates have also been seen with the advent of newer drugs, such as FK506 and rapamycin.[33] Although some studies have suggested a correlation between the Quilty effect and acute rejection or even lymphomas, our own studies and those of several others have not shown a good correlation with these entities. The Quilty effect does cause diagnostic difficulty when it is cut tangentially and appears to be arising from the middle of the myocardium. Our policy is to cut through the block to see whether this infiltrate in fact reaches the endocardium, in which case we often designate it "Quilty" and do not treat the patient further. If the relationship with the endocardium cannot be made, it

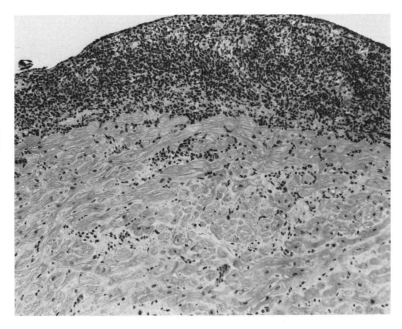

Figure 5–10. Endomyocardial biopsy from a cardiac recipient showing Quilty effect: wide lymphocytic infiltrate of the endocardium. (Hematoxylin & eosin, × 200)

is safer to treat the patient for acute rejection. In our institution, the Quilty effect is observed in over 20 per cent of adult cardiac biopsy specimens and up to 60 per cent of biopsy material from pediatric patients treated with cyclosporine. Quilty effect is not related to lymphoproliferative, EBV (Epstein-Barr virus), CMV, or acute rejection episodes or treatment. It has been found to be slightly more prevalent in patients transplanted for cardiomyopathies than for other diseases. Graft coronary disease appears to be less in Quilty-positive patients.

Humoral and Vascular Rejection in Cardiac Transplants

Patients usually present with clinical symptoms and signs similar to that of acute rejection, although the endomyocardial biopsy shows only interstitial edema with very sparse mixed inflammatory cells. The interstitial material may show proteinaceous fluid or fibrin as well. Myocyte damage is minimal in our experience. Hemorrhage may also accompany this type of humoral rejection. The biopsy may also demonstrate evidence of endothelial cell swelling in capillaries, venules, and/or arterioles, although these findings may be quite subtle on light microscopy. At a later stage, the biopsy specimen may show evidence of vascu-

litis. The vascular damage will lead to immunofluorescent evidence of vascular injury, with immunoglobulin deposition as described by Hammond[34-36] in Chapter 6. It is our opinion that vascular rejection or humoral rejection is relatively rare.

Infectious Myocarditis

Because of the degree of immunosuppression in cardiac transplant recipients, they are prone to a variety of systemic and myocardial infections. The most common of the cardiac infections are those caused by cytomegalovirus (CMV) and *Toxoplasma gondii*. We have seen one case of *Pneumocystis carinii* in a cardiac biopsy, but this is quite unusual. If a fungal infection is rampant, then *Aspergillus* or other fungal hyphae may be seen in vascular spaces in the biopsy material. If the inflammatory infiltrate in the biopsy is mixed and contains eosinophils as well as neutrophils, then an infectious diagnosis should always be suspected (Fig. 5–11). Occasionally, the typical features of CMV may be seen, and this may evoke an adjacent inflammatory infiltrate and edema (Fig. 5–12), or occasionally CMV can occur with no infiltrate. Likewise, unruptured cysts of *Toxoplasma gondii* may not be accompanied by an inflammatory reaction, and these cysts,

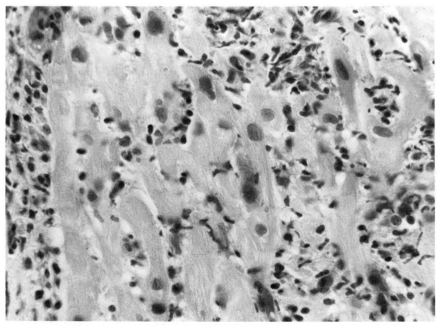

Figure 5–11. Endomyocardial biopsy from a cardiac recipient with cytomegalovirus (not seen), showing the mixed inflammatory infiltrate (neutrophils and eosinophils). (Hematoxylin & eosin, × 360)

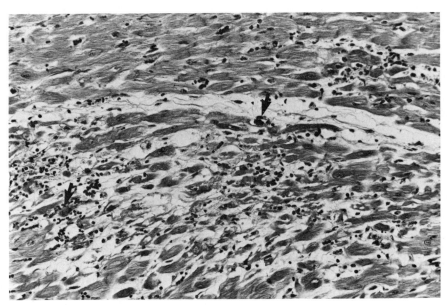

Figure 5–12. Autopsy myocardium showing edema and myocyte loss in a focus of cytomegalovirus (arrows). (Hematoxylin & eosin, × 250)

of course, are more difficult to see. Pathologists should be warned not to use periodic acid–Schiff (PAS) stain to highlight *Toxoplasma* in the myocardium, since the myocardium is full of glycogen and PAS positivity will only make it more difficult to see the organism.

At Stanford, where almost 700 cardiac transplants have been performed, the overall infection rate was 30 per cent prior to the advent of cyclosporine and is 5 per cent since cyclosporine. These figures are based on actuarial figures for freedom from infection. The pathologist should be particularly alert not to miss infectious myocarditis when ruling out acute rejection. It is obviously important to distinguish infection from rejection since the treatments for each are radically different. It is often useful to use immunoperoxidase or polymerase chain reaction (PCR) to establish viral infections.[37] Occasionally, acute rejection and infectious myocarditis are found in the same biopsy, in which case the clinicians must make a judgment as to which condition is worse. In our hospital, it has been possible to treat both at the same time with good results.

Immunophenotype of the Cellular Infiltrate in Acute Rejection

There have been many attempts to characterize the phenotypic cell of acute rejection for target-selective immunosuppression. Many centers quantify T cell subsets in serial endomyocardial biopsies for this reason.[38, 39] In our experience at Stanford, we found that T cell subset demonstration did not help in the management or prediction of acute rejection, and this has also been the finding of some other centers. The infiltrating cells are not a true marker for rejection, since they may be influenced by varying types of immunosuppression and the amount of absorbed immunosuppression. Newer observations suggest that the staining of activation markers of infiltrating mononuclear cells may have some relevance in determining the severity of acute rejection; however, we have not found this to be a problem: the more severe the rejection, the easier it is to diagnose on simple histologic grounds. Kemnitz[38] and Wijngaard[10] have shown a correlation with the number of infiltrating T cells and the severity of acute rejection. They also found that the number of CD3+ T cells tended to decline and the number of macrophages to increase in the resolving stages of acute rejection, as might be expected. Neither group has been able to rely on these trends alone in the evaluation of biopsy samples. These two groups also found that the NK (leu-7) cells were increased in the worst grades of acute rejection and decreased following treatment. Other cells, monocyte macrophages (CD36 and OKM5+), were not useful and did not not show significant trends. Further studies should be encouraged; although not useful at this time, they may contribute to our understanding of the mechanisms of allograft rejection.

Pitfalls and Morphologic Mimics of Acute Cellular Rejection

Those responsible for the management of cardiac allograft recipients following transplantation should be aware of several pitfalls in the endomyocardial biopsy diagnosis of acute rejection.

1. The most common pitfall of the biopsy is *insufficient or inadequate tissue* to rule out acute rejection. Tissue adequacy has been dealt with earlier in this chapter; however, it is felt that three good pieces with at least 50 per cent of the pieces of myocardium (not fat or hemorrhage) that can be evaluated should be obtained in order to rule out acute rejection.

2. *Previous biopsy sites* can be a nuisance—anyone who reads biopsy results knows they occur very frequently. If a recent biopsy site is present, fibrin and granulation tissue will be present (Fig. 5–13). Later biopsy sites will show fibrous replacement with a distinctive disarray of the subjacent myocardium (Fig. 5–10). Craters in the endocardium may also be seen. If several of the pieces of tissue obtained in one biopsy procedure contain previous biopsy site, this may render the material inade-

quate to rule out acute rejection. Lymphocytic infiltrates trapped in old biopsy sites may remain for years and should not be counted as acute rejection. Occasional foreign body granulomas can be seen in an old biopsy site.

3. Another pitfall previously described is the *Quilty B effect,* in which there is "spillover" into the myocardium that may in some cases cause myocyte damage (see Fig. 5–8). Treatment for acute rejection may cause the rejection to disappear; however, the Quilty effect may persist.

4. *Infectious myocarditis* has been described earlier. The difference in the type of infiltrate—a mixed infiltrate rather than a monomorphous lymphocytic one, as seen in most cases of acute rejection—should be helpful in this particular pitfall.[5] Instrumentation into the right ventricle, such as the placement of a pacemaker, is not always reported to the pathologist. Obviously, if the biopsy is taken in the region of a pacemaker implantation or similar instrumentation, then changes of inflammation in the surrounding myocardium confuse the diagnosis of acute rejection. This particular pitfall is quite rare, however.[6] If tissue resembling chordae tendineae is seen in a biopsy specimen, this should be reported to the clinicians as a complication of an endomyocardial biopsy. In biopsy material containing epicardial fat, mesothelial cells may be seen, and these too should be reported as they indicate perforation of the epicardium such that hemopericardium may ensue.

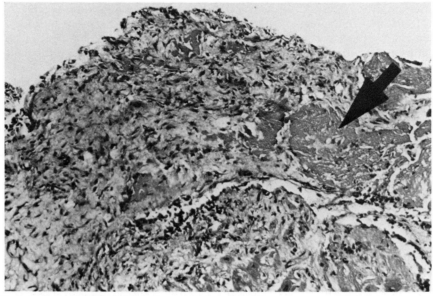

Figure 5–13. Endomyocardial biopsy showing a recent, previous biopsy site with fibrin (arrow) and surrounding infiltrate, which should not be confused with acute rejection. (Hematoxylin & eosin, × 360)

THE PATHOLOGY OF LONG-TERM CARDIAC TRANSPLANTATION

To date, the longest cardiac allograft survivor lived for 22 years. Now many other patients are surviving between 10 and 20 years. The pathologic changes that can be expected in long-term survivors include occasional acute rejection (although this is much more rare than in the first 3 months following transplantation), fibrosis and hypertrophy of the allograft, and, of course, graft coronary disease, which is the single most discouraging aspect of long-term survival.

Acute rejection and infectious episodes are diminished after 1 year; however, episodes of acute rejection may develop following a CMV infection or reduction in immunosuppressive therapy to combat osteoporosis, nephrotoxicity, or hypertension. Occasionally a patient will reduce intake of prescribed drugs to mitigate the unwanted side effects of moon face or hirsutism. The development of opportunistic infections is a problem inherent in cardiac transplantation and can occur at any time, including in long-term survivors. The range of organisms responsible for infections in long-term cardiac survivors is quite extensive.

Hypertrophy and Fibrosis

All long-term survivors of cardiac transplantation show an increase in interstitial fibrosis with compensatory hypertrophy of the myocardium. Within a week of cardiac transplantation, the donor heart becomes hypertrophied; this is noticed in children and infants as well as in adults. The hypertrophy continues into late survival. A morphometric study of cardiac allografts at 3 years after cardiac transplantation showed that myocyte hypertrophy was typical regardless of ischemic time or differences in immunosuppressive treatment.[40] It was also shown that myofibril volume fraction is often reduced. Overall, myocardial vascularity was no greater in most cases, but a few patients did have marked reductions (this is hypothesized to be due to damage to small vessels at the reperfusion level following transplantation). For those surviving more than 1 year, hypertrophy and fibrosis were almost universal. The hypertrophy appears to correlate with the degree of fibrosis and is therefore thought to be compensatory in type. Fibrosis, which may be patchy in type due to scar tissue from previous rejection episodes or previous ischemic epi-

sodes, may also be of a fine perimyocytic type. The latter was noticed particularly in the early days of cyclosporine use (1981) when much larger doses were being administered. This type of fibrosis seems to be less frequent now, although it is seen occasionally.

The etiology of the fibrosis is unclear, but one possible explanation is that it is the result of damage to capillaries and reperfusion injury at the time of transplantation, documented by electron microscopy, in the same way that fine interstitial fibrosis occurs following radiation damage in which capillaries and small vessels are injured. The reduction in small myocardial vessels has been documented at 3 years post-transplantation.[40] Endocardial fibrosis may be increased focally as a result of multiple, repeated endomyocardial biopsies, but these biopsy sites are usually difficult to see grossly at autopsy.

The other feature of fibrosis in long-term recipients involves the pericardium. The pericardium is usually left open following transplantation, but it may have become adhesive to the epicardium and thickened to the point at which it may cause constrictive pericarditis. Many donor hearts, however, do not show any evidence of chronic pericarditis even after many years of the graft in situ.

There is no significant difference between cyclosporine-treated groups and noncyclosporine-treated groups, as might be expected because of the increased hypertension prevalent in cyclosporine-treated patients. The significant reduction of myofibril volume fraction in cardiac allografts is characteristic of the chronic hypertrophy and has been associated with impaired ventricular contraction. A gradual decline of cardiac index has been observed in cardiac transplant recipients over a period of years, which might be attributed to the gradual loss of myofibrils with time.

Graft Coronary Disease

This lesion has been termed *chronic rejection, accelerated atherosclerosis,* and other names. *Graft coronary disease* is a less confusing term. This condition occurs more frequently in long-term survivors,[41–43] although it has been recognized as early as 5 months post-transplantation, including in infants. This disease also affects cardiac allografts in combined heart-lung transplantation. Many centers have reported an incidence of graft coronary disease (evaluated angiographically) of between 4 per cent and

47 per cent at 3 years following transplantation. Nitkin and Schroeder reported an incidence of 40 per cent of graft coronary disease by angiography at 5 years post-transplant.[44] Many studies have been undertaken with regard to the etiology of graft coronary disease. In general, it can be said that graft coronary disease is apparently not affected by donor heart ischemic time nor by HLA mismatches; episodes of acute rejection, whether or not the patient had coronary disease originally; or the type of immunosuppression. Although a few centers have indicated some correlations, these have not always been upheld.

The pathology of graft coronary disease is different from that of naturally occurring atherosclerosis and has been described many times. The typical changes consist of a concentric intimal proliferation along the full length of the epicardial coronary vessels, affecting also the small branches and intramyocardial vessels (Fig. 5–14). These changes are quite unlike those occurring as asymmetric plaques with grumous atherosclerotic material containing cholesterol crystals and associated with calcification. The latter lesions are usually associated with disruption of the internal elastic lamina. In contrast, in graft coronary disease the internal elastic lamina is usually almost intact. The intimal proliferation in graft coronary disease consists of modified smooth muscle cells and lipid-filled macrophages, although some lymphocytes may be seen. Endothelialitis is often seen in acute rejection (Fig. 5–15), but vasculitis is not the rule. Graft coronary disease in the donor hearts leads to all the consequences of ordinary coronary atherosclerosis, such as arrhythmias, heart failure, and myocardial infarcts. The usual warning signs of angina pectoris are lacking in cardiac recipients because of denervation of the allograft. Treating patients with antiplatelet aggregating agents and diets has failed to influence substantially the development of graft coronary artery disease. A recent study using diltiazem appears to delay the time of onset of graft coronary disease.[45]

Many studies are being undertaken in many different medical centers on the etiology and prevention of graft coronary disease, but so far none of them has been successful. It has been reported that pediatric cardiac transplantation at Loma Linda University in California and at Harefield in England results in less graft coronary disease, since the staff does not treat routinely with steroids unless the patient is actually rejecting. The transplanted proximal segments of the great arteries, the pulmonary artery, and the aorta have also been shown to develop intimal proliferation and thickening of the wall of the vessel, as well as occlusion of the adventitial vessels.[46] This is not noted so readily grossly because of the large diameter of these vessels (see Chapter 7).

Treatment. The only successful treatment for graft coronary disease is retransplantation.

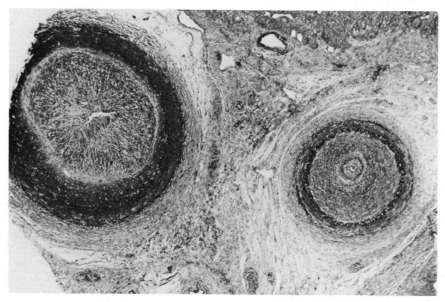

Figure 5–14. Explanted heart showing sections of coronary artery and branch with graft coronary disease (intimal proliferation) 14 months after cardiac transplantation. (Elastic van Gieson, × 20)

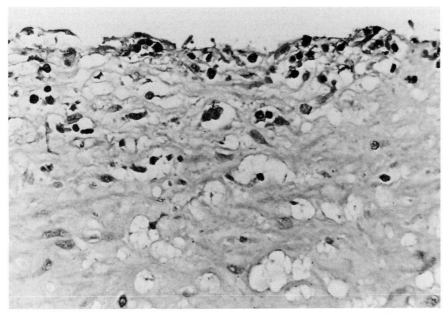

Figure 5–15. Section showing "endothelialitis" on the intimal surface of coronary arteries from the same patient as in Figure 5–14. (Immunoperoxidase Pan T, L22 [CD43] × 400)

Because the small intramyocardial branches are affected, coronary artery bypass grafts are ineffective. There have been sporadic reports of partially successful balloon angioplasty and atherectomies being performed in transplant recipients to remove focal coronary lesions (presumably occurring from the original donor). Long-term cardiac survivors—more than 10 years—may begin to show changes similar to those seen in naturally occurring coronary artery disease of asymmetric atherosclerotic plaques.[47] In both diseases, thrombosis may occur.

The Conduction System and Reinnervation in the Transplanted Heart

Although there have been some indications of reinnervation, as shown by electrophysiologic changes, and a few reports of cardiac recipients feeling cardiac pain, there has been no good morphologic evidence of reinnervation of the myocardium in the transplanted heart. Reinnervation of the sympathetic nerves has not been demonstrated either morphologically or pharmacologically. The postganglionic nerves of the parasympathetic system are known to retain their viability following transplantation, since the ganglia are left intact in the atrioventricular groove. It is most likely the parasympathetic nerves that can be

seen on electron microscopy of the transplanted heart. A morphometric study counting nerves per unit area within the transplanted heart has shown a marked decrease in the usual number of nerves by the end of the first year (suggesting loss of sympathetic innervation). These studies have been continued up to 12 years post-transplantation and do not show any increase in the number of nerves per unit area within the myocardium, which would be expected if reinnervation occurred.[48]

As has been pointed out, the conduction system in the transplanted heart is subject to the inflammatory infiltrate of acute rejection. The small vessels to the sinus and AV node may be affected by graft coronary disease. The conduction system itself remains largely morphologically intact following cardiac transplantation, and there is little evidence of permanent structural damage.[49] It has been reported that there is about a 50 per cent chance of surgical or procurement damage to both the recipient and the donor tissue around the conduction system (SA and AV nodes).[50]

Lymphoproliferative Disease in Cardiac Transplantation

Post-transplant lymphoproliferative disorder is a frequently fatal complication of immunosuppression following transplantation.[51] The lymphoproliferative disorders occurring in heart transplantation consist of the usual abnormal proliferations of lymphocytes. One of the primary pathogenic influences is believed to be the Epstein-Barr virus (EBV). More recently, some of the tumors have been shown to express EBV DNA virus. The incidence of lymphoproliferative disease in heart transplants is 1.8 per cent, which is slightly higher than that in the kidney but less than the incidence in the liver and combined heart-lung transplantation.[51] Transplant recipients tend not to have cancers that are common in the general population, but lymphoma constitutes 22 per cent of the neoplastic disease. An interesting feature of lymphoproliferative disease in cardiac allografts is that in some cases the lesions regress with reduction or cessation of immunosuppression (cyclosporine); this was first demonstrated by Starzl and coworkers in 1984.[52]

Transplant recipients tend to have a higher proportion of lymphomatous lesions within the central nervous system. Early on, when rabbit antithymocyte globulin (RATG) was being used at Stanford by intramuscular injection, some patients developed lymphoma at the injection site. The lymphomatous lesions may occur in the gastrointestinal tract or present with isolated solitary organ masses that can involve the liver, the lungs, the kidney, or virtually any organ. There is also a higher incidence of lymphoma in the pediatric post-transplantation group. It is felt that the duration of immunosuppression and the drug dosage are the most significant risk factors.

One study suggests that the introduction of OKT3 for rejection increased the incidence of lymphoma.[53] This study concluded that the use of OKT3 is associated with a statistically significant increase in the risk of lymphoma after heart transplantation, and it was concluded that the increased incidence of lymphoma was not due to a specific effect of OKT3, but rather to the amount and duration of immunosuppression. It has also been suggested that lymphoma should be treated by stopping all immunosuppression and then reintroducing it in a step-wise fashion when allograft rejection begins to occur. Lymphoma has also been reported in a trial of FK506 at the University of Pittsburgh. Multicenter studies have demonstrated that lower cyclosporine doses reduce lymphoma occurrence, and the addition of cyclosporine to existing immunosuppressive regimens increases the incidence of lymphoma. It was also suggested that OKT3 may induce the release of cytokines that might promote growth and malignant transformation of EBV-infected cells. (The data in this portion of this chapter are extrapolated from the Cincinnati Transplant Tumor Registry by Dr. Penn and his coworkers, who have collected data from transplant centers throughout the world for nearly 25 years.[54]) See Chapter 13.

Cutaneous malignancies also tend to occur with increased frequency in organ transplant recipients. Kaposi's sarcoma is fairly rare. Other tumors occur in a frequency similar to that of the general population. The results of the Clinical Transplantation Interactive Multicenter Workshop in Orlando in October, 1991, showed that, although there was no difference in graft survival or graft function between groups treated with antilymphocyte globulin (ALG) for induction and OKT3 for treatment of rejection, the risk of developing lymphoma was six times greater in patients who had received ALG and 22 times greater in patients who had received both ALG and OKT3.

Pathology of Transplantation in Children

Although cyclosporine became available in 1981, between 1980 and 1983 very few children underwent cardiac transplantation. By 1984, however, 50 children had been transplanted, and the numbers doubled annually until, by 1990, 206 children under the age of 10 years had been transplanted. Neonates are transplanted for hypoplastic left heart and other complicated congenital anomalies at birth. Later, children are transplanted for difficulty in revising the original corrective procedures for congenital heart lesions, as well as for cardiomyopathies and myocarditis. In other words, children also are transplanted only for end-stage cardiac disease. As in adults, the limits of pediatric heart transplantation are bounded by graft rejection and postinfection. Rejection occurs with a mean frequency of 1.0 to 2.5 episodes per patient in pediatric heart transplant recipients. It is therefore important to make the diagnosis of acute rejection. Endomyocardial biopsies can be performed (using a modified smaller size of bioptome) on neonates and very young children; however, they are more hazardous. In most centers, endomyocardial biopsy is not performed routinely on very young children, but only when it is absolutely necessary.

The disadvantages of endomyocardial biopsy in children include (1) sampling error, which is increased in the smaller pieces obtained; and (2) it is an invasive technique that has obvious disadvantages in young children and sometimes requires anesthesia or sedation to prevent crying, with possible air embolus. Anesthesia is an added risk in itself. On the other hand, in a group of 521 endomyocardial biopsies performed at Stanford in children ranging in age from 1 to 15 years (mean, 8.1 years) only 8 of 521 (1.5 per cent) of the biopsy specimens were inadequate for diagnosis, and 121 of 521 (23.2 per cent) were positive for acute rejection. The grading of endomyocardial biopsy in children is similar to that in adults.

Interpretive Differences Between Endomyocardial Biopsies of Children and Adults

1. The sampling error because of the smaller pieces of tissue obtained has already been alluded to.

2. The increased cellularity of the myocardium in infants, due to the smaller size of the myocyte nuclei, approximates to the size of intracellular lymphocytes. The tissue should be very carefully screened, therefore, so as not to miss the lymphocytes. Immunoperoxidase markers that will stain the cytoplasm of the infiltrating lymphocytes are more desirable in the identification of activated immune cells in children.

3. Based on the Stanford experience of examining more than 500 endomyocardial biopsy specimens in children and almost 20,000 from adults, it appears that larger arteries are more prominent in children's biopsies.

4. Endomyocardial biopsy specimens from children who have been treated with triple therapy and cyclosporine show an increased amount of Quilty lesions (60 per cent, as opposed to 20 per cent in adults). Many children have pronounced Quilty effect without any other evidence of acute rejection.

5. The myocardium of children is more prone to dystrophic calcification, so undue amounts of pressor agents can cause foci of calcification, as can ischemic areas or old rejection sites or biopsy sites.

Cardiac biopsies should be performed in infants of 1 year or younger only when clinically indicated, and it is probably not justified to use the biopsy for routine surveillance. Characteristic echocardiographic and other changes should be used for the management and diagnosis of acute rejection whenever possible. Despite the high prevalence of infections that may occur equally in children, infectious deaths in infants are infrequent, representing less than 5 per cent of perioperative mortality. In some centers, such as Loma Linda, prophylactic strategies of antibiotic, antiviral agents, and active and passive immunization are currently in use for children and infants to protect them from infection.[55]

Lymphoproliferative disease occurs with greater frequency in children. However, children respond rapidly to reduction or removal of immunosuppression[52] and also to irradiation.

Unfortunately, graft coronary disease also occurs in infants and children (see Figure 5–14). We know of an infant of 5 months who died of severe three-vessel coronary disease after being successfully transplanted at birth for hypoplastic left heart syndrome. One of the main problems in treating children is to ensure proper growth by reducing the amounts of steroids they are given for immunosuppression. In most cases, the reduction of steroids and the introduction of growth hormone have been successful in restoring children to their normal growth percentile for age, and these techniques also reduce the risk of graft coronary disease.

When children reach adolescence, there is often a problem with compliance for taking their immunosuppressive drugs because of the natural rebelliousness of this age group. The problems of adolescence and cardiac transplantation have been addressed elsewhere.

CONCLUSION

The results of cardiac allograft transplantation continue to improve over the years, and there are increasing numbers of survivors between 10 and 20 years postcardiac transplantation. Cardiac transplantation is now a routine procedure being performed successfully on infants and young children for congenital or acquired heart disease. Cardiac transplantation is also being performed successfully in older age groups in the 7th decade of life. The leading causes of death in the first postoperative year continue to be infection or acute rejection and in the later years graft coronary disease. Over 22,000 cardiac allografts have been performed worldwide; the pathology remains approximately the same with minor variations whether it is for young children or adults. It is hoped that the next decade will lead to new and improved immunosuppressive agents with fewer side effects. It is also hoped that a reliable noninvasive technique will be found to monitor acute rejection and infection in cardiac allografts.

REFERENCES

1. Barnard CN. A human cardiac transplant: An interim report of a successful operation performed at Groote Schuer Hospital, Capetown. S Afr Med J 41:1271, 1967.
2. Reitz BA, Wallwork JL, Hunt SA, et al. Heart-lung transplantation: Successful therapy for patients with pulmonary vascular disease. N Engl J Med 306:557, 1982.
3. Kaye MP. The Registry of the International Society for Heart and Lung Transplantation: Tenth official report—1993. J Heart Lung Transplant 12:1, 1993.
4. Caves PK, Stinson EB, Billingham ME, Shumway NE. Percutaneous transvenous endomyocardial biopsy in human heart recipients (experience with a new technique). Ann Thorac Surg 16:325, 1973.
5. Keren A, Gillis AM, Freedman RA, et al. Heart transplant rejection monitored by signal-averaged electrocardiography in patients receiving cyclosporine. Circulation 70(Suppl 1):1, 1984.
6. Dawkins KD, Oldershaw PJ, Billingham ME, et al. Changes in diastolic function as a noninvasive marker of cardiac allograft rejection. J Heart Transplant 3:286, 1984.
7. Yee E, et al. Cardiac allograft rejection: Comparative evaluations by magnetic resonance imaging vs. cine computed tomograms. J Heart Transplant 5:366, 1986.
8. McKillop JH, McDougall IR, Goris ML, et al. Failure to diagnose cardiac transplant rejection with Tc-99m-PYP images. Clin Nucl Med 6:375, 1981.
9. Fieguth H-G, Haverich A, Schaffers H-J, et al. Cytoimmunologic monitoring in early and late acute rejection. J Heart Transplant 7:95, 1988.
10. Wijngaard PLJ, Heyn A, Van der Meulan A, et al. Cytoimmunologic monitoring following heart transplantation. Bibl Cardiol 43:173, 1988.
11. Wijngaard PLJ. Immunological aspects of heart transplantation in man. Thesis for PhD, Heart Transplant Center, Ultrecht/Gronigen, 1992.
12. Jutte NPHM, Hesse CJ, Balk AHMM, Mochtar B, Weimer W. Sequential measurements of soluble IL-2 receptor levels in plasma of heart transplant recipients. Transplantation 50:328, 1990.
13. Sakakibara S, Konno S. Endomyocardial biopsy. Jpn Heart J 3:537, 1962.
14. Konno S, Sekiguchi M, Sakakibara S. Catheter biopsy of the heart. Radiol Clin North Am 9:491, 1971.
15. Caves PK, Schulz WP, Dong E Jr, Stinson EB, Shumway NE. A new instrument for transvenous cardiac biopsy. Am J Cardiol 33:264, 1974.
16. Richardson PJ. King's endomyocardial bioptome. Lancet 1:660, 1974.
17. Kawai C, Matsumori A. Myocardial biopsy. Am Rev Med 31:139, 1980.
18. Mason JW. Techniques for right and left endomyocardial biopsy. Am J Cardiol 41:887, 1978.
19. Tilkian AG, Daily EK (eds). Cardiovascular procedures. St. Louis, CV Mosby, 1986, pp 180–203.

20. Valantine HA, Billingham ME. Recurrence of amyloid in a cardiac allograft four months after transplantation. J Heart Transplant 8:337, 1989.
21. Kong G, Madden B, Spyrou N, Pomerance A, et al. Response of recurrent giant cell myocarditis in a transplanted heart to intensive immunosuppression. Eur Heart J 12:554, 1991.
22. Gries W, Farkas D, Winters GL, et al. Giant cell myocarditis: First report of disease recurrence in the transplanted heart. J Heart Lung Transplant 11:370, 1992.
23. Spiegelhalter DJ, Stovin PGI. An analysis of repeated biopsies following cardiac transplantation. Stat Med 2:33, 1983.
24. Zerbe TR, Arena V. Diagnostic reliability of endomyocardial biopsy for assessment of cardiac allograft rejection. Hum Pathol 19(11):1307, 1988.
25. Myles JL, Ratliff NB, McMahon JT, Golding LR, Hobbs RE, Rincon G, Sterba RW, Stewart R. Reversibility of myocyte injury in moderate and severe acute rejection in cyclosporine-treated cardiac transplant patients. Arch Pathol Lab Med 111:947, 1987.
26. Trento A, Hardesty RL, Griffith BP, Zerbe T, Kormos RL, Bahnson HT. Role of the antibody to vascular endothelial cells in hyperacute rejection in patients undergoing cardiac transplantation. J Thorac Cardiovasc Surg 95:37, 1988.
27. Jennings RB, Wartment WB. Reactions of the myocardium to obstruction of the coronary arteries. Med Clin North Am 46:3, 1962.
28. Billingham ME. Diagnosis of cardiac rejection by endomyocardial biopsy. J Heart Transplant 1:25, 1982.
29. Billingham ME. Endomyocardial biopsy detection of acute rejection in cardiac allograft recipients. *In* Sekiguchi M, Olsen J, Goodwin E, (eds). *Myocarditis and Related Disorders.* New York, Springer-Verlag, 1985, pp 86–90, and J Heart Vessels 1:86, 1985.
30. Billingham ME. The postsurgical heart. The pathology of cardiac transplantation. Am J Cardiovasc Pathol 1:319, 1988.
31. Billingham ME. Dilemma of variety of histopathologic grading systems for acute cardiac allograft rejection by endomyocardial biopsy. Presented at the International Society of Heart Transplantation Meeting, Colorado Springs, July 1989. J Heart Transplant 9:272, 1990.
32. Billingham ME, Cary NRB, Hammond ME, Kemnitz J, Marboe C, McAllister HA, Snovar DC, Winters GL, Zerbe A. A working formulation for the standardization of nomenclature in the diagnosis of heart and lung rejection: Heart Rejection Study Group. J Heart Lung Transplant 9:587, 1990.
33. Mohacsi PJ, Joshi A, Wang J, Morris RE, Billingham ME. Endocardial mononuclear cell infiltrates (Quilty effect) in heterotopic cardiac allografts in rapamycin-treated rats. Submitted to Circulation.
34. Hammond EH, Yowell RL, Nunoda S, Menlove R, Renlund DG, Bristow MR, Gay WA, Jones KW, O'Connell JB. Vascular (humoral) rejection in heart transplantation: Pathologic observations and clinical implications. J Heart Transplant 8:430, 1989.
35. Ensley RD, Hammond EH, Renlund DG, et al. Clinical manifestations of vascular rejection in cardiac transplantation. Transplant Proc (Suppl 1)23:1130, 1991.
36. Jambores G, et al. Acute humoral rejection after heart transplantation. Transplantation 46:603, 1988.
37. Weiss LM, Movahed LA, Berry GJ, Billingham ME. *In situ* hybridization studies for viral nucleic acids in heart and lung allograft biopsies. Am J Clin Pathol 93:675, 1990.
38. Kemnitz J, Haverich A, Uysal A, Heublein B, Wahlers T, Schafers HJ, Borst HG. Correlation of histopatho-

logic findings in endomyocardial biopsies from heart-transplanted patients with the positivity pattern of the immunophenotype of the cellular infiltrates. *In* Kemnitz J (ed). *Diagnosis of Rejection in Biopsy Material of Cardiac Allografts.* Berlin, Wolfgang Pabst Verlag, 1991, pp 11–30.

39. Marboe CC, Buffaloe A, Fenoglio JJ Jr. Immunologic aspects of rejection. Prog Cardiovasc Dis 32:419, 1990.

40. Rowan RA, Billingham ME. Pathologic changes in the long-term transplanted heart: A morphometric study of myocardial hypertrophy, vascularity and fibrosis. Hum Pathol 21:768, 1990.

41. Billingham ME. Cardiac transplant atherosclerosis. Transplant Proc, Vol XIX, 4(5):19, 1987.

42. Billingham ME: Graft vascular disease in heart transplants: Histopathology and results of retransplantation. *In* Touraine JL, et al (eds). *Transplantation and Clinical Immunology XXI.* New York, Excerpta Medica/Publishers, 1990, pp 27–41.

43. Billingham ME. Histopathology of graft coronary disease. J Heart Lung Transplant 11:S38–S44, 1992.

44. Nitkin RS, Schroeder JS. Accelerated coronary artery disease risk in heart transplant patients. J Am Coll Cardiol 5(Suppl):II-535, 1985.

45. Schroeder J, Gao S-Z, Aldeman E, et al. A preliminary study of Diltiazem in the prevention of coronary artery disease in heart transplant recipients. N Engl J Med 328:164, 1993.

46. Russell ME, Fujita M, Masek MA, Rowan RA, Billingham ME: Cardiac graft vascular disease: Nonselective involvement of large and small vessels. Transplantation 56:762, 1993.

47. Pucci AM, Forbes C, Billingham ME. Pathologic features in long-term cardiac allografts. J Heart Transplant 9(4):339, 1990.

48. Rowan R, Billingham ME. Myocardial innervation in long-term cardiac transplant survivors: A quantitative ultrastructural survey. J Heart Transplant 7:448, 1988.

49. Bahrati S, Billingham M, Lev M. The conduction system in transplanted hearts. Chest 102:1182, 1992.

50. Stovin PGI, Hewitt S. Conduction tissue in the transplanted human heart. J Pathol 149:183, 1986.

51. Penn I. Malignant lymphoma in organ transplantation recipients. Transplant Proc 13:736, 1981.

52. Starzl TE, Porter KA, Iwatsuki S, et al. Reversibility of lymphomas and lymphoproliferative lesions developing under cyclosporine steroid therapy. Lancet 1:583, 1984.

53. Swinnen LJ, Costanzo-Nordin MR, Fisher SG, O'Sullivan EJ, Johnson MR, Heroux AL, Dizikes GJ, Pifarre R, Fisher RI. Increased incidence of lymphoproliferative disorder after immunosuppression with the monoclonal antibody OKT3 in cardiac transplant recipients. N Engl J Med 323:1723, 1990.

54. Penn I (ed). Roundtable report on immunosuppression and lymphoproliferative disorders. University of Cincinnati. Raritan, New Jersey, OrthoBiotech, 1992.

55. Bailey L. Personal communication, 1992.

6

PATHOLOGY OF CARDIAC VASCULAR (MICROVASCULAR) REJECTION

ELIZABETH H. HAMMOND, MD

Pathologic descriptions of allograft rejection of all solid organs have long recognized vascular involvement in the rejection process. Renal allografts, the earliest allografts to be studied, commonly display vasculitis involving the arteries and arterioles of the cortex of the kidney, with or without cellular infiltrates invading tubules.[1-3] This vascular inflammatory process, termed *acute vascular rejection*, is often associated with allograft loss unless immunosuppressive therapy is begun, and often in spite of it.[2, 3] Similarly, arteritis has been identified in the heart on endomyocardial biopsy and has been associated with poor allograft survival.[4, 5] In all these studies, emphasis has been placed on involvement of the arterioles and arteries rather than on capillaries or venules. Since venules and capillaries are the sites of lymphocyte trafficking as well as being the most important sources of tissue oxygenation, it is also important to consider the changes in these vascular structures in allograft rejection.[6, 7]

Studies of allograft rejection in animals have shown that the microvasculature is the earliest structure to be destroyed during rejection.[8, 9] Destruction of the microvasculature of skin allograft in humans has also been shown to be the central event in first-set rejection; in fact, the destruction of the capillary bed is likely more damaging to the graft than piecemeal destruction of the graft parenchyma.[10] Al-

though endothelialitis of venules is considered evidence of rejection in the liver and capillaritis is considered an important component of allograft rejection in the lung, the importance of microvascular changes in cardiac allografts has been ignored until recently.[11, 12]

We and others have studied capillaries, venules, and arterioles of endomyocardial biopsy material to evaluate microvascular parameters of rejection.[13-16] Since 1985, we have studied endomyocardial biopsy specimens from cardiac transplant recipients by light microscopy, immunofluorescence, and electron microscopy. As of November, 1993 we have reviewed approximately 15,900 endomyocardial biopsies by light microscopy, 7300 endomyocardial biopsies by immunofluorescence, and approximately 410 endomyocardial biopsies by electron microscopy.[16]

In this chapter, the vascular changes of the microvasculature (capillaries and venules) are described in patients, most of whom were treated with immunoprophylactic protocols, including antilymphocyte globulin (ALG) and OKT3.[17, 18] The morphologic observations detail the types of microvascular changes that can be encountered in endomyocardial biopsies, explanted hearts, and autopsies from such patients.[14, 16, 19] Acute cellular rejection will not be discussed in this chapter since it is the subject of Chapter 5 by Dr. Billingham; cardiac vasculopathy involving the coronary arteries is not included since it is the focus of Chapter 7 by Dr. Marboe.

In all histologic observations, it is important to remember that our observations are static and that the process is dynamic. The types of infiltrating cells in a biopsy, the presence of immune complexes, and so on, though important, may not be relevant to the mechanism by which microvessels are altered. Many publications have focused on the relevance of CD8+ or CD4+ cells in the rejection process involving vessels.[20–22] These observations are flawed because the observers are trying to relate human vascular changes to those of well-characterized animal models and because the relevance of any finding, isolated in time, to long-term outcome of a graft must be shown with clinical correlative studies. Of course, the impact of immunosuppression, and its effectiveness in the treatment of rejection, must also be taken into account. This is a particular problem in relating the experience in untreated experimental allografts to those of treated human ones.[8, 9, 22–24]

IMMUNOCYTOCHEMICAL DETERMINANTS OF MICROVASCULAR REJECTION

Initial emphasis of immunopathologic studies of microvessels has focused on the detection of microvascular immune complexes (co-localization of immunoglobulin and complement components), which were found to correlate with subsequent hemodynamic compromise of the allograft in the absence of cellular infiltrates.[13, 14, 19] Frequently the biopsies also exhibited vascular and interstitial fibrin accumulation.[13–16, 25] Patients with endomyocardial immune complexes in microvessels were more likely to have had positive panel-reactive antibodies and positive cross-matches; however, many patients (more than half) did not have these predisposing factors.[13, 14, 19] Since persistent demonstration of these microvascular immune complexes correlated with poor allograft survival in three separate evaluations of our patients at 1, 3, and 5 years of follow-up, these features are now used as criteria to diagnose microvascular rejection and to classify patients as to rejection type.[13, 14, 25]

For a complete classification of microvascular rejection, alterations of other markers of endothelial activation or damage should also be included, and a composite score of these changes should be made. This is the approach advocated by Faulk and Labarrere and their colleagues.[15, 25] In Chapter 4, Drs. Faulk and Labarrere discuss the relevance of immunocytochemical studies of anticoagulant and fibrinolytic pathways in assessing microvascular damage. They note that antithrombin-III (ATT), a marker of the natural anticoagulant pathway expressed by the microvasculature of the heart, is lost in instances of microvascular damage. Furthermore, tissue plasminogen activator (tPA), normally present in smooth muscle cells of arterioles, is similarly lost in allograft microvascular injury.[15, 25] Whether these changes of anticoagulant and fibrinolytic pathway expression are results of or precursors to a vascular endothelium specific immune response is unknown. However, the alteration of the expression of these molecules clearly precedes permanent microvascular injury of cardiac allografts and has been correlated with cardiac allograft survival.[15, 25] We have been able to confirm these observations in our cardiac allograft population and therefore have incorporated them into the schema to classify microvascular rejection. This is presented as Table 6–1.

In the following description, both the light microscopic and immunocytochemical findings will be detailed, since both are used to arrive at the appropriate classification. The methodology used for immunocytochemistry by immunofluorescence is the standard methodology used for investigation of renal biopsies. Included are direct immunofluorescent examination of frozen, unfixed endomyocardial biopsy sections with IgG, IgM, C3, C1q, and fibrin and indirect determination of the presence of HLA-DR (MHC class II), ATT, and tPA.[13, 15, 25, 26] Antibodies, suppliers, and dilutions are shown in Table 6–2 and in Chapter 4, page 50. It is not recommended that the sections be stained with antibody directed against the MHC class I backbone determinates since they are so pervasively present.[27] We do not recommend that biopsies be routinely evaluated for immunophenotyping of lymphocytes, since studies of this type have not yielded clinically useful information.[20–22]

Other immunocytochemical studies may prove useful in the future. It has been suggested that the evaluation of biopsies for macrophage markers (CD14), markers of activation, IL-2R (CD25) on T lymphocytes, and FcgRII expression by macrophages and endothelial cells yields important information rele-

Table 6–1. Vascular Rejection Criteria Using Immune Complexes, Fibrin, ATT, and tPA

ISHLT Grade	Microvascular Grade	LM*	ATT/tPA†	Fibrin	Ig/C‡
0	negative	Negative	1/1	none	none
0	equivocal	Endothelial activation, edema, hemorrhage	1–2/1–2	none	Ig or C
0	mild	Endothelial activation, edema, hemorrhage or focal vasculitis	1–2/1–2	0–1 +	Ig and C in blood vessels, 1 +
0	moderate	Endothelial activation, edema, hemorrhage, *or* vasculitis	3/3	1–3 +, also interstitial	Ig and C in vessels, 2 +
4	severe	Diffuse aggressive polymorphous ± infiltrate, ± edema, ± hemorrhage, ± vasculitis, with necrosis	3/3	2–3 +, vessel and interstitial	Ig and C in vessels, Interstitial Ig and C

*Light microscopy.
†Antithrombin-III/tissue plasminogen activator.
(Patterns are given: 1 = normal, 3 = most abnormal; see text.)
‡Immunoglobulin/complement.

vant to rejection.[28, 29] Others have evaluated vascular adhesion marker expression in cardiac allografts and have suggested that increased expression of vascular cell adhesion molecule (VCAM) and intercellular adhesion molecule-1 (ICAM-1) but not endothelial leukocyte adhesion molecule (ELAM) on the microvasculature is found in association with lymphocytic infiltration.[30] In animal models of allograft rejection, antibodies to leukocyte adhesion molecules were efficacious in reducing the rejection.[31] This finding confirms the relationship of lymphocyte adhesion and infiltration but is not diagnostically useful. If upregulation of these adhesion molecules can be demonstrated before infiltration or can be correlated with the need for treatment, the molecules may become important monitoring criteria. Archival frozen tissue on all endomyocardial biopsies will be crucial to this approach.

Immunocytochemical markers to establish

Table 6–2. Antibodies Used for Cardiac Transplant Immunofluorescence Assay

Antibody	Supplier	Usual Dilution	Catalog No.
IgG-FITC	Protos	1:5	311
IgM-FITC	Protos	1:10	313
C3c, d-FITC	Dako	1:2, combined	c: F201
			d: F323
			F254
C1q-FITC	Dako	straight	350
Fibrin-FITC*	American Diagnostics	1:20	
HLA–DR–PE*	Becton-Dickinson	1:5	7367
Mouse IgG–FITC	Protos	1:10	346

*Monoclonal antibody; others, rabbit polyclonal. FITC = fluorescein; PE = phycoerythrin.

Addresses of Suppliers:
American Diagnostics, American House, 49 East 68th Street, New York, New York 10021
Becton-Dickinson, 2375 Garcia Avenue, Mountain View, California 94043
Dako, 6392 Via Real, Carpinteria, California 93013
Protos, 1485 Bayshore Boulevard, Suite 388, San Francisco, California 94124

that the microvasculature has been destroyed have only recently been described. Antibody to the microvasculature of the kidney has been used in this way: loss of the antibody activity, like loss of MHC II expression, can be associated with destruction of these vessels.[22-24] Factor VIIIra, a marker of intact vascular endothelium, can be shown to have altered morphologic expression in cardiac allograft microvascular injury.[16, 32] Patients with long-standing microvascular injury show loss of factor VIIIra or alteration of its expression, but this loss is only a confirmation of severe damage.[16]

CLASSIFICATION OF VASCULAR (MICROVASCULAR) REJECTION

Microvascular rejection can be evaluated descriptively or semiquantitatively by immunocytochemistry. The following categories are described on the basis of histologic and immunocytochemical findings.

No Evidence of Microvascular Rejection

In this category are included all biopsy specimens that show no light or immunofluorescent evidence of vascular rejection/alteration. By light microscopy, such sections show no endothelial cell swelling, endothelial cell necro-

sis, thrombosis, or inflammatory infiltrates in the walls of microvessels. Interstitial edema and hemorrhage are not present (Fig. 6–1).

By immunofluorescence, negative biopsies show no significant MHC class II expression by endothelial cells. Furthermore, no vascular accumulation of immunoglobulin or complement components is detected. Leakage by fibrin and albumin, which would indicate increased vascular permeability and endothelial cell activation or injury, is not seen. Examination of the biopsy material for evidence of anticoagulant pathway expression shows strong, uniform ATT expression of arterioles and venules without expression by capillaries. This is the normal pattern of expression in the heart and is called pattern 1 by Faulk and Labarrere.[15, 25] tPA is expressed exclusively by smooth muscle cells of the arterioles. This is the normal pattern of expression, also known as pattern 1. The site of these substances in allografts without rejection has been confirmed by double-labeling experiments. See Chapter 4 and illustration on page 60.

Equivocal Evidence of Microvascular Rejection

By light microscopy, equivocal biopsies show histologic endothelial cell activation or dam-

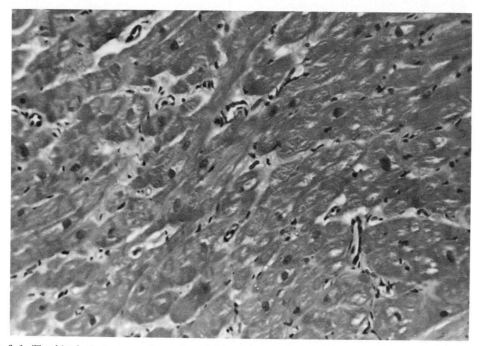

Figure 6–1. The histologic features of an allograft biopsy without rejection or microvascular alteration. Note that capillaries possess flat, continuous endothelium. (Hematoxylin & eosin, × 250)

age with or without associated edema or hemorrhage. No inflammation or thrombosis is demonstrated in the walls of any capillaries, venules, or arterioles within the sample. Histologically, such biopsies are considered to be ISHLT 0. Since these features are very subjective, microvascular rejection can only be suspected on this basis. Only immunofluorescent findings are diagnostic of microvascular rejection in such cases (see following) (Fig. 6–2). Similar equivocal findings can be seen in patients with systemic viral illnesses, especially those caused by cytomegalovirus.[16, 26]

By immunofluorescence, such equivocal biopsies may show microvascular accumulation of immunoglobulin or complement components but not both. Furthermore, vascular leakage may be demonstrated by seeing extravasated albumin in the absence of vascular immune complexes.[26] These features indicate that diffuse endothelial cell permeability is present. Thus, these features are quite nonspecific and cannot be used specifically to diagnose vascular rejection or vascular damage. MHC class II antigen expression may be upregulated on the microvasculature. These changes are ubiquitous in the first weeks posttransplant in patients undergoing induction immunosuppression with monoclonal anti-

CD3 (OKT3), which has been shown to produce transient lymphocytic activation and release of cytokines such as tumor necrosis factor (TNF) and interleukin-1 (IL-1).[33, 34] Since these factors lead to vascular permeability and endothelial activation, it is not surprising that patients show these findings during OKT3 therapy.[35–38] We have also seen these features early after transplant in a patient receiving a heart from a pregnant patient dying of cerebral vascular accident during delivery (personal unpublished data).

Expression of ATT is of equivocal significance if loss of ATT from venules but not arterioles is seen (pattern 2 of Faulk and Labarrere). Tissue plasminogen activator may show focal loss from arteriolar smooth muscle (pattern 2 of Faulk and Labarrere).[15, 25] See Chapter 4, page 60.

Mild Microvascular Rejection

In this category, light microscopic evidence of vasculitis may be demonstrated (Fig. 6–3). Alternatively, the biopsy may be deceptively innocuous, showing only evidence of interstitial edema or hemorrhage, with endothelial cell activation and no inflammation at all (see Fig-

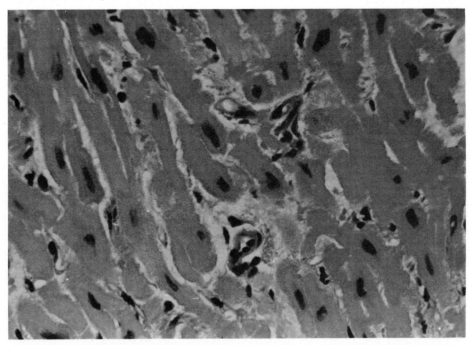

Figure 6–2. Equivocal histologic evidence of microvascular rejection or damage. Biopsy specimen shows endothelial activation and swelling of the capillary endothelium. Diffuse interstitial edema is present. No cellular rejection is seen. (Hematoxylin & eosin, × 250)

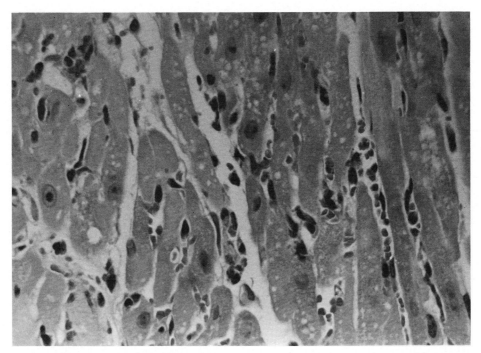

Figure 6–3. In addition to endothelial activation, capillaries in this biopsy specimen show vasculitis. No cellular rejection is seen. (Hematoxylin & eosin, × 250)

ure 6–2). This is the type of biopsy in which immunofluorescence is particularly useful, since one can be misled by the light microscopic appearance. The presence of light microscopic vasculitis, which is often leukocytoclastic, qualifies the biopsy for a diagnosis of mild vascular rejection. Venules and capillaries may be involved. Such vessels may show prominent accumulation of nuclear dust, and the invading inflammatory cells are commonly neutrophils as well as lymphocytes (see Fig. 6–3).

By immunofluorescence, the majority of such biopsies will show co-localization of immunoglobulin and complement components in capillaries and venules, occasionally with intravascular localization of small amounts of fibrin. Rarely, such vasculitis can be caused by cellular immune mechanisms; in such cases, immune complexes in vessel walls are not demonstrated. We have seen this pattern of findings in only 3 of 75 patients with vascular rejection, but it has been more frequent in the experience of others, especially in the absence of immunoprophylactic therapy.[15, 39, 40] This group of patients consistently demonstrates alterations of the natural anticoagulant and fibrinolytic pathways. The microvasculature exhibits partial loss of ATT (on venules) and tPA (in smooth muscle cells of arterioles) or com-

plete loss of ATT, so-called pattern 3, and loss of smooth muscle tPA, also known as pattern 3. Either of these patterns may be present.[15, 25] See Chapter 4, page 60. Upregulation of MHC class II is also uniformly seen.[16, 41]

Moderate Microvascular Rejection

In this category, vasculitis may be extensive and arteriolitis may be found (Fig. 6–4). Alternatively, patients with moderate microvascular rejection may show no vasculitis and only severe interstitial edema with a blue fibrillar appearance of the interstitium, which has been shown to be associated with fibrin accumulation (Fig. 6–5). In such patients, it is critical to review the previous biopsy to see whether or not the process is worse or better, in order to make an adequate assessment. By immunofluorescence, moderate microvascular rejection usually shows large accumulations of immunoglobulin and complement components within capillaries and venules (Fig. 6–6). In some cases, particularly in long-standing vascular rejection, only intravascular and interstitial fibrin is detected.[14, 16] In biopsies of patients with moderate microvascular rejection, ATT and tPA are usually completely lost. This pattern of expression (pattern 3) is often asso-

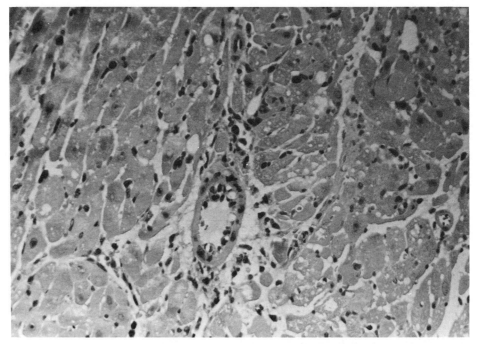

Figure 6–4. Biopsy specimen with moderate vascular rejection. Capillaries, venules, and arterioles such as this one had vasculitis. Interstitial edema and hemorrhage were also present. No cellular rejection is present. (Hematoxylin & eosin, ×250)

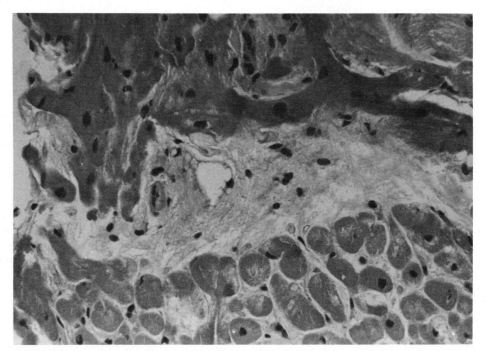

Figure 6–5. Moderate microvascular rejection was diagnosed on the basis of immunofluorescent findings of vascular localization of immunoglobulin and complement with fibrin accumulation (see Figure 6–6). Histologically, the biopsy shows only diffuse, severe interstitial edema and endothelial activation. (From Hammond EH, Hansen J, Spencer LS, et al. Vascular rejection in cardiac transplantation: Histologic, immunopathologic, and ultrastructural features. Cardiovasc Pathol 2:21, 1993. Copyright 1993 by Elsevier Science Publishing Co., Inc.)

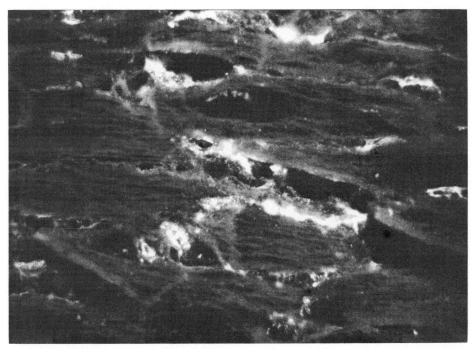

Figure 6–6. Immunofluorescent findings in moderate vascular rejection. Capillaries showed co-localized IgG and C3. The IgG is shown here. Antithrombin III was not found on arterioles or venules, a pattern 3 distribution consistent with moderate vascular rejection. (× 250) (From Hammond EH, Hansen J, Spencer LS, et al. Vascular rejection in cardiac transplantation: Histologic, immunopathologic, and ultrastructural features. Cardiovasc Pathol 2:21, 1993. Copyright 1993 by Elsevier Science Publishing Co., Inc.)

ciated with hemodynamic compromise clinically[15, 25] (Figs. 6–7 and 6–8). Immunofluorescence is extremely helpful in this setting because the light microscopy may merely show interstitial edema without evidence of vasculitis. Such biopsies may show piecemeal myocyte necrosis or subendocardial infarction, either of which is evidence that larger vessels, not included in the biopsy, may have vascular compromise. This is particularly true in the early months post-transplant, when it is very unlikely that the process could be related to epicardial coronary vasculopathy. As mentioned in Chapter 5, myocyte necrosis without inflammation, detected in the first few weeks post-transplant, may be caused by prolonged ischemic time or perisurgical hypoxia (Fig. 6–9). See Chapter 5, pages 74–75.

Severe Microvascular Rejection

Severe microvascular rejection is identical to severe cellular rejection and should be regarded as the end result of any severe rejection process. The endomyocardial biopsy shows a diffuse, mixed leukocytic infiltration, including neutrophils and eosinophils (Fig. 6–10). Myocyte necrosis and interstitial edema and hemorrhage may be prominent. Vasculitis is obvious. Immunocytochemically, biopsies with severe cellular/vascular rejection often will have vascular deposits of immunoglobulin and complement, as well as interstitial and vascular accumulation of fibrin. Complement components may also be distributed in the interstitium. Examination of such biopsies for ATT and tPA will show loss of these reactants (pattern 3).[15, 25] In addition, such vessels may paradoxically show lack of MHC class II expression owing to the prominent vascular injury that may be present in such biopsies. This can be highlighted by immunoperoxidase staining of such vessels with factor VIIIra.[16] In severe rejection, these vessels are ragged or frayed or may show missing endothelium[14, 16] (Fig. 6–11).

RELATIONSHIP OF MICROVASCULAR REJECTION TO ISHLT GRADING

The current ISHLT grading scheme for cardiac allograft rejection does not include provi-

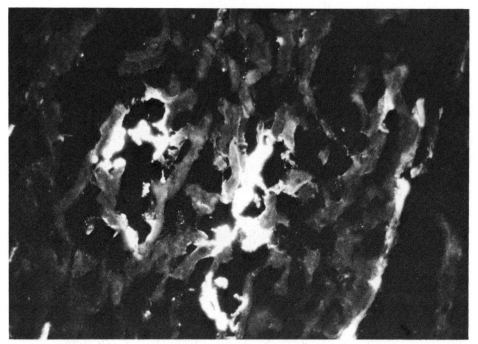

Figure 6–7. Fibrin localized by immunofluorescence. This is the same biopsy specimen as shown in Figure 6–6. (× 250)

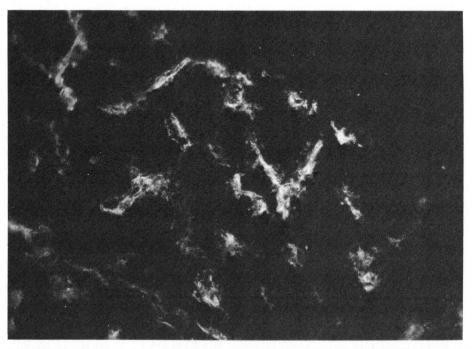

Figure 6–8. MHC class II antigen detected on microvasculature with anti–HLA-DR labeled with phycoerythrin. MHC class II was diffusely present (2+) on all microvessels. (× 250) (From Hammond EH, Hansen J, Spencer LS, et al. Vascular rejection in cardiac transplantation: Histologic, immunopathologic, and ultrastructural features. Cardiovasc Pathol 2:21, 1993. Copyright 1993 by Elsevier Science Publishing Co., Inc.)

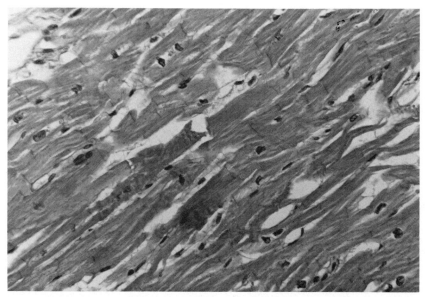

Figure 6–9. Biopsy specimen from a patient with persistent vascular rejection for several weeks, showing contraction band necrosis of myocytes without surrounding inflammation. (Hematoxylin & eosin, × 400)

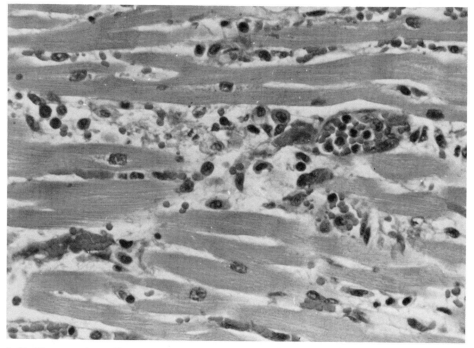

Figure 6–10. Biopsy specimen illustrating the histologic appearance of severe cellular and vascular rejection. Vasculitis, a mixed cellular infiltrate with myocyte necrosis, and prominent intercellular edema are seen. Immunofluorescence showed loss of antithrombin and extensive fibrin, immunoglobulin, and complement in vessel walls. (Hematoxylin & eosin, × 400)

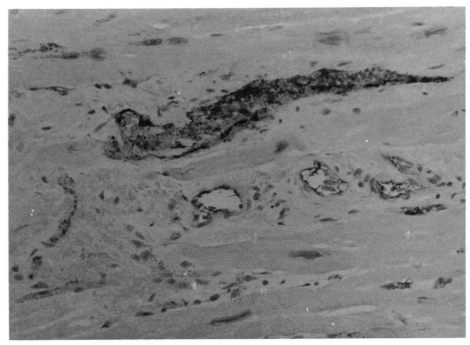

Figure 6–11. In this case of moderate microvascular rejection, vessels show ragged endothelial surfaces. (Factor VIIIra stained section. Immunoperoxidase method. Counterstained with hematoxylin. × 400)

sion for the aforementioned processes.[42] Since these microvascular rejection types have been found in up to 25 per cent of cardiac allografts, it will be important to revise ISHLT criteria to incorporate these findings. The relationship of the microvascular grades and the ISHLT grades was described in Table 6–1. The specific features of the ISHLT grading scheme are described and tabulated in Chapter 5, page 77.

CLASSIFICATION OF MIXED (CELLULAR AND VASCULAR) REJECTION

Mixed cellular and microvascular rejection may be seen in biopsy material and is independently graded but simultaneously demonstrated.[13, 14, 16] Independent grades of each process are assigned. The cellular grading criteria are shown in Table 6–3, along with the corresponding ISHLT grades. Vascular grades are assigned according to the criteria described in Table 6–1. Mixed rejection as defined in this chapter is not recognized in the ISHLT schema; such biopsies are called by

their cellular grade. Vasculitis is often ignored in the ISHLT schema except in severe rejection (grade 4), in which it is the rule[42] (Fig. 6–12).

Table 6–3. Comparison of UCTP and ISHLT Grades*

UCTP Cellular Rejection:	ISHLT Grades
Focal mild rejection:	ISHLT IA or 2, depending on damage
Mild rejection:	ISHLT 1B or 2, depending on presence of myocyte damage
Moderate rejection:	ISHLT 3A or 3B, depending on extent of myocyte damage and infiltrate
Severe rejection:	ISHLT 4, identical criteria

UCTP Vascular Rejection:	ISHLT Grades
Mild vascular rejection:	ISHLT 0
Moderate vascular rejection:	ISHLT 0
Severe vascular rejection:	ISHLT 4

UCTP Mixed Rejection:	All considered as corresponding ISHLT cellular grade. Simultaneous occurrence of various UCTP cellular and vascular grades as defined above.

*UCTP = UTAH Cardiac Transplant Program. ISHLT = International Society of Heart and Lung Transplantation.

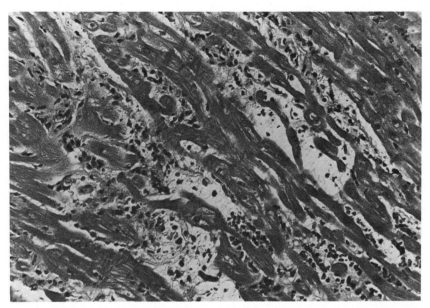

Figure 6–12. Histologic picture of moderate mixed rejection. Vasculitis and a space-occupying infiltrate of cells are seen associated with myocyte damage. (Hematoxylin & eosin, × 250)

DESIGNATION OF DOMINANT PATHOLOGIC REJECTION PATTERN

We have found it prognostically useful to designate patients according to their predominant form of histologic rejection.[13, 14, 16] Three separate clinical correlation evaluations of our patients have shown that these designations are prognostically important. Patients with vascular rejection have a significantly worse survival rate than patients with cellular or mixed rejection patterns, prospectively assigned in the first 3 months post-transplant (Fig. 6–13).[14, 16, 19] It is interesting that although patients with mixed rejection have a survival rate like that of the cellular rejection patients, they have a fourfold higher risk of developing allograft coronary artery disease; vascular rejection patients have an eight- to ninefold greater risk (Fig. 6–14). These risks are irrespective of the time post-transplantation.[14] Assignment of the rejection type of the patient is done in the following manner:

Cellular Rejection Patients

Cellular rejecting patients had only cellular rejection, as defined by the ISHLT criteria after July, 1990, and by the Utah criteria before that time.[42]

Vascular Rejection Patients

Vascular rejecting patients were those who developed features of vascular rejection defined immunocytochemically in the absence of any cellular rejection during the first 8 weeks post-transplant. Criteria for the grades of vascular rejection are summarized in Table 6–1,

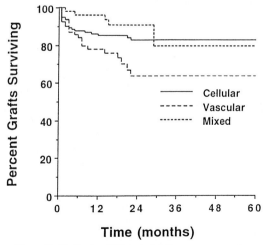

Figure 6–13. Kaplan-Meier graft failure curves are shown for each type of rejection group. Tarone-Ware test was significant (p = .027) only when OKT3-sensitized patients were included in the analysis. (From Hammond EH, Yowell RL, Price GD, et al. Vascular rejection and its relationship to allograft coronary artery disease. J Heart Transplant 11:S111, 1992.)

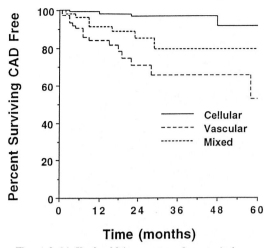

Figure 6–14. Kaplan-Meier coronary free survival curves are shown for each type of rejection group. Tarone-Ware test was significant among groups regardless of whether OKT3-sensitized patients were included. The proportional hazard regression model showed that patients with the vascular pattern (p = .0001), as well as those with the mixed pattern (p = .014), were significantly different from cellular pattern patients. (From Hammond EH, Yowell RL, Price GD, et al. Vascular rejection and its relationship to allograft coronary artery disease. J Heart Transplant 11:S111, 1992.)

including the corresponding ISHLT grade. These criteria now include evaluation of ATT and tPA, which further refine the criteria. At least three separate episodes of pure microvascular rejection (no simultaneous cellular rejection) had to occur for the patient to be considered a microvascular rejection patient. A few patients were classified as microvascular rejection based on constant vascular rejection for 4 or more weeks.

In a retrospective review of our data, we found that 25 of 268 prospectively followed patients had two episodes of mild microvascular rejection but no subsequent episodes of pure vascular rejection (unpublished data). In all other episodes, these patients had only cellular rejection. We therefore require three episodes in order to consider a patient as a pure vascular rejector. Now that the ATT and tPA findings are utilized, this requirement may change; Faulk and Labarrere have found that persistent loss of ATT and tPA are always associated with clinical instability of the allograft, a sign of significant microvascular damage.[15, 25] If immunoglobulin and complement are demonstrated in vessels without concomitant loss of ATT and tPA, it may be that these immune complexes are pathologically unimportant.

Mixed Rejection Patients

Independent grades of microvascular and cellular rejection have always been assigned. The grading criteria are shown in Table 6–3 along with the corresponding ISHLT grades. Patients were considered to be of the mixed rejection type if they had at least three episodes of simultaneous cellular and vascular rejection. In the aforementioned retrospective study, we found 40 of 268 patients who had two episodes of mild vascular rejection, after which they developed episodes of mixed rejection composed of cellular and vascular rejection. These patients were considered to be mixed rejectors for subsequent analysis (unpublished personal data).

ALLOGRAFT CORONARY ARTERY VASCULOPATHY (GLOBAL MYOCARDIAL ISCHEMIA)

In patients undergoing long-standing microvascular compromise or allograft coronary vasculopathy, a distinctive group of morphologic features is demonstrated on endomyocardial biopsy. Patients show focal areas of myocyte dropout in which myocytes are replaced by loose connective tissue. Surrounding myocytes are often hypertrophied. In these areas, focal inflammatory cells may remain. Capillaries are difficult to find, and no endothelial activation is present (Fig. 6–15).[14, 16, 43–45]

The patchy nature of this process and its subendocardial distribution suggest that the myocyte loss is due to generalized microvascular damage, which includes small arteries and arterioles outside the field of examination. This observation has been documented on autopsy and explant evaluation of such hearts.[14, 16] These changes have also been described in hearts showing allograft coronary vasculopathy[43–45] (see Chapter 7, page 111). If these changes are encountered on endomyocardial biopsy in patients with slowly worsening cardiac function, they are an ominous sign. Such patchy myocyte loss is distinctive from that loss usually associated with myocardial infarction in which large zones of myocyte necrosis are ultimately replaced by dense scarring. When we recognize this ischemic change at intervals after the first month post-transplant, we note it in our reports as evidence of ischemia. When these patients come to allograft replacement or autopsy, they usually

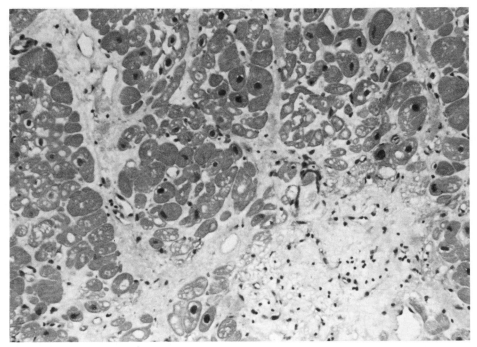

Figure 6–15. Histologic findings in a biopsy specimen with ischemic changes. Irregular areas of scarring surrounded by hypertrophied myocytes are seen. (Hematoxylin & eosin, × 250)

show uniformly narrowed coronary or epicardial arteries with or without inflammation in such vessels.[14, 16]

In immunocytochemistry studies, patients with global myocardial ischemia or allograft coronary vasculopathy usually show generalized increased MHC class II (HLA-DR) staining of microvasculature of endomyocardial biopsy (2 to 3+) in the absence of other pathologic evidence of acute rejection (see Figure 6–8).[14, 16] The immunocytochemical findings of microvascular immunoglobulin and complement components may be decreased from previous biopsies or may be totally absent. ATT is often absent in the microvasculature, and tPA is undetectable in smooth muscle. This pattern of ATT and tPA expression was detected in 7 of 11 hearts examined at autopsy in which global ischemic changes were the predominant cause of heart failure (personal unpublished observations). We have examined biopsy samples from several patients who lack microvascular damage but have coronary vasculopathy; ATT and tPA staining were not diminished. The amount of fibrin staining is often decreased over that of previous biopsies. We believe that these altered morphologic expressions in the microvasculature may be the results of attempted repair of chronic damage of the microvasculature. In

such patients, only the observation of serial biopsies plus a careful examination of the light microscopic findings will lead to the correct pathologic diagnosis of chronic global ischemia. Other immunopathologic features with presumed pathogenic significance are described in Chapter 7 by Dr. Marboe, page 122.

Ultrastructural observations of biopsy specimens from patients with histologic evidence of chronic damage of large and small blood vessels have shown changes analogous to those found in ischemic hearts of experimental animals; these hearts show a prominent loss of actin over myosin in myofilament bundles that are intact, giving a coarse appearance to the myofilaments (Fig. 6–16).[16, 46] In addition, large numbers of myocyte cytoplasmic organelles are scattered around in the interstitium, associated with a patchy and haphazard collection of collagen fibrils. The vessels usually have irregular profiles and may show irregular endothelial cell swelling (see Figure 6–16).[16, 46]

DRUG-INDUCED VASCULAR PROCESSES SIMULATING VASCULAR REJECTION

In patients treated with antibodies raised in various animal species such as horses, rabbits,

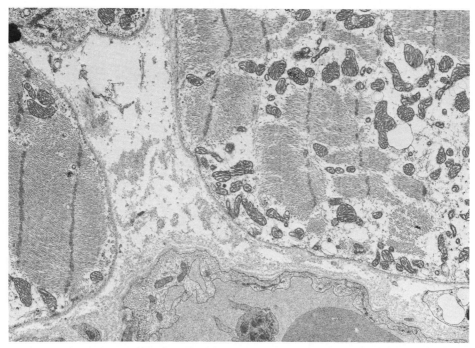

Figure 6–16. Ultrastructural appearance of myocytes and microvasculature from a biopsy specimen showing histologic evidence of ischemia. The myofilament structure appears coarse, owing to the predominant loss of actin filaments. The basal lamina around the capillary is reduplicated, and the vessel profile is irregular. ($\times$ 6250)

sheep, or mice, an immune complex–mediated response to these foreign proteins may develop.[47–49] In patients who develop these reactions, the immunosuppressive function of the monoclonal antibody is abrogated by the production of antibodies against the immunosuppressive agent. Such patients may show early rejection because of lack of immunosuppression.[50] Alternatively, they may show a serum sickness–like process within their cardiac vessels, related to the deposition of immune complexes of the monoclonal antibody and the host antibody directed against it. Usually these antibodies are anti-idiotypic antibodies directed against the foreign protein.[51]

In our institution, in which the great majority of patients have been treated with OKT3, a mouse monoclonal antibody, all patients are routinely evaluated by immunocytochemistry for the accumulation of mouse immunoglobulin (the antigen) in cardiac vessels.[52] Typically, the efficacy of OKT3 therapy is monitored by following total daily T lymphocyte counts or, in the case of OKT3, CD3 lymphocyte counts. This method is an insensitive way to detect early anti-idiotypic antibody accumulation; a better method is the flow cytometric assay described by Wittwer and colleagues, which detects declines in steady state plasma levels of

the OKT3 1 to 3 days earlier than the return of CD3-positive cells.[53] The value of early detection is that the patient can be immediately withdrawn from OKT3 therapy and placed on alternative immunosuppression.

We have demonstrated that maintaining the patient on OKT3 in the presence of anti-idiotypic antibodies leads to humorally mediated microvascular alterations in every case.[52] Since this is associated with severe hemodynamic consequences, it should be avoided. A subsequent study, in which therapy was promptly aborted in patients sensitized to OKT3, has led to dramatic improvement in allograft survival.[54] Eleven of twelve patients shown to be sensitized and removed from therapy at the time of sensitization have not lost their allografts. In this study, patients without sensitization during induction treatment with OKT3 did not develop sensitization if retreatment was necessary. This is another situation in which routine immunocytochemical monitoring is very helpful in understanding the nature of the immunologic response.

Morphologically, such heart biopsies are identical to those found in vascular rejection patients. The only different feature is the presence of mouse, horse, or rabbit immunoglobulin in a distribution identical to the human immunoglobulin and complement components, which serves to distinguish this process from vascular rejection. There are no direct data concerning the distribution of altered ATT and tPA expression in these patients. Fibrin was found in an interstitial and vascular distribution in all of them; in view of the fibrin deposition, ATT would be expected to be missing from the microvasculature.[15]

PATHOGENESIS OF MICROVASCULAR REJECTION

The changes described in this chapter suggest that endothelial cell activation, permeability, and subsequent myocyte degeneration are prominent features in patients displaying light microscopic and immunocytochemical alterations associated with microvascular rejection. These morphologic features suggest that the endothelial cell plays an important role in this rejection process. In-depth investigations of endothelial cell biology have shown that rather than being nonspecific targets of injury, endothelial cells are capable of many important functions that can be altered in the allograft.[35–38]

Endothelial cells provide a natural anticoagulated surface through their binding of ATT-III and thrombomodulin, although the evidence in cardiac transplants suggests that the former pathway is more important than the latter.[15, 25] Endothelial cells produce diverse cytokines that can modulate the biologic behavior of cells in the myocardial tissue. These cytokines are produced in inflammation, ischemia, and many other circumstances commonly operative in transplantation, such as infection and lymphocyte activation.[35–38] There is good evidence that endothelial activation can be the result of immunosuppression or immunoprophylaxis utilizing monoclonal anti–T cell antibodies. The therapy can generate T cell activation, as a result of interaction of the antibody and the CD3 or T cell receptor antigen on the lymphocyte surface.[33, 34, 50] Recent reports suggest that such lymphocyte activation leads to increased release of IL-2 and interferon-gamma, which promotes further endothelial cell activation, as has been elegantly shown by the in vitro studies of Pober and colleagues.[35–38]

We have observed that the morphologic pattern of vascular rejection includes patients sensitized to OKT3 while undergoing immunoprophylaxis. This type of vascular rejection is related to humoral immune responses with probable altered B lymphocyte immune regulation or polyclonal B lymphocytic activation.[52, 54] The morphologic changes are very similar to those described in reports detailing humorally mediated vascular rejection in renal transplant recipients, patients with serum sickness, and experimental animals with leukocytoclastic vasculitis, or the Arthus phenomenon.[48, 49, 55–57]

The pathogenetic mechanisms responsible for these vascular inflammatory processes (in which an antigen-antibody complex process is definitely implicated) involve complement activation, cytokine release and chemotaxis, and activation of neutrophils and macrophages.[57–59] The pathogenesis of the vasculitis and deposition of immune complexes demonstrated in vascular rejection and allograft coronary artery vasculopathy is unclear. Although the pathogenesis could result from humoral immune mechanisms to defined or undefined transplantation antigens, the possibility that this process is caused by delayed hypersensitivity and enhanced vascular permeability related to cytokine release cannot be differentiated by the present or previous studies.[58, 60–64] We have consistently seen upregulation of HLA-DR on the large and small vessels of the allograft, which, at least in experimental situations, is produced exclusively by interaction of endothelial cells with interferon-gamma.[58] This finding, as well as the prominent fibrin deposition and endothelial activation, suggests that delayed-type hypersensitivity may be implicated in this process.[10, 65]

The consequence of either a humoral or cellular immune response directed against the vascular endothelium would be compromised myocardial oxygenation. Important inflammatory participants in this process include neutrophils and macrophages that can be activated by complement components, endotoxin, and platelet-activating factor.[66–68] Such activation can result in the production of various leukotrienes, arachidonic acid metabolites, and a variety of cytokines that lead to vascular permeability, leukocyte adherence via various specifically induced adhesion molecules, and the activation of proteolytic enzymes such as protein kinase C.[28–31, 33, 50] The ability of endothelial cells to express adhesion molecules (ELAM, ICAM, VLAM) in response to inflammatory stimuli or cytokine release such as IL-1 can create the morphologic expression of vascular rejection, including endothelial activation and capillaritis. Furthermore, complement components are similarly capable of inducing expression of such adhesive molecules, which can lead to the adherence and migration of polymorphonuclear leukocytes through vessels, with consequent destruction of adjacent cells such as myocytes by the above-described mechanisms.[30, 31, 35, 60, 61]

Thus it appears likely that the manifestations of vascular rejection, as well as severe rejection, represent the consequences of endothelial cell activation, secretion of cytokines, increased endothelial cell adherence of leukocytes, migration of such leukocytes, and ischemic damage to the myocardium.

The long-term consequence of long-standing or intermittent vascular rejection, if it does not lead to acute allograft loss or demise of the patient, appears in our studies to be allograft coronary artery disease in most patients.[14] In a previous prospective study, we have shown a significant and independent correlation with the vascular and mixed patterns of rejection diagnosed in the early post-transplant period and the subsequent development of chronic allograft vasculopathy.[14, 16] The light microscopic and immunofluorescent findings that allow patient stratification into these patterns of rejection are therefore important to recognize, because they may lead to allograft loss in a slow and insidious way that is largely untreatable.[14, 16]

REFERENCES

1. Jeannet M, Pinn V, Flax M, Winn HJ, Russell PS. Humoral antibodies in renal allotransplantation in man. N Engl J Med 282:111, 1970.
2. Farnsworth A, Hall BM, Ng ABP, et al. Renal biopsy morphology in renal transplantation. Am J Surg Pathol 8:243, 1984.
3. Salmela KT, von Willebrand EO, Kyllonen LEJ. Acute vascular rejection in renal transplantation; Diagnosis and outcome. Transplantation 54:858, 1992.
4. Herskowitz A, Soule LM, Ueda K, Tamura F, Baumgartner WA, Borton AM, Reitz BA, Achuff SC, Traill TA, Baughman KL. Arteriolar vasculitis on endomyocardial biopsy: A histologic predictor of poor outcome in cyclosporine-treated heart transplant recipients. J Heart Transplant 6:127, 1987.
5. Smith SH, Kirklin JK, Geer JC, Caulfield JB, McGiffin DC. Arteritis and cardiac rejection after transplantation. Am J Cardiol 59:1171, 1987.
6. Butcher EC. The regulation of lymphocyte traffic. Curr Top Microbiol Immunol 128:85, 1986.
7. Berg EL, Goldstein LA, Jutila MA, et al. Homing receptors and vascular addressins: Cell adhesion molecules that direct lymphocyte migration. Immunol Rev 108:5, 1989.
8. Forbes RDC, Guttman RD, Gomersall M, Hibberd J. A controlled serial ultrastructural tracer study of first set cardiac allograft rejection in the rat. Am J Pathol 111:184, 1983.
9. Leszcynski D, Laszcyska M, Halttunen J, Hayry P. Renal target structures in acute allograft rejection: A histochemical study. Kidney Int 31:1311, 1987.
10. Dvorak HF, Mihm MC, Dvorak AM, et al. Rejection of first set skin allografts in man: The microvasculature is the critical target of the immune response. J Exp Med 150:322, 1979.
11. Snover DC, Freese DK, Sharp HL, et al. Liver allograft rejection: An analysis of the use of biopsy in determining outcome of rejection. Am J Surg Pathol 11:1, 1987.
12. Stewart S. Pathology of lung transplantation. Semin Diagn Pathol 9:210, 1992.
13. Hammond EH, Yowell RL, Nunoda S, et al. Vascular (humoral) rejection in heart transplantation: Pathologic observations and clinical implications. J Heart Transplant 8:430, 1989.
14. Hammond EH, Yowell RL, Price GD, et al. Vascular rejection and its relationship to allograft coronary artery disease. J Heart Transplant 11:S111, 1992.
15. Faulk WP, Labarrere CA, Pitts, D, Halbrook H. Laboratory-clinical correlates of time associated lesions in the vascular immunopathology of human cardiac allografts. J Heart Lung Transplant 12:S125, 1993.
16. Hammond EH, Hansen J, Spencer LS, et al. Vascular rejection in cardiac transplantation: Histologic, immunopathologic, and ultrastructural features. Cardiovasc Pathol 2:21, 1993.
17. Woodley SL, Renlund DG, O'Connell JB, Bristow MR. Immunosuppression following cardiac transplantation. J Heart Transplant 8:83, 1990.
18. Renlund DG, O'Connell JB, Gilbert EM. A prospective comparison of murine monoclonal CD-3 (OKT3) antibody-based and equine antithymocyte globulin-based rejection prophylaxis in cardiac transplantation. Transplantation 47:599, 1989.
19. Ensley RD, Hammond EH, Renlund DG, et al. Clinical manifestations of vascular rejection in cardiac transplantation. Transplant Proc 23:1130, 1991.
20. Marboe CC, Schierman SW, Rose E, et al. Characterization of mononuclear cell infiltrates in human cardiac allografts. Transplant Proc 16:1598, 1984.
21. Colvin RB. Diagnostic use in transplantation; Clinical applications of monoclonal antibodies in renal allograft biopsies. Am J Kidney Dis 11:2, 1988.
22. Bishop AG, Hall BM, Duggin GG, Horvath JS, Sheil AG, Tiller DJ. Immunopathology of renal allograft rejection analyzed with monoclonal antibodies to mononuclear cell markers. Kidney Int 29:708, 1986.
23. Bishop GA, Waugh JA, Landers DV, et al. Microvascular destruction in renal transplant rejection. Transplantation 48:408, 1989.
24. Hayry P, Renkonen R, Leszcynski D, et al. Local events in graft rejection. Transplant Proc 21:3716, 1989.
25. Labarrere CA, Pitts D, Halbrook H, Faulk WP. Natural anticoagulant pathways in normal and transplanted human hearts. J Heart Transplant 11:342, 1992.
26. Hammond EH, Hansen LK, Spencer LS, et al. Immunofluorescence of endomyocardial biopsy specimens: Methods and interpretation. J Heart Lung Transplant 12:S113, 1993.
27. Sell KW, Talaat T, Wang YC, et al. Studies of major histocompatibility complex class I/II expression on sequential human heart biopsy specimens after transplantation. J Heart Transplant 7:407, 1988.

28. Wijngaard PLJ, Tuijnman WB, Meyling FHJ, et al. Endomyocardial biopsies after heart transplantation. The presence of markers indicative of activation. Transplantation 55:103, 1993.
29. Gassel AM, Hansmann ML, Radzun HJ, Weyland M. Human cardiac allograft rejection. Correlation of grading with expression of different monocyte/macrophage markers. Am J Clin Pathol 94:274, 1990.
30. Briscoe DM, Schoen FJ, Rice GE, et al. Induced expression of endothelial-leukocyte adhesion molecules in human cardiac allografts. Transplantation 51:537, 1991.
31. Sadahiro M, McDonald TO, Allen MD. Reduction in cellular and vascular rejection by blocking leukocyte adhesion molecule receptors. Am J Pathol 142:675, 1993.
32. Rand JH, Wu XX, Potter BJ, et al. Co-localization of von Willebrand factor and type VI collagen in human vascular subendothelium. Am J Pathol 142:843, 1993.
33. Breisblatt WM, Schulman DS, Stein K, et al. Hemodynamic response to OKT3 in orthotopic heart transplant recipients: Evidence of reversible myocardial dysfunction. J Heart Lung Transplant 10:359, 1991.
34. Abramowicz D, Schandene L, Goldman M, et al. Release of tumor necrosis factor, interleukin-2, and gamma-interferon in serum after injection of OKT3 monoclonal antibody in kidney transplant recipients. Transplantation 47:606, 1989.
35. Cotran RS. New roles for the endothelium in inflammation and immunity. Am J Pathol 129:407, 1987.
36. Cotran RS, Pober JS, Gimbrone MA, Springer TA, Wiebke EA, Gaspari AA, Rosenberg SA, Lotze MT. Endothelial activation during interleukin-2 immunotherapy: A possible mechanism for the vascular leak syndrome. J Immunol 139:1883, 1987.
37. Pober JS. Cytokine-mediated activation of vascular endothelium. Am J Pathol 133:426, 1988.
38. Pober JS, Collins T, Gimbrone MA, et al. Inducible expression of class II major histocompatibility complex antigens and the immunogenicity of vascular endothelium. Transplantation 41:141, 1986.
39. Miller LW, Wesp A, Jennison SH, et al. Vascular rejection in heart transplant recipients. J Heart Lung Transplant 12:S147, 1993.
40. Heroux AL, Costanzo-Nordin MR, Radvany R, et al. The enigma of acute allograft dysfunction without cellular rejection: Role of humoral alloimmunity. J Heart Lung Transplant 12:S91, 1993.
41. Carlquist JF, Hammond ME, Yowell RL, et al. Correlation between class II antigen (DR) expression and interleukin-2–induced lymphocyte proliferation during acute cardiac allograft rejection. Transplantation 50:582, 1990.
42. Billingham ME, Cary NRB, Hammond ME, et al. A working formulation for the standardization of nomenclature in the diagnosis of heart and lung rejection: Heart Rejection Study Group. J Heart Transplant 9:587, 1990.
43. Rowan RA, Billingham ME. Pathologic changes in the long-term transplanted heart: A morphometric study of myocardial hypertrophy, vascularity and fibrosis. Hum Pathol 21:768, 1990.
44. Billingham ME. Histopathology of graft coronary disease. J Heart Lung Transplant 11:S38, 1992.
45. Neish AS, Loh E, Schoen FJ. Myocardial changes in cardiac transplant–associated coronary arteriosclerosis: Potential for timely diagnosis. J Am Coll Cardiol 19:586, 1992.
46. Hammond EH, Yowell RL. Ultrastructural findings in cardiac transplant recipients. Ultrastruct Pathol 18:203, 1993.
47. Vaughan JH, Barnett EV, Leadley PJ. Serum sickness: Evidence in man of antigen-antibody complexes and free light chains in the circulation during the acute reaction. Ann Intern Med 67:596, 1967.
48. Lawley TJ, Bielory L, Gascon P. A prospective clinical and immunologic analysis of patients with serum sickness. N Engl J Med 311:1407, 1984.
49. Andres G, Brentjens JR, Caldwell PRB, et al. Biology of disease: Formation of immune deposits and disease. Lab Invest 55:510, 1986.
50. Suthanthiran M, Fotino M, Riggio RR, et al. OKT3-associated adverse reactions: Mechanistic basis and therapeutic options. Am J Kidney Dis 14:39, 1989.
51. Jaffers GJ, Fuller TC, Cosimi B, et al. Monoclonal antibody therapy: Anti-idiotypic and non anti-idiotypic antibodies to OKT3 arising despite intense immunosuppression. Transplantation 41:572, 1986.
52. Hammond EH, Wittwer CT, Greenwood J, et al. Relationship of OKT3 sensitization and vascular rejection in cardiac transplant patients receiving OKT3 rejection prophylaxis. Transplantation 50:776, 1990.
53. Wittwer CT, Knape WA, Bristow MR, Gilbert EM, Renlund DG, O'Connell JB, DeWitt CW. Quantitative flow cytometric plasma OKT3 assay: Potential application in cardiac transplantation. Transplantation 48:533, 1989.
54. Hammond E, Yowell R, Greenwood J, et al. Monitoring of patients for OKT3 sensitization prevents adverse outcome. Transplantation 55:1061, 1993.
55. Talbot D, Given AL, Shenton BK, et al. Rapid detection of low levels of donor-specific IgG by flow cytometry in renal transplantation. J Immunol Methods 112:279, 1988.
56. Brasile L, et al. Clinical significance of the vascular endothelial cell antigen system/evidence for genetic linkage between the endothelial cell antigen system and the major histocompatibility complex. Transplant Proc 17:6, 2318, 1985.
57. Hugli TE. Complement and cellular triggering reactions: Introductory remarks. Minisymposium presented by the American Association of Immunologists at the 67th Annual Meeting of the Federation of American Societies for Experimental Biology, Chicago. FASEB J 43:2540, 1983.
58. Pober JS, Cotran RS. The role of endothelial cells in inflammation. Transplantation 50:537, 1990.
59. Cines DB, Lyss AP, Bina M, Corkey R, Kefalides NA, Friedman HA. Fc and C3 receptors induced by herpes simplex virus on cultured human endothelial cells. J Clin Invest 69:123, 1982.
60. Yasuda M, Takeuchi K, Hiruma M, Iida H, Tahara A, Itagane H, Toda I, Akioka K, Teragaki M, Hisao O, Yoshiharu K, Takeda T, Kolb WP, Tamerius JD. Complement system in ischemic heart disease. Circulation 81:156, 1990.
61. Mannik M. Mechanisms of tissue deposition of immune complexes. J Rheumatol 13:35, 1987.
62. Miltenburg AM, et al. Induction of antibody-dependent cellular cytotoxicity against endothelial cells by renal transplantation. Transplantation 48:681, 1989.
63. Oluwole SF, Tezuka K, Wasfie T, Stegall MD, Reemtsma K, Hardy MA. Humoral immunity in allograft rejection. Transplantation 48:751, 1989.

64. Martin S, Morris D, Dyer PA, et al. Association between cytomegalovirus specific antibody, lymphocytotoxic antibody, HLA-DR phenotype and graft outcome in renal transplant recipients. Transplantation 51:1303, 1991.

65. Dvorak HF, Galli SJ, Dvorak AM. Cellular and vascular manifestations of cell-mediated immunity. Hum Pathol 17:122, 1986.

66. Mason DW, Morris PJ. Effector mechanisms in allograft rejection. Annu Rev Immunol 4:119, 1986.

67. Hall BM. Cellular infiltrates in allografts. Transplant Proc 19:50, 1987.

68. Braquet P, Hosford D, Braquet M, et al. Role of cytokines and platelet activating factor in microvascular immune injury. Int Arch Allergy Appl Immunol 88:88, 1989.

Chapter

7

CARDIAC TRANSPLANT VASCULOPATHY

Charles C. Marboe, MD

INCIDENCE

Methods for Diagnosis

The development of vascular lesions in the grafted organ is the leading cause of graft failure and patient death more than 1 year after cardiac transplantation.[1] The frequency of this complication of transplantation depends on the time post-transplant, the method used to assess the vessels, and the diagnostic criteria for significant vessel disease. Histopathologic studies have been the most sensitive way to assess coronary disease, and direct comparison with prior coronary angiography has shown that the latter technique severely underestimates the extent and severity of vasculopathy.[2] The prevalence of vascular lesions of epicardial coronary arteries has been described histologically as 95 per cent, with concentric fibrointimal thickening by 1 year and universal thickening after 1 year. Eighty per cent of epicardial coronary arteries also show foam cell lesions or mixed fibrointimal and foam cell lesions.[3] Angiographic studies have shown an incidence of coronary arterial disease in 10 to 20 per cent of patients per year[4] and significant disease in 19 to 36 per cent of cardiac transplants at 1 year, increasing to 45 per cent at 3 years and 50 per cent at 5 to 7 years following transplantation.[5–7] The application of intravascular ultrasound imaging to the coronary arteries has provided qualitative descriptions and quantitative measurements of vessel wall morphology and luminal dimensions. This technique can provide extremely sensitive

evaluation of the early stages of intimal hyperplasia in these vessels and will make possible the study of therapies directed at slowing or preventing arteriopathy.[8, 9]

Noninvasive tests, such as stress electrocardiography, ambulatory electrocardiographic (ECG) monitoring, planar stress thallium scintigraphy, or oral persantine stress thallium SPECT scintigraphy, which are sensitive and specific for detecting silent or symptomatic atherosclerotic coronary artery disease, have shown low sensitivity for detecting allograft vasculopathy. Newer techniques using the technetium-based myocardial perfusion tracers sestamibi and teboraxime in combination with new imaging approaches like tomographic perfusion scintigraphy or high count rate cameras may provide useful information on myocardial perfusion.[10] The assessment of perfusion as well as measures of myocardial function will be critical in the study of patients whose arteriopathy primarily compromises small vessels that are inaccessible to the intravascular ultrasound catheter.

The endomyocardial biopsy is not a sensitive means of directly demonstrating vasculopathy since the involved vessels are generally too large to be present in the biopsy tissue. Proliferative arteriolar occlusion has been noted on endomyocardial biopsies and can predate arteriographically detectable large vessel disease.[11] Arteriolar vasculitis in an endomyocardial biopsy has also been associated with progressive cardiac rejection and poor outcome.[12] Histopathologic changes may, however, be present in the biopsy tissue to predict

111

vasculopathy or a poor outcome. The most extensively described lesion is "humoral rejection," defined as linear deposits of immunoglobulin and complement in capillaries in endomyocardial biopsy specimens.[13] This pathologic finding, and its clinical correlates, are discussed in Chapter 6.

Histologic alterations, reflecting the effect of vessel lesions on myocardial perfusion, have been described in myocytes. These include (1) subendothelial myocyte vacuolation ("myocytolysis"), which is a potentially reversible change indicating severe chronic ischemia;[14] (2) interleukin-6 expression in myocytes as a response to hypoxia and reoxygenation;[15] (3) lipid accumulation in myocytes, reflecting ischemia-induced alterations in fatty acid metabolism in myocytes; (4) focal coagulation necrosis, which heals in an altered and delayed time course due to immunosuppressive therapy; and (5) healing granulation tissue and scar resulting from repair following myocardial infarction. This last lesion may be impossible to distinguish from a focus of healed cellular rejection, as the areas of myocyte damage can be small, reflecting small vessel involvement. When the lesion is a broad patch or band of healing that spares the immediate subendocardium, it may be more readily recognized as ischemic in origin.

Clinical Manifestations

The clinical presentation of cardiac transplant vasculopathy is insidious, with nonspecific complaints of fatigue or cough. Congestive heart failure, silent myocardial infarction on the electrocardiogram, or ventricular arrhythmia and sudden death may be presenting signs. Acute myocardial infarction in heart transplant recipients is generally unaccompanied by chest pain,[16] but most centers with a large number of long-term survivors have experience with rare patients with typical anginal pain. Recent experience at the University of Michigan has demonstrated that variable sympathetic reinnervation, as determined by norepinephrine release in response to tyramine, occurs in no patient within 5 months of transplantation but in 78 per cent of patients more than 1 year after transplantation.[17, 18] Sensory function is thus more likely in long-term survivors; the effect of reinnervation on coronary artery tone is being studied.[19]

IMMUNOPATHOLOGY

Lymphocytes and Macrophages

Whereas the initial studies of transplant vasculopathy in the early post-operative period in renal grafts focused on the presence of immunoglobulin deposits in the affected vessels, T lymphocytes have subsequently been identified in the vessel lesions in allografted kidneys,[20] livers,[21] and hearts.[22, 23] In the vessels of transplanted hearts, lymphocytes initially accumulate beneath the endothelium but are also found deeply within thicker intimal lesions as well as in the media.

The presence of mononuclear cells in vessels of grafts is now widely recognized, but the phenotypes of the infiltrating cells and their relationship to the development of the vasculopathy is the subject of current debate. The intimal lesions contain predominantly T lymphocytes and macrophages, primarily in a zone immediately beneath the endothelium; variable numbers of smooth muscle cells are found deeper in the lesions, adjacent to the media. B lymphocytes are not present in significant numbers. The ratios of CD4+ to CD8+ T lymphocytes in the lesions have varied widely. One study finds a ratio of approximately 1, in grafts from 4.5 to 46 months after transplant; three of these seven hearts also showed acute cellular rejection.[23] Another group found predominantly CD8+ cells and very few CD4+ cells in a single graft, with a survival of 55 months and very severe vasculopathy.[22] In the intima of grafts in place for more than 3 months, our group has found an average CD4/CD8 ratio of approximately 1.6.[24] It is of note that we found the average CD4/CD8 ratio in the intima of vessels in grafts surviving less than 3 months to be 0.67.

An explanation for the different CD4/CD8 ratios in early and late transplant vasculopathy lesions is that the CD4/CD8 ratio of less than 1 in the short-term (less than 3 months) survivors reflects a state of acute cellular rejection. We have previously shown that the CD4/CD8 ratio in the myocardium is less than 1 in acute cellular rejection.[25] Six of our short-term survivors showed some acute rejection in the myocardium. In this regard it is interesting that we have found that the CD4/CD8 ratio in the myocardium mirrors the ratio in the intima of epicardial arteries. In the short-term survivors (less than 3 months), the CD4/CD8 ratio in the vascular intima was 0.67 and in the myocardium it was 0.70. In our group of longer-surviving grafts (4.5 to 57 months), the CD4/CD8 ratio was greater than 1.0 in the vascular intima in 10 of 11 cases (average value, 1.61) and in 8 of 11 cases in the myocardium (average value, 2.09).

The T lymphocytes present in the transplant lesions tend to be activated (HLA-DR+) and lie, with HLA-DR+ macrophages, subjacent to the HLA-DR+ endothelium.[23] This close association of lymphocytes with endothelial cells has also been seen in ultrastructural studies.[26] This proximity of activated CD8 and CD4 cells with activated endothelium is the basis of the suggestion that transplant vasculopathy may be the result of a chronic delayed-type hypersensitivity (DTH) reaction. Under normal circumstances, the inflammation in DTH subsides over days as the antigen is cleared from the site of contact or injection. In transplanted vessels, however, the antigenic stimulus (HLA-DR+ endothelial cells) persists. The persistent activation of endothelial cells could result from the recognition by CD8+ T lymphocytes of foreign MHC class I antigen found constitutively on the allogeneic endothelium; release of cytokines by these lymphocytes induces the endothelial expression of class II molecules. This HLA-DR expression by endothelial cells can activate CD4+ cells,[23] which typically mediate DTH. In some circumstances, CD8+ T lymphocytes may themselves mediate DTH.[27] This interpretation is consistent with our finding of CD8+ lymphocyte predominance in the early postoperative period and CD4+ predominance in later months following transplantation.

The cytokine cascade resulting from this activation of T lymphocytes could lead to stimulation of macrophages in the lesions to produce interleukin-1 (IL1), tumor necrosis factor (TNF), platelet-derived growth factor (PDGF), and transforming growth factor α.[28-30] These factors are stimulants to smooth muscle proliferation, and interleukin-1 and tumor necrosis factor will prompt interleukin-1 production by endothelial cells[31] and smooth muscle cells, amplifying the immune and inflammatory responses.

The role of macrophages in atherosclerosis and transplant vasculopathy is a complex one. The macrophage-derived foam cell is an early and prominent component of the atherosclerotic lesion, and macrophage products play important roles in the progression of the atherosclerotic lesion. However, the initial recruitment and accumulation of monocytes in the arterial wall most likely depends on factors from endothelial and smooth muscle cells.[reviewed in 32] The chemotactic factors that recruit monocytes to the intima include hyperlipidemia, factors from endothelial cells (oxidized low density lipoprotein—LDL), an interleukin-1–induced factor, other monocyte chemotactic factors, adhesion glycoproteins such as GP-90, GP-155, and GP-160, substances from smooth muscle cells (oxidized LDL, monocyte chemotactic protein-1), and factors from macrophages already present in the lesions (oxidized LDL).

Once present, macrophages take up lipid in the form of oxidized LDL via a scavenger receptor. This scavenger receptor is not downregulated and will continue to fill the cell with modified LDL, creating the typically plump foam cell. The continued expansion of the cell may eventually lead to its rupture, with the attendant release of oxidized LDL, free radicals, elastase, and collagenase. These latter factors can be cytotoxic or damaging to endothelium or contribute to the disruption and alteration of the atherosclerotic plaque. In addition, activated macrophages in the early lesions can secrete a mitogenic factor, a macrophage-derived growth factor (similar to PDGF) that can induce smooth muscle cell proliferation.[reviewed in 32, 161] Cytokines from T lymphocytes can also induce macrophages to secrete other mitogenic factors as already noted.

Endothelium

In addition to being HLA-DR+, the endothelium of grafted vessels also expresses vascular cell adhesion molecule-1 (VCAM-1) and intercellular adhesion molecule-1 (ICAM-1). In our experience, expression of all these molecules is weak within the first 3 weeks after transplantation and very strong thereafter. Both ICAM-1 and VCAM-1 are known to be expressed on vascular endothelial cells (VEC) after cytokine stimulation or at sites of inflammation, as is MHC class II.[33-35] ICAM-1 and VCAM-1 mediate lymphocyte adhesion to VEC and thereby play an important role in recruitment of lymphocytes to the site of inflammation. There is very little adhesion molecule expression on normal, nonactivated VEC. We have previously shown ICAM-1 to be upregulated during acute rejection in endomyocardial biopsies from human cardiac allografts.[36] Other studies have shown that VCAM-1 is also upregulated during acute rejection.[37, 38] After in vitro stimulation of VEC with cytokines, ICAM-1 and VCAM-1 are detectable after 2 to 6 hours and remain stable for 48 to 72 hours.[33] This might suggest that the adhesion molecules are part of a delayed hypersensitivity reaction in which the mononuclear cell infiltrate is present for about 72 hours.[39] Both ICAM-1 and VCAM-1 are also adhesion molecules for macrophages that are prominent in atherosclerotic plaques.

These adhesion molecules are also expressed in "typical" atherosclerosis. ICAM-1 is expressed on various cells in human atherosclerotic lesions;[40, 41] another study of a homolog to human VCAM-1 in a rabbit model found VCAM-1 expressed on endothelial cells overlying early atherosclerotic lesions.[42] This latter study suggests that VCAM-1 (entitled "athero-ELAM") in rabbits may play a role in the lymphocyte and monocyte recruitment and adhesion seen as one of the earliest events in atherosclerosis. ELAM-1 has been seen to be upregulated on endothelial cells in human atherosclerotic lesions, adjacent to subendothelial infiltrates of T lymphocytes and macrophages.[43]

One possible reason transplant vasculopathy in epicardial vessels may proceed apparently independently from cellular rejection extending from microvasculature and venules in the myocardium is the antigenic heterogeneity of vascular endothelium. One study has suggested that normal coronary artery endothelium, unlike other large vessels, constitutively expresses MHC class II and VCAM-1 molecules.[44] Capillary endothelium, including that of the myocardium, strongly expresses MHC class I and II molecules as well as ICAM-1 and the monocyte/endothelial marker OKM5. Except as noted earlier for coronary arteries, these molecules are weakly expressed or undetectable on large vessels. In contrast, large vessel endothelium strongly expresses von Willebrand factor and constitutively expresses ELAM-1.

The process by which leukocytes traverse the vascular endothelium to mount an inflammatory response to target tissues is multistep and combinatorial.[reviewed in 45] The endothelial side of the initial low-affinity rolling interaction is mediated by E-selectin (ELAM) and P-selectin (granule membrane protein of molecular weight 140 kD [GMP-140]; platelet activation-dependent granule external membrane protein [PADGEM]). In the second phase of the process, leukocyte activation is mediated by

concentration gradients of various chemotactic factors from endothelial cells and tissues, including interleukin-8–like molecules, the chemotactic fragment of complement protein C5, and leukotrienes. Finally, there is a high affinity adhesion with change in leukocyte shape and extravasation, which is mediated by the binding of β1, β2, and β7 integrins on leukocytes with ICAM-1, -2, and -3 and VCAM-1 on endothelial cells.

This complex, multifactorial process allows different combinations of mediators and interactions to induce different types of leukocyte subpopulations to migrate to a given type of tissue during various inflammatory processes.[reviewed in 46, 47] An additional factor in the ability of endothelium to induce varied responses to different stimuli is the ability of some of the "adhesion" molecules to serve as costimulatory signals to lymphocytes. These costimulatory signals are necessary to augment the T cell receptor/CD3 interaction with the peptide presented by MHC antigens to insure maximal T cell stimulation.[48] The absence of this second, costimulatory message may lead to anergy.[49] One such message is delivered by CD28 on endothelial cells to B7 on leukocytes[50] and is crucial to avoiding clonal anergy.

The importance of this interaction has been recently shown in experiments that block the interaction of B7 with CD28 and suppress T cell–dependent antibody responses[51] or provide tolerance to human pancreatic islet cell transplants into mice.[52] Similar blocking of CD28 in rats has prolonged the survival of heart allografts.[53] We have had preliminary success in delaying cardiac allograft rejection in the baboon (*Papio anubis*) with the administration of LFA3-TIP, a fusion protein composed of the first domain of LFA3 with human IgG1, to block the interaction of another costimulatory set of molecules: CD2 on lymphocytes and LFA3 on endothelial cells.[54, 55]

Smooth Muscle Cells

Smooth muscle cells are prominent in the intimal lesions of transplant vasculopathy. As noted earlier, multiple cytokines may stimulate smooth cell proliferation, including the cells' own production of IL-1.[56–61] One cytokine not mentioned earlier is basic fibroblast growth factor (bFGF), which has been identified as a factor in ordinary atherosclerosis and in some proliferations following injury.[62, 63] Whereas many monocytes and macrophages are sources of PDGF,[64] smooth muscle cells themselves are a reservoir for bFGF.[65] Preliminary studies of transplant vasculopathy have demonstrated PDGF and bFGF in lesions.[59, 66] Despite the presence of these factors, the rate of cell proliferation in transplant vasculopathy is less than 1 per cent of cells,[66] similar to the low rates seen in both ordinary human atherosclerosis and the hypercholesterolemic swine model of atherosclerosis (0 to 5 per cent range).[67, 68] Thus, while the stimuli for the predominance of smooth muscle cells in transplant vasculopathy are present, the apparent rate of cell proliferation does not reach that seen in vitro, nor is it significantly higher than that seen in the more slowly progressive lesions of ordinary atherosclerosis. Other controls on cell proliferation are apparently active in vivo. Indeed, the initial smooth muscle cell replication (following balloon injury) is not inhibited by antibodies to bFGF or PDGF.[62] It has been shown, however, that PDGF plays a role in the migration of smooth muscle cells into the endothelium.

We have found ICAM-1 expressed on spindle-shaped cells in the intimal lesions of transplants. These cells may be smooth muscle cells; other studies have shown ICAM-1 expressed on smooth muscle cells in atherosclerotic plaques.[40, 41] Similarly, we have found intimal smooth muscle cells to express MHC class II antigens. This expression has also been noted in atherosclerotic plaques but not in normal arteries.[69]

Immunoglobulin and Complement

The possible roles of humoral immunity in rejection and its association with transplant vasculopathy will be discussed in detail later. The direct role of immunoglobulin in endothelial cytotoxicity in coronary arteries has been difficult to establish. The presence of a diffuse mural staining for IgM accompanied by IgG and albumin, without the specific colocalization of complement, is usually interpreted as a nonspecific leakage across damaged endothelium. Although there have been a few reports of endothelial cell necrosis and denudation,[70, 71] the prominent change in transplant vasculopathy is an intimal proliferation.

Nonlytic damage to endothelial cells could certainly alter their anticoagulant and permeability characteristics.[72] Indeed, endothelial binding and degranulation of platelets have been seen in animal models of transplant vasculopathy,[73, 74] and thrombosis of vessels is seen in human allografts.[22] Nonlytic injury might also lead to changes in lipid uptake and transport across endothelium, as well as production and release of growth factors as noted earlier. Recent evidence suggests that binding of anti-HLA antibodies to human aortic endothelium can upregulate expression of ICAM-1 by the endothelium.[75] This is a potentially important mechanism to link alloantibody production to subsequent cellular rejection in vessels of cardiac transplants.

ANTIBODIES

Anti-HLA

The involvement of HLA antigens as a stimulus of cardiac allograft rejection is suggested by the inverse correlation between actuarial survival and the degree of HLA disparity between recipient and donor.[76] A correlation of the development, following transplantation, of cytotoxic anti-B cell antibodies and irreversible graft failure was another suggestion that anti-HLA antibodies might be present in chronic rejection.[77, 78] These initial documentations of cytotoxic antibodies in recipients' sera did not determine specificity of the antibodies for donor HLA antigens. Suciu-Foca's group has extended these studies to show, in heart allograft recipients, an actuarial survival at 4 years of 90 per cent in recipients who do not form anti-HLA antibodies and a survival of only 38 per cent in antibody producers.[79]

HLA antigens from the injured graft are released into the serum and can be found free or complexed with anti-HLA antibodies much more frequently in patients who subsequently died with graft failure than in patients with successful grafts more than 1 year after transplantation. If the soluble HLA antigens are depleted from the serum, anti-HLA antibodies become detectable in 53 per cent and 74 per cent of sera obtained in the first and second years post-transplantation, respectively, from patients suffering graft failure. Long-term survivors have a significantly lower frequency (16 per cent in the first year; 18 per cent in the second year) of anti-HLA antibodies in sera depleted of HLA antigens. Studies of anti-anti-HLA A2 and -A3 suggest that graft acceptance may be aided by the presence of anti-idiotypic antibodies, an observation also made in renal transplantation.[79-81] Patients who form anti-HLA antibodies in the first 6 months post-transplantation but cease antibody production have a better 3-year survival rate than do patients who produce antibodies throughout the first year post-transplantation (91 per cent versus 70 per cent). The time of antibody production in the first year is also correlated with differences in survival: patients forming antibody in the first 6 months have a poorer 4-year survival rate than do patients who form anti-HLA antibodies starting in the second half of the first year (69 per cent versus 91 per cent).

The relationship of anti-HLA antibody production to the development of graft coronary artery disease has been studied only in preliminary fashion, due to the lack of sensitive means of identifying vessel disease in vivo. Once such study used quantitative cinevideo-densitometry and defined coronary artery disease as either a discrete stenosis of more than 50 per cent or a diffuse tapering of vessels that was hemodynamically significant. With this definition, coronary artery disease was detected significantly more often in the first 2 years in anti-HLA antibody producers than in non-producers (12 of 66 angiograms versus 1 of 33).[82] More recently, intravascular ultrasound has been used to evaluate a small series of patients treated with photochemotherapy in addition to their standard immunosuppression (steroids, azathioprine, cyclosporine).[83] Patients treated with photochemotherapy were less likely to form anti-HLA antibody and were also less likely to develop intimal proliferation in the proximal left anterior descending coronary artery. This is another association of anti-HLA antibody production with graft vasculopathy, but no etiologic or pathogenetic link between the two events has been proved.

Vascular (Humoral) Rejection

A distinctive form of antibody-associated pathology in human heart allografts has been best described by Dr. Hammond and her colleagues in Utah.[13, 84, 85] Termed *vascular* (or *humoral*) *rejection*, this immunohistologic entity shows plump, swollen vascular endothelium and, rarely, vasculitis by light microscopic examination of the endomyocardium. The diagnostic immunofluorescent studies show linear deposits of immunoglobulin and complement in vessel walls (including capillaries). Cellular lymphoid infiltrates are generally absent when these vascular changes are detected. Patients whose biopsies show this pattern of vascular (humoral) rejection have clinical courses that are different from those of patients who exhibit only typical (cellular) rejection or whose biopsies may show either or both types of rejection (mixed). The vascular rejection pattern usually occurs in the first 4 to 6 weeks after transplantation and is associated with diminished actuarial survival at 5 years (62 per cent versus 83 per cent for cellular rejection or 80 per cent for mixed rejection).[13]

There has been concern that the use of OKT3 induction therapy or antithymocyte globulin (ATG) induction therapy might predispose to vascular rejection.[85] Proof of a causative relationship between OKT3 induction and vascular rejection has not been possible. No center has reported a concurrent trial of OKT3 induction therapy versus no induction therapy in which biopsy sections were also studied for vascular rejection. Non-simultaneous trials at one center or comparisons of trials between centers are difficult to interpret due to the frequent and multiple changes in post-transplant therapeutic regimen. Hammond and associates, however, have demonstrated that sensitization to OKT3 (shown as a decline in plasma OKT3 levels before the conclusion of therapy, associated with development of human antimouse antibody) is associated with the development of vascular rather than cellular rejection.[86] The high incidence of vascular rejection in this group was related to the use of a 21-day course of OKT3 rejection prophylaxis rather than the 14-day mode of treatment. A subsequent report by the Utah group shows 24 per cent of patients with vascular rejection to be OKT3-sensitized and 8 per cent and 0 per cent of mixed and cellular rejection patients, respectively, to be sensitized. When the sensitized patients are deleted from survival analysis, the times to graft failure changed slightly; survival differences between the patients based on type of rejection were no longer significant.[87]

We have corroborating evidence on the potential importance of sensitization to mouse immunoglobulin from our smaller study of anti-HLA antibodies and humoral rejection.[88] Seven of our patients received OKT3 induction therapy; 68 per cent of their biopsies showed vascular rejection, compared with 38 per cent of biopsies from nine patients not receiving OKT3. Thus, sensitization to mouse immunoglobulin is the factor predisposing to vascular rejection in some patients. This underscores the importance of different therapeutic regimens in determining the immunologic phenotype of rejection.

The clinical significance of vascular rejection must be considered in the care of heart allograft recipients. Vascular rejection is more often associated with hemodynamic compromise and lower echocardiographic fractional shortening than is cellular rejection.[85] Retreatment with antilymphocyte preparations (e.g., OKT3 or ATG) is required more often in humoral than in cellular rejection episodes and, as noted earlier, long-term survival is diminished. These factors suggest that the standard antirejection regimens are tailored to treat cellular rejection, and that the control of vascular rejection will require new therapies.

Vascular rejection is associated with a trend to a greater incidence of coronary arteriopathy as detected by angiogram. Actuarial survival free of vasculopathy (defined as more than 20 per cent luminal narrowing) at 60 months after transplant was significantly different for vascular versus cellular or mixed rejection.[86] The vasculopathy-free survival was 55 per cent in vascular rejection patients, 80 per cent in mixed rejection patients, and 95 per cent in cellular rejection patients. Among patients with vasculopathy, there is a trend to earlier development of lesions in those with vascular rejection (7.9 months versus 14.2 months).[85] When explanted and postmortem hearts are examined, all patients with vascular rejection (except those dying of acute vascular rejection in the first month post-transplant) show acute vascular rejection (immunofluorescence-positive), acute vasculitis, or chronic vasculopathy of epicardial or penetrating coronary arteries. Patients with cellular rejection show only extremely rare immunofluorescence positivity in these vessels and only rare acute vasculitis.[84] The presence of chronic vascular changes, it should be noted, is similar between cellular and vascular rejection groups.

The relationship of vascular (humoral) rejection to anti-HLA antibody production has been studied in only a very few patients.[87] There was no significant relationship between the presence of anti-HLA antibody in the serum and the simultaneous presence of linear immunoglobulin and complement deposits in myocardial capillaries. There are many possible explanations for the presence of tissue deposits of immunoglobulin and complement in the apparent absence of anti-HLA antibody in the plasma: formation of immune complexes of anti-HLA antibody with HLA antigens from the graft, inhibition of anti-HLA antibody by anti-idiotypic antibody, the complete clearance of antibody from the circulation into the extensive endothelial surface of the graft, sensitization by OKT3 mouse monoclonal antibody, and the presence of other antibodies directed against non-HLA antigens on endothelial cells. There is early evidence that some of these events do occur in human heart transplantation.[79] This study has shown that seemingly negative sera do in fact contain anti-HLA antibodies that escape detection because they are complexed with soluble antigens from the graft. The same study demonstrated that anti-HLA antibodies can also be complexed with anti-idiotypic antibodies, and that the presence of anti-idiotypic antibody has a strong correlation with graft survival. None of the 15 sera from five patients who rejected their grafts had anti-idiotypic antibody, whereas 17 of 26 sera from five patients with functional grafts had anti-idiotypic antibody. The complex relationship between shed histocompatibility antigens, anti-HLA antibody, and anti-idiotype antibody must be better defined, but it appears that the ability to develop anti-idiotypic antibody may greatly determine graft survival.

The relationship of humoral rejection to cellular rejection (diagnosed by cellular infiltrates and myocyte damage in biopsy tissue) is not well defined. Hammond and associates observed nine patients who showed linear deposits of immunoglobulin, complement, and fibrinogen in their biopsy material either prior to (seven patients) or concomitant with (two patients) the presence of cellular infiltrates of the "classic" type.[13] This observation suggests that humoral rejection may precede, or be simultaneous with, cellular rejection. These examples of a mixed immunofluorescence "vascular" pattern and cellular infiltrates occurred later after transplantation than in patients with a purely "vascular" rejection. Suciu-Foca and colleagues have also shown a strong statistical correlation between the biopsy diagnosis of acute cellular rejection and the presence of circulating anti-HLA antibody.[79] It is noteworthy that this association was even stronger for serum samples drawn in the 30 days prior to the biopsy than for serum from the 30 days after the biopsy. This suggests that humoral rejection may not be just a byproduct of graft damage or enhanced donor antigen expression in the wake of cellular rejection.

We have additional observations which suggest that anti-HLA antibodies precede, rather than result from, vascular rejection.[88] Twenty-seven biopsies demonstrating linear deposits of immunoglobulin were selected. None of the biopsies displayed cellular rejection. We found that 85 per cent of the biopsies were preceded by circulating anti-HLA antibody ($p = 0.194$), whereas only 77 per cent were followed by circulating antibody ($p = 44$). The same held true for 16 biopsies showing vascular rejection. In this instance, 94 per cent were preceded by a positive anti-HLA antibody test ($p = 0.077$), but only 81 per cent were followed by a positive test ($p = 0.303$). This suggests that humoral (vascular) rejection not only is capable of occurring independently of cellular rejection of the "classic" type but also is more likely to be preceded by circulating anti-HLA antibody.

Antiendothelial Cell Antibodies

The role of antibodies directed against endothelial cell antigens that are not HLA or ABO blood group antigens in the development of transplant vasculopathy has not been defined. Some of these vascular endothelial cell (VEC) antigens may also be expressed on peripheral blood monocytes, making prospective monocyte cross-matching possible.[89] Such testing shows a 7 per cent incidence of positive monocyte cross-matches with negative cross-matches by traditional techniques. It has been suggested this could explain much of the graft loss in renal transplants from HLA-identical, living related donors (loss is 10 to 15 per cent).[89–91] This VEC antigen system has been implicated in acute cardiac allograft dysfunction occurring in recipients with negative donor-specific lymphocyte cross-matches.[92] Its importance in chronic vasculopathy has not been determined.

Other approaches have more recently been employed to search for humoral responses to endothelium. A technique of SDS-PAGE and Western immunoblotting has been used to detect the presence and specificity of anti-endothelial cell antibodies.[93] Proteins from cultured human umbilical vein endothelial cells were probed with serum from transplant patients. Patients with angiographically detected coronary disease at 1 or 2 years after transplant were more likely to have antiendothelial antibodies than were patients without vessel disease. Of the antibody-positive patients, 75 per cent of the antibodies reacted with a doublet of polypeptides at 62 and 60 kDa, a size suggesting they are not products of the MHC. Future identification of these peptides may be useful for diagnostic and therapeutic purposes.

We have used a whole cell ELISA technique to screen heart transplant recipient's serum IgG for binding to human omental endothelial cells (matched to MHC of the patient's donor). Significantly increased levels of binding of IgG to endothelium were found to correlate with graft vasculopathy as determined by angiography, intravascular ultrasound, or autopsy.[94]

Panel-Reactive Antibodies

The panel-reactive antibody (PRA) analysis is a lymphocytotoxicity assay in which lymphocytes from randomly chosen individuals are exposed to the prospective recipient's serum. The antibodies causing cytotoxicity are presumed to be anti-HLA; unless the serum is depleted of IgM (usually by treatment with dithiothreitol—DTT), autoantibodies may be included. These autoantibodies are probably irrelevant to graft survival. If the PRA is positive (the "positive" value is set by each center—most centers use demonstrated cytotoxicity against more than 10 per cent of the random members of the panel), most centers require a donor-specific lymphocytotoxic cross-match (LCM). The importance of prior sensitization in determining renal graft survival and short-term cardiac graft survival has been noted.[95, 96] The relationship of PRA and LCM to long-term cardiac allograft survival is slowly emerging. At the Pittsburgh Center, the 5-year actuarial freedom from death (by all forms of rejection—hyperacute, acute, and graft atherosclerosis) was 85 per cent for patients with PRA of 0 to 10 per cent, 68 per cent for PRA of 11 to 25 per cent, and 68 per cent for PRA over 25 per cent ($p < 0.005$). A negative LCM does not reduce the risk of death by rejection in any of these groups.[97] A more recent study of the time to onset of angiographically determined epicardial coronary disease, and of the histologically determined luminal narrowing of epicardial coronaries in failed grafts, showed no significant difference in these end points for patients with PRAs of 0, 1 to 10 per cent, or greater than 10 per cent.[98] At the London and Harefield Centers, lymphocytotoxic antibody status does not have a significant effect on cardiac allograft survival at 2 years. A negative LCM does, however, predict a better survival at 2 years.[99] This is at variance with their experience in heart-lung recipients in whom there is a significant effect of a positive PRA but not of a positive LCM.

If there is an effect of PRA or LCM on graft survival, it would be expected to be mediated by vascular (humoral) rejection. The Utah group has reported the relationship of some clinical characteristics (age at transplant, pretransplant diagnosis, sex, LCM) to the type of rejection in individual patients. The strongest correlation was for 83 per cent of patients with a positive LCM to manifest vascular rejection, whereas only 26 per cent of patients with negative LCM showed vascular rejection. Women were also more likely to have vascular rejection than were men (43 per cent versus 26 per cent),[87] presumably reflecting sensitization during pregnancy.

CYTOMEGALOVIRUS INFECTION

Cytomegalovirus (CMV) infection in renal transplant recipients has been associated with an increased incidence of graft failure[100, 101] and recipient mortality.[102] An association with cardiac allograft rejection, patient survival, and vasculopathy has also been noted.[103–105] The incidence of angiographically defined vasculopathy has been reported as being higher in patients who have had CMV infection diagnosed by serology or culture,[106] although this experience has not been shared by all centers.[107] It has been suggested that persistent viremia for at least 4 months is the significant factor in determining the development of vasculopathy.[108]

There are multiple direct and indirect mechanisms through which CMV infection might promote vasculopathy in the cardiac allograft. Direct attack of endothelial cells with subsequent cell death and denudation of the basement membrane and exposure of the subendothelial collagen matrix could lead to platelet aggregation and incite events in Ross' "response to injury" hypothesis for atherosclerosis.[109] Nonlytic, nondenuding injury by latent CMV infection could alter endothelial cell anticoagulant properties,[110, 111] change the permeability of the endothelial cell barrier, promote leukocyte adhesion, or stimulate endothelial cell production of growth factors and cytokines.

Vascular smooth muscle cell infection by CMV could also accelerate transplant vasculopathy. The virus may induce the proliferation of smooth muscle cells either directly[112] or indirectly by cytokine secretion acting on endothelial cells.[113] Herpesviruses have been shown capable of stimulating lipid accumulation in smooth muscle cells.[114, 115]

Cytomegalovirus infection has been associated with increased expression of MHC class II antigens on renal endothelial and tubular cells[116] and on T lymphocytes[117] following renal transplantation. This viral infection has also been associated with the induction of MHC class II antigens on bile duct epithelium and hepatocytes and rarely on vascular endothelium in human hepatic allografts.[118] Human aortic smooth muscle cells can be induced to regulate MHC class I antigen expression by CMV infection.[113] This upregulation of MHC expression is apparently mediated by soluble factors, most likely interferon-gamma from activated T lymphocytes, since CMV infection of vascular endothelium in vitro, in the absence of interferon-gamma, does not induce MHC class II antigen expression.[119] The increased expression of MHC antigens may stimulate the process of allograft rejection and vasculopathy.

The recognition that human CMV and the HLA-DRβ chain show sequence homology and immunologic cross-reactivity[120] allows speculation that a patient's appropriate response to CMV infection will also cross-react with MHC class II antigen of the allograft. Presumably, cross-reacting antibodies will bind to allograft vessels and stimulate or potentiate cell-mediated rejection. One additional factor that must be considered in the linking of CMV with vascular disease is organ tropism. Murine CMV isolates from one mouse organ replicate preferentially in endothelial cells from that same organ.[121] Different susceptibilities of endothelium in different organs may determine the pathogenicity of certain strains of CMV and the distribution of vascular and parenchymal lesions.

Although it is not clear which of these potential mechanisms links CMV infection with allograft rejection, extensive clinical experience recognizes the correlation of the two events. A patient who has been previously free of rejection develops CMV infection and shortly thereafter suffers a first rejection episode. At the same time, vasculopathy may have been initiated.

The possibility that viruses may cause or may be a cofactor in the pathogenesis of atherosclerosis is not of recent derivation. Some athero-sclerotic lesions may be induced in chickens with herpesviruses,[114, 115, 122] and herpes simplex virus DNA has been demonstrated in human aortic tissue by in situ hybridization.[123] There is now a statistical association of CMV infection with transplant vasculopathy: CMV DNA has been demonstrated in coronary arteries of transplanted hearts by in situ hybridization[124] and CMV antigens similarly have been dem-onstrated in transplanted hearts.[125–127] These associations do not, however, establish CMV infection as a cause of atherosclerosis or trans-plant vasculopathy. Indeed, a high percentage (55 per cent) of aortas and femoral arteries from normal individuals appear to contain CMV nucleic acids in atherosclerotic and non-atherosclerotic segments.[128, 129] By polymerase chain reaction (PCR), the percentage of CMV nucleic acid positive vessels is higher in athero-sclerotic patients than in patients with virtually normal vessels (90 per cent versus 53 per cent).[130]

Additional support for an association of CMV with transplant vasculopathy could come from a trial of CMV prophylaxis, as with DHPG (dihydroxyphenylglycerol), in an attempt to modify the rate of graft rejection and vasculop-athy. A trial of vaccination of renal transplant recipients with a Towne live virus vaccine has shown a significant reduction of graft loss, but the effect on graft pathology was not de-tailed.[131] Further trials of antiviral prophylaxis or therapy in cardiac allografts will help define the role of CMV in cardiac rejection and vas-culopathy.

OTHER FACTORS

HLA Mismatch

Histocompatibility antigen matching, as well as negative T cell cross-match and low PRA level, are associated with increased renal allo-graft survival.[132] Some studies of cardiac allo-graft survival have not shown an effect of HLA mismatching on patient survival,[133–135] while others have shown an association of HLA-DR mismatches with more frequent and more se-vere rejection episodes[136–138] and decreased survival.[76, 139, 140]

Studies of the relationship of HLA incom-patibility and the development of vasculopathy have generated extremely varied results. Some studies have shown a higher incidence of HLA

incompatibility, particularly HLA-DR, among patients who develop vasculopathy than in those who do not,[6, 141] while other studies[142, 143] have not found this difference. One of the latter studies,[143] in fact, found that patients with two HLA-A matches were more likely to develop vasculopathy than were recipients with one or no match. This finding is reminiscent of the observation in liver transplant recipients that the incidence of vanishing bile duct syn-drome is higher in patients with more HLA-A matches.[144] The presumed explanation is that HLA-A matching promotes the interaction of antigen-presenting cells and graft target cells with the host's effector cells.

The analysis of this relationship of HLA incompatibility with vasculopathy has been hampered by the relatively small number of heart transplants, the continuous refinement of serologic reagents that makes interpretation of historical data depend too much on as-sumptions and speculations, the existence of minor histocompatibility systems that are not assayed, variability of immunosuppressive regi-mens over time, and multiple other host fac-tors that affect graft acceptance and suscepti-bility to infection. For these reasons, we will not have enough reliable data to determine the relationship of HLA incompatibility and vasculopathy until studies are performed util-izing standardized methods of DNA typing of histocompatibility antigens and standardized immunosuppressive therapy in large multicen-ter trials.

Cellular Rejection Episodes

The presence of angiographically deter-mined vasculopathy has been associated with a history of cellular rejection episodes in some centers[6, 98, 142, 145] but not in others.[5, 77, 87] The association between the two events does not identify a causal relationship. The Utah expe-rience in the study of "vascular" rejection in the myocardium, as well as our experience with anti-HLA antibodies, suggests that vascu-lar (humoral) rejection is capable of occurring independently of cellular rejection. Vasculop-athy and cellular rejection are different mani-festations of immunologic response to the al-lograft; each may be augmented by additional factors (histocompatibility, CMV infection, hy-perlipidemia), and the variable presence of these factors may determine which form of re-jection predominates in an individual patient.

Hyperlipidemia

Of the nonimmunologic factors that are associated with, and may predispose to, vasculopathy, the most frequently described is hyperlipidemia. Most reports have shown hypercholesterolemia, hypertriglyceridemia, and increased low density lipoproteins to develop in the first 1.5 years after heart transplantation.[146] High density lipoprotein (HDL) alterations are more variable; some centers have reported increased or unchanged HDL,[146] whereas in one report, three patients showed decreased HDL.[147] Most studies suggest a relationship between hypercholesterolemia and vasculopathy; only about half the studies of hypertriglyceridemia and vasculopathy have found a direct relationship.

The pathophysiology of post-transplant hyperlipidemia is complex and multifactorial. Among the contributing factors are obesity,[148] prednisone,[147, 149, 150] and cyclosporine.[151, 152]

It is most likely that, in the development of transplant vasculopathy, hyperlipidemia is an important cofactor to immunologic events. Animal studies have shown the synergy of immunologic injury with high-fat or high-cholesterol diets in producing vascular lesions in graft coronary arteries.[94, 153–155] A similar interaction of cytotoxic anti-B cell antibodies with hypercholesterolemia has been suggested in human heart transplant recipients.[77]

Recipient Age

Of six studies of the relationship of recipient's age to the development of transplant vasculopathy, three showed no association.[146] One study showed an increased incidence of vasculopathy in patients under 20 years of age.[156] The largest study found an increased incidence of vasculopathy in recipients over 50 years of age but increased graft loss from coronary disease in patients younger than 30 or older than 40 years.[157] In a recent abstract, patients with vasculopathy diagnosed late (more than 2 years after transplant) were older than patients in whom no vasculopathy was seen.[158]

These studies require careful pathologic study of the lesions to attempt to distinguish transplant vasculopathy from "usual" atherosclerosis. This distinction is also crucial in considering the heart from the older donor. Could the lesion be progression of prior usual atherosclerosis that was present in the heart at the time of transplantation?

Donor Age

In light of the shortage of organ donors, many centers are hoping to extend their formal or informal age limits for donors. The methods of evaluation of donor hearts for preexisting atherosclerosis vary between centers, and the degree of "acceptable" atherosclerotic coronary disease and the actual amount of coronary disease present in the donor hearts certainly varies between centers. One center has reported an increased risk of vasculopathy developing in hearts from donors over 40 years of age compared with donors younger than 40 years.[157] Other studies have found no relationship of vasculopathy with donor age.[146]

Sex of Donor and Recipient

One study has looked at the effect of sex mismatch between donor and recipient.[157] Compared with transplants between donor and recipient of the same sex, female recipients of a male donor heart had a relative risk of 1.56 of graft loss from transplant vasculopathy, whereas a male recipient of a female donor heart had a relative risk of 3.33.

Recipient's Pretransplant Heart Disease

The largest study to address this question showed a relative risk of developing vasculopathy of 2.71 for recipients with ischemic heart disease, compared with recipients with other cardiomyopathies.[157] Other studies have shown only a trend to more frequent development of vasculopathy in patients with ischemic disease,[147] or no difference,[6] or a diminished frequency of vasculopathy[158] compared with patients whose own heart showed idiopathic cardiomyopathy.

Immunosuppressive Therapy

Immunosuppressive regimens developed to better control acute cellular rejection also might have reduced the incidence of vasculopathy. This has not been the case. No decrease in vasculopathy has been seen with triple therapy (azathioprine, prednisone, cyclosporine) versus double therapy (azathioprine, prednisone),[158] or with the use of cyclosporine and prednisone versus azathioprine and prednisone.[5] No decrease in vasculopathy has been seen in association with higher doses of prednisone[159] or cyclosporine.[148] The failure of better inhibition of cellular immunity and acute cellular rejection to diminish transplant vasculopathy also suggests different mechanisms for the two processes.

Coagulation Factors

One change in endothelial cells that occurs apparently independently of cellular infiltrates is vascular disease associated with deposits of fibrin. In addition to their barrier, vascular tone, and immunologic functions, endothelial cells show a balance of procoagulant and anticoagulant properties that does not depend solely on immunologic mechanisms.[160, 161] Some of these properties have been studied in human cardiac allografts.

Hemostatic pathways have been preliminarily investigated by staining for fibrin on microvascular endothelium. Fibrin deposits are not seen in stable grafts but are present in and around vessels of rejecting allografts.[162] The presence of these deposits is not strictly associated with cellular infiltrates, but biopsies of grafts with cellular infiltrates often contain fibrin deposits. Although tissue factor–containing cells are rarely seen in normal or transplanted hearts, the experience in renal allografts shows a loss of tissue factor from glomeruli in rejecting allografts.

There is additional information to show that hemostasis is impaired after heart transplantation, with a net increase in procoagulant activity.[163] Compared with age-matched healthy controls or age-matched patients with ischemic heart disease, heart transplant recipients have increased levels of fibrinogen, factor VIIC, and von Willebrand factor antigen. Heart transplant recipients with graft vasculopathy tend to have higher levels of all coagulation factors, with a significant difference for factor IX. These recipients with vasculopathy did not have significantly different values for fibrinolytic factors or naturally occurring inhibitor values from recipients without graft vasculopathy. However, heart transplant recipients as a group have increased antithrombin III and protein kC activity compared with normal controls (but not compared with ischemic heart

disease patients). The increase in plasma antithrombin III may be a post-transplant phenomenon related to immunosuppressives. The euglobulin clot lysis time (ECLT) test is a global test of fibrinolytic activity and is prolonged in patients with ischemic heart disease and those patients transplanted for ischemic heart disease. This prolongation in the ECLT is in spite of increased levels of tPA, suggesting that the decreased fibrinolytic activity is due to the increased levels of total plasminogen activator inhibitor also reported in these persons.[163]

Fibrinolytic pathways, as represented by tissue plasminogen activator, are depleted from arteriolar smooth muscle cells in cellular, vascular, and mixed forms of rejection.[164] Urokinase is not present in detectable amounts in human hearts. In dysfunctional kidney allografts, urokinase is progressively depleted from proximal tubular epithelial cells.

Anticoagulant pathways are also altered in situ in rejecting cardiac allografts. Thrombomodulin is uniformly distributed on cardiac endothelium. It appears to be sensitive to the presence of macrophages and is diminished in capillary endothelium in biopsies of allografts with vasculopathy.[162] Antithrombin III is normally present in the heart on the endothelial cells of medium-sized veins, and its presence appears to be less sensitive (than is the presence of thrombomodulin) to soluble factors from macrophages. This venous anticoagulant pathway is progressively depleted during rejection. Antibodies to antithrombin III also react with smooth muscle cells of small arterioles in normal hearts and in the intima and media of arteries with transplant vasculopathy.

The exact relationship of these alterations in coagulant activity in vascular endothelium to the development of transplant vasculopathy is not certain. Some grafts include lesions with thrombi. If the alterations in microvascular endothelium of biopsy specimens are predictors of epicardial vasculopathy, it will provide a useful diagnostic tool. Similarly, the study of plasma fibrinogen level as a possible predictor of vasculopathy might provide useful information. Fibrinogen levels are independent predictors of cardiovascular disease death among men who have not received transplants.[165] The mechanisms by which cytokines can influence endothelial cell coagulant properties have been studied; the possibility that antiendothelial cell or anti-HLA antibodies can induce similar changes needs additional study. Thus, the immune response with the release of cytokines and the effects of immunosuppressive therapy with cyclosporine and prednisone act together to create a procoagulant environment on the endothelial cells of the graft. With coexisting hyperlipidemia and cellular and humoral immune attack on the endothelium, there are multiple factors for the initiation and progression of atheromas.

Vascular Tone

Endothelium can profoundly affect vascular tone by releasing relaxing factors, such as prostacyclin and nitric oxide (EDRF, endothelium-derived relaxing factor), and constriction factors, such as endothelin-1.[61, 166, 167] These relaxing factors also inhibit platelet deposition. Damage to the endothelium could cause increases in vasoconstrictors or loss of vasodilators. There is evidence that arteries with typical atherosclerosis have elevated vascular tone and a paradoxic vasoconstrictor response to acetylcholine.[168] A similar endothelial dysfunction has been seen in coronary arteries of heart transplant patients.[169, 170] Local secretion of EDRF also appears diminished in typical atherosclerosis in human coronary arteries.

Vascular tone may also be influenced by factors previously discussed as growth factors that promote the intimal lesions of vasculopathy. Platelet-derived growth factor and epidermal growth factor also have vasoconstrictor properties.[171] Growth factors and vasoactive agents share common intracellular signaling pathways,[172, 173] which most likely accounts for these shared functions. This intracellular cross-talk is therefore the probable explanation for the observation that vasoconstrictors (such as endothelin, angiotensin II, norepinephrine) stimulate vascular smooth muscle growth in vitro,[174, 175] and that vasodilators (EDRF, prostaglandins) inhibit smooth muscle growth.[176–178] This interrelationship of vascular tone with cell proliferation provides the rationale for including agents that alter vascular tone and promote the release of vasodilators in the treatment or prevention of transplant vasculopathy.

TREATMENT

The apparent multifactorial etiology of vasculopathy and the many factors suspected to contribute to its pathogenesis can suggest a variety of potential therapeutic interventions. Unfortunately, no trial has yet had an adequate number of patients with sufficient follow-up to demonstrate benefit from any one agent.

Coronary artery bypass grafting is not useful in typical transplant vasculopathy due to the diffuse involvement of large and small vessels. The results of percutaneous transluminal coronary angioplasty will be discussed later. In the absence of a proven prophylaxis or treatment (other than retransplantation), most centers make efforts to have patients control hyperlipidemia[179] and not smoke cigarettes; some centers have tried to decrease or eliminate prednisone. Lovastatin, a 3-hydroxy-3-methylglutaryl-coenzyme A reductase inhibitor, has been used to manage hypercholesterolemia after transplantation.[180] Although rhabdomyolysis and acute renal failure have been reported in transplant recipients receiving lovastatin,[181] the drug seems to be safe and effective therapy in low doses and with careful monitoring of drug levels.

With the severe shortage of donor organs and up to 30 per cent of transplant candidates dying before an initial graft can be procured, candidates with an expected survival substantially below that of the "ideal" candidate have been denied transplantation. Some centers, in light of the generally poor outcome of repeat transplantation, have decided not to retransplant. This is an extremely difficult decision when emotional bonds have formed between the patient, the family, and the transplant team and all have invested considerable time and effort in the patient's care.

The failure of traditional methods of dealing with coronary disease has underlined the need to find new therapies for transplant vasculopathy. Some of the old and newer approaches will be reviewed.

Retransplantation

The results of retransplantation have been disappointing, with 1-year survival rates of only 40 per cent to 75 per cent. A recent review of 449 second allografts reported to the registry of the International Society for Heart and Lung Transplantation and of 125 repeat transplants recorded in a multicenter database has shown 1-year survival rates of 48 per cent and 60 per cent, respectively.[182] Much of the mortality (15 per cent) is very early and apparently related to surgical complications and the added risk to patients on mechanical assist devices. There is little difference in survival rates once patients reach 6 months after retransplantation. The incidence of rejection, infection, and coronary vasculopathy is not different between primary and secondary allograft recipients. Recipients of a second graft are more likely to have major surgical complications, to have a higher level of sensitization to MHC antigens, to have a positive donor-specific cross-match, and to develop nonskin malignancies. The best predictors of survival after repeat transplantation are longer interval between transplants, coronary vasculopathy as a cause of graft loss, and lack of preoperative mechanical assistance. Unfortunately, even the ideal candidate for repeat allografting has an expected survival rate significantly less than that anticipated for a recipient's initial graft.

Percutaneous Transluminal Coronary Angioplasty (PTCA)

Palliative therapy for vasculopathy using PTCA has been tried at many centers. The experience of 11 centers (with treatment of 95 lesions in 35 patients) has been reported, with two thirds of patients having no adverse outcome (death, retransplant, myocardial infarct) in the first year after the procedure.[183] These results, in a selected group of transplant patients, are similar to those of routine angioplasty. Restenosis may occur more frequently (50 per cent at median 6-month follow-up) than with angioplasty in nontransplant patients. The ability of angioplasty to prolong allograft survival seems unlikely, given the diffuse nature of transplant vasculopathy, but remains to be tested in a prospective trial.

Calcium Channel Blockers

As noted earlier, vasoconstrictors have growth-promoting effects while vasodilators appear to inhibit vascular smooth muscle growth. The signal transduction pathways regulating cell contraction and cell growth seem to be shared, and the common mediator appears to be the modulation of intracellular calcium and calcium-dependent kinases. Studies in several types of animal models, particularly cholesterol-fed rabbits, have shown that calcium competitors, calcium chelators, anticalci-

fying agents, and calcium channel blockers can inhibit the progression of atherosclerotic lesions.[184, 185] The dihydropyridine calcium channel blockers appear to be more potent antiatherosclerotic agents than other classes of calcium channel antagonists.[186] This action of calcium channel blockers may involve not only the inhibition of smooth muscle growth but also the amelioration of hypercholesterolemia-induced dysfunction and inhibition of lipid accumulation by inhibiting the transcription of hydroxymethylglutaryl-coA (HMG-coA) reductase.[187] This latter effect would interfere with the action of PDGF, which stimulates transcription of the genes for the LDL receptor and HMG-coA.[188] There is the additional suggestion that smooth muscle cell migration, as well as proliferation, in vessel walls may be inhibited by some calcium channel blockers. Calcium channel blockers may also act to block immunologic responses in ways that are not necessarily the result of calcium channel inhibition.[189]

With this experimental background, trials in typical atherosclerosis have been initiated, with one study (INTACT) demonstrating a decrease in the appearance of new, angiographically defined coronary artery disease in patients treated with the vasodilator nifedipine.[190] Another study showed no influence of nicardipine on the overall rate of progression or regression of coronary lesions, but it did inhibit the progression of minimal lesions (stenosis less than 20 per cent).[187] Thus, initial evidence from these two studies suggests that calcium channel blockers may slow the progression of early atherosclerotic lesions but do not influence the evolution of established coronary atherosclerosis. A retrospective review by the Virginia group suggests that calcium antagonists may retard the development of graft vasculopathy.[191] Preliminary evidence from the Stanford group suggests that the calcium channel blocker diltiazem can attenuate the progression of vasculopathy, as assessed by angiography at 1 and 2 years after transplantation.[192]

Angiopeptin

Angiopeptin is a somatostatin analog that is a cyclic octapeptide with antiproliferative effects against several tumor cell lines as well as against vascular smooth muscle cells. In a rabbit heart transplant model, it inhibits myointimal proliferation, and in the FK506 rat heart allograft model, it reduces vasculopathy.[193, 194] A multicenter trial of angiopeptin to prevent restenosis after coronary angioplasty has been initiated. Preliminary results indicate that subcutaneous injections of angiopeptin significantly decrease restenosis following PTCA compared with placebo treatment.[195] Studies are in progress in Germany to assess efficacy in preventing transplant vasculopathy.

Heparin

Heparin has immunosuppressive and antiproliferative properties independent from its anticoagulant function. It blocks smooth muscle proliferation, retards cell migration, and alters the extracellular matrix made by the cell.[196] It is possible that these effects can be augmented by combining heparin with a vasodilator with additional antiproliferative effects.[197]

Photochemotherapy

Photochemotherapy involves the reinfusion of autologous lymphocytes following treatment with 8-methoxypsoralen and ultraviolet A light. This treatment renders the lymphocytes incapable of division but appears to stabilize their surface membrane and allows them to recirculate in the patient, inducing a host autoregulatory T cell response.[198] Our preliminary results from a clinical trial of the addition of monthly photochemotherapy to standard triple drug therapy suggest that photochemotherapy results in the early return of anti-HLA antibodies to baseline levels and reduces coronary artery intimal thickening, as assessed by intravascular ultrasound or histologic examination.[83] The treatment is well tolerated and does not increase the morbidity of triple drug immunosuppression. This trial continues, and additional trials in cardiac and renal transplantation are planned.

Antiplatelet Agents

Antiplatelet agents, including aspirin and dipyridamole, are used routinely in the postoperative care of most transplant patients despite the absence of a controlled clinical trial demonstrating the ability of these agents to reduce the incidence or progression of transplant vas-

culopathy. An early uncontrolled clinical trial[199] and the ability of dipyridamole in combination with cyclosporine to prevent vasculopathy in a rat allograft model[200] form the rationale for the use of these agents. It has been observed that platelets of heart transplant recipients exhibit a marked hyperaggregation in response to adenosine diphosphate when compared with platelets of nontransplanted controls.[201] These platelets from transplant recipients also appear to be resistant to the inhibitory effects of aspirin. The use of other approaches to modify the interaction between platelets and endothelium[202] will depend on a better understanding of the role of platelets in transplant vasculopathy.

SUMMARY

Cardiac transplant vasculopathy is a stark reflection of the multiple factors that initiate and promote atherosclerotic coronary artery lesions. Transplant vasculopathy is distinguished from nontransplant atherosclerosis by its accelerated course, its diffuse distribution through the vascular bed, and the frequency of its appearance in children. These features are reminders of the importance of immunologic responses to the graft in the pathogenesis of the lesion.

The initiating factor in the process is not obvious. It could be a "typical" risk factor, such as hypercholesterolemia promoting macrophage attachment to vascular endothelium, or the hypertension which so frequently accompanies cyclosporine therapy. It is possible that immunologic factors are just powerful promoters of the process, becoming important only after some nonimmunologic damage. This seems unlikely, however, in light of the statistical associations of vasculopathy with HLA mismatch, anti-HLA antibody and "vascular"-type rejection, and the failure of the vasculopathy to occur in the native heart when a heterotopic transplant is placed. The potential importance of immunologic factors in the creation of vasculopathy was indeed shown in the early 1970s by Laden[153] and Minick and associates[74, 154] before this process was seen to be the major contributor to late mortality in human cardiac allografts.

The primary mediator of the immunologic damage that engenders, or promotes, graft vasculopathy is also not defined. In most models, allograft rejection is primarily mediated by cellular, rather than humoral, factors. Our observations on infiltrating lymphocytes in the epicardial vessels of grafts are consistent with a delayed-type hypersensitivity reaction, as noted. Persistent immunologic attack on the vessel wall leads to a transmural inflammation; the process is not limited to the intima as is more frequently the case in "usual" atherosclerosis. The general assumption has been that cell-mediated damage to the graft microvascular endothelium promotes increased expression of HLA antigens and releases free HLA and endothelial cell antigens into the serum, promoting an antibody response. It may not be necessary for the amount of cellular infiltrate and damage to reach the severity of a biopsy-diagnosed or clinically diagnosed cellular rejection episode. There is not a good correlation at all centers between the number of cellular rejection episodes and the subsequent development of antigraft antibody or graft vasculopathy. There are also instances when antibody appears prior to a known rejection episode. The importance of humoral immunity is underscored by the observation that improved therapies for the prevention and treatment of cellular rejection have not led to any real decline in the incidence of transplant vasculopathy.

Once antibodies are formed, they react with HLA or other endothelial antigens that are not necessarily uniformly distributed on the coronary vascular bed. This reaction may be complement fixing and directly cytolytic, may direct cell-mediated cytotoxicity, or may alter endothelial cell function to increase antigen expression, promote the release of various cytokines, or alter endothelial permeability or transport of lipids or other molecules.

Additional damage to the vascular endothelium and vessel wall can be the result of cytomegalovirus infection. This may be by direct viral cytotoxicity, or it may be indirect by the virus' upregulation of HLA antigen expression on cells of the graft or by its stimulation of antibodies that cross-react with the HLA-DRβ chain.

The "risk" factors that promote "typical" atherosclerosis work synergistically with the immunologic or infectious damage to the vessel wall. Some of these factors, such as hypertension, hypercholesterolemia, glucocorticoid-induced metabolic changes, and coagulation abnormalities, are prominent among heart transplant recipients. As noted earlier, these factors collaborate with oxidation of LDL and release of multiple cytokines from the endo-

thelium and smooth muscle cells, as well as macrophages, to cause the progression of the intimal lesion. In transplant vasculopathy, this process is augmented by the release of cytokines from infiltrating cells bent on cellular rejection; their promotion of this vasculopathy can be a byproduct of their initial role in graft rejection. Cytokines from the atherosclerotic process as well as from the rejection process stimulate the ingrowth and proliferation of smooth muscle cells in these intimal lesions; CMV can stimulate smooth muscle proliferation directly or through cytokine action and may also stimulate lipid accumulation by smooth muscle cells.

Cardiac transplant vasculopathy is a manifestation of allograft rejection, influenced by the pathogenetic factors that cause atherosclerosis. The challenge is to identify the factor in the immune response that is the most powerful inciting agent for this form of rejection. If this factor is indeed an antibody, new treatments to control humoral immunity are clearly necessary. In the meantime, continued dissection of the immune response and factors that promote "typical" atherosclerosis will suggest multiple new ways to slow the progression of these vascular lesions. Advances in the understanding of the pathologic process in these cardiac vessels will not only carry over to other vascularized organ grafts but also will provide insights into the roles of inflammatory cells and cytokines in other vascular and immunologic disorders.

REFERENCES

1. Jamieson SW, Oyer PE, Baldwin J, et al. Heart transplantation for end-stage ischemic heart disease: The Stanford experience. Heart Transplant 3:224, 1984.
2. Dressler FA, Miller LW. Necropsy versus angiography: How accurate is angiography? J Heart Lung Transplant 11:S56, 1992.
3. Johnson DE, Gao SZ, Schroeder JS, et al. The spectrum of coronary artery pathology in human cardiac allografts. J Heart Transplant 8:349, 1989.
4. O'Neill BJ, Pflugfelder PW, Singh NR, et al. Frequency of angiographic detection and quantitative assessment of coronary arterial disease one and three years after cardiac transplantation. Am J Cardiol 63:1221, 1989.
5. Gao SZ, Schroeder JS, Alderman EL, et al. Prevalence of accelerated coronary artery disease in heart transplant survivors: Comparison of cyclosporine and azathioprine regimens. Circulation 80:III-100, 1989.
6. Uretsky BF, Murali S, Reddy PS, et al. Development of coronary artery disease in cardiac transplant patients receiving immunosuppressive therapy with cyclosporine and prednisone. Circulation 76:827, 1987.

7. Pascoe EA, Barnhart GR, Carter WH Jr., et al. The prevalence of cardiac allograft arteriosclerosis. Transplantation 44:838, 1987.

8. St. Goar FG, Pinto FJ, Alderman EL, et al. Intravascular ultrasound imaging of angiographically normal coronary arteries: An in vivo comparison with quantitation angiography. J Am Coll Cardiol 18:952, 1991.

9. Valentine H, Pinto FJ, St. Goar FG, et al. Intracoronary ultrasound imaging in heart transplant recipients: The Stanford experience. J Heart Lung Transplant 11:S60, 1992.

10. Rodney RA, Johnson LL. Myocardial perfusion scintigraphy to assess heart transplant vasculopathy. J Heart Lung Transplant 11:S74, 1992.

11. Palmer DC, Tsai CC, Roodman ST, et al. Heart graft arteriosclerosis: An ominous finding on endomyocardial biopsy. Transplantation 39:385, 1985.

12. Herskowitz A, Soule LM, Ueda K, et al. Arteriolar vasculitis on endomyocardial biopsy: A histologic predictor of poor outcome in cyclosporin treated heart transplant recipients. J Heart Transplant 6:127, 1987.

13. Hammond EH, Yowell RL, Nunoda S, et al. Vascular (humoral) rejection in heart transplantation: Pathologic observations and clinical implications. J Heart Transplant 8:430, 1989.

14. Neish AS, Schoen FJ. Myocardial changes in cardiac transplant–associated arteriosclerosis (abstract). Lab Invest 62:73A, 1990.

15. Leavy JA, Marboe CC, Barr ML, et al. Myocardial interleukin-6: A marker for accelerated graft atherosclerosis following cardiac transplantation (abstract). Circulation 84:II-486, 1991.

16. Gao SZ, Schroeder JS, Hunt SA, et al. Acute myocardial infarction in cardiac transplant recipients. Am J Cardiol 64:1093, 1989.

17. Wilson RF, McGinn AL, Johnson TH, et al. Sympathetic reinnervation after heart transplantation in human beings. J Heart Lung Transplant 11:S88, 1992.

18. Stark RP, McGinn AL, Wilson RF. Chest pain in cardiac transplant recipients: Evidence of sensory reinnervation after cardiac transplantation. N Engl J Med 324:1791, 1991.

19. McGinn AL, Meyer SM, Christiansen BV. Can sympathetic reinnervation affect coronary resistance after human cardiac transplantation? Circulation 84:493, 1991.

20. Sanfilippo F. Renal transplantation. *In* Sale GE (ed). *The Pathology of Organ Transplantation.* Boston, Butterworths, 1990, p 51.

21. Oguma S, Belle S, Starzl TE, et al. A histomorphometric analysis of chronically rejected human liver allografts. Insights into the mechanism of bile duct loss: Direct immunologic and ischemic factors. Hepatology 9:204, 1989.

22. Hruban RH, Beschorner WE, Baumgartner WA, et al. Accelerated arteriosclerosis in heart transplant recipients is associated with a T-lymphocyte-mediated endothelialitis. Am J Pathol 137:871, 1990.

23. Salomon RN, Hughes CCW, Schoen FJ, et al. Human coronary transplantation–associated arteriosclerosis: Evidence of a chronic immune reaction to activated graft endothelial cells. Am J Pathol 138:791, 1991.

24. Nielsen H, Symmans F, Marboe CC. Arteriopathy in human cardiac allografts: An immunopathologic study: Cell phenotyping and expression of adhesion molecules. Submitted to Am J Pathol, 1993.

25. Marboe CC, Schierman SW, Rose E, et al. Characterization of mononuclear cell infiltrates in human cardiac allografts. Transplant Proc 16:1598, 1984.

26. Chomette G, Aurior MK, Delcourt A, et al. Human cardiac transplants. Diagnosis of rejection by endomyocardial biopsy. Causes of death. Virchows Arch (A) 407:295, 1985.

27. Doherty PC, Allen JE, Lynch F, et al. Dissection of an inflammatory process induced by CD8+ T cells. Immunol Today 11:55, 1990.

28. Libby P, Warner SJC, Friedman GB. Interleukin-1: A mitogen for human vascular smooth muscle cells that induces the release of growth-inhibitory prostanoids. J Clin Invest 88:487, 1988.

29. Raines EW, Dower SK, Ross R. Interleukin-1 mitogenic activity for fibroblasts and smooth muscle cells is due to PDGF-AA. Science 243:393, 1989.

30. Fellstrom B, Dilmeny E, Larsson E, et al. Importance of PDGF receptor expression in accelerated atherosclerosis–chronic rejection. Transplant Proc 21:3689, 1989.

31. Dinarello CA, Ikejima T, Warner SJC, et al. Interleukin-1 induces interleukin-1. I. Induction of circulating interleukin-1 in rabbits in vivo and in human mononuclear cells in vitro. J Immunol 139:1902, 1987.

32. Badimon JJ, Fuster V, Chesebro JH, et al. Coronary atherosclerosis: A multifactorial disease. Circulation 87(Suppl II):II-3, 1993.

33. Dustin ML, Rothlein R, Bahn AK, et al. Induction by IL-1 and interferon gamma: Tissue distribution, biochemistry and function of a natural adhesion molecule (ICAM-1). J Immunol 137:245, 1986.

34. Rice GE, Munro JM, Bevilacqua MP. Inducible cell adhesion molecule 110 (INCAM-110) is an endothelial receptor for lymphocytes. A CD11 ± 18-independent adhesion mechanism. J Exp Med 171:1369, 1990.

35. Osborn L, Hession LC, Tizard R, et al. Direct expression cloning of vascular cell adhesion molecule-1, a cytokine-induced endothelial protein that binds lymphocytes. Cell 59:1203, 1989.

36. Nielsen H, Marboe CC, Hamby C, et al. Induction of HLA and intercellular adhesion molecule-1 expression in acute rejection of human cardiac allografts. FASEB J 4:A1023, 1990.

37. Briscoe DM, Schoen JF, Rilce GE, et al. Induced expression of endothelial leukocyte adhesion molecules in human cardiac allografts. Transplantation 51:537, 1991.

38. Carlos T, Gordon D, Fishbein D, et al. Vascular cell adhesion molecule-1 is induced on endothelium during acute rejection in human cardiac allografts. J Heart Lung Transplant 11:1103, 1992.

39. Dvorak HF, Galli SJ, Dvorak AM. Cellular and vascular manifestations of cell-mediated immunity. Hum Pathol 17:122, 1986.

40. Poston RN, Haskard DO, Coucher JR, et al. Expression of intercellular adhesion molecule-1 in atherosclerotic plaques. Am J Pathol 140:665, 1992.

41. Printseva OY, Pecle MM, Gown AM. Various cell types in human atherosclerotic lesions express ICAM-1. Further immunocytochemical and immunochemical studies employing monoclonal antibody 10F3. Am J Pathol 140:889, 1992.

42. Cybulsky MI, Gimbrone MA. Endothelial expression of a mononuclear leukocyte adhesion molecule during atherogenesis. Science 251:788, 1991.

43. van der Wal AC, Das PK, Tigges AJ, et al. Adhesion molecules on the endothelium and mononuclear cells in human atherosclerotic lesions. Am J Pathol 141:1427, 1992.

44. Page C, Rose M, Yacoub M, et al. Antigenic heterogeneity of vascular endothelium. Am J Pathol 141:673, 1992.
45. Lasky LA. Selectins: Interpreters of cell-specific carbohydrate information during inflammation. Science 258:964, 1992.
46. O'Rourke AM, Mescher MF. Cytotoxic T-lymphocyte activation involving a cascade of signalling and adhesion events. Nature 358:253, 1992.
47. Shimizu Y, Newman W, Tanaka Y, et al. Lymphocyte interactions with endothelial cells. Immunol Today 13:106, 1992.
48. van Seventer GA, Shimizu Y, Shaw S. Roles of multiple accessory molecules in T cell activation. Curr Opin Immunol 3:294, 1991.
49. Harding FA, McArthur JG, Gross JA, et al. CD28-mediated signalling co-stimulates murine T cells and prevents induction of anergy in T-cell clones. Nature 356:607, 1992.
50. Linsley PS, Brady W, Grosmare L, et al. Binding of the B cell activation antigen B7 to CD28 costimulates T cell proliferation and IL-2 MRNA accumulation. J Exp Med 173:721, 1991.
51. Linsley PS, Wallace PM, Johnson J, et al. Immunosuppression in vivo by a soluble form of the CTLA-4 T cell activation molecule. Science 257:792, 1992.
52. Lenschow DJK, Zeng Y, Thistlethwaite JR, et al. Long-term survival of xenogeneic pancreatic islet grafts induced by CTLA4Ig. Science 257:789, 1992.
53. Turka LA, Linsley PS, Lin H, et al. T-cell activation by the CD28 ligand B7 is required for cardiac allograft rejection in vivo. Proc Natl Acad Sci USA 89:11102, 1992.
54. Moingeon P, Chang H, Wallner BP, et al. CD2-mediated adhesion facilitates T lymphocyte recognition function. Nature 339:312, 1989.
55. Hochman PS, Majeau GR, Miller GT, et al. Structure-function analysis of inhibition of in vitro human T cell responses by LFA3-Ig fusion proteins. Submitted to Transplantation, 1993.
56. Warner SJC, Auger KR, Libby P. Interleukin-1 induces interleukin-1. II. Recombinant human interleukin-1 induces interleukin-1 production by adult human vascular endothelial cells. J Immunol 139:1911, 1987.
57. Warner SJC, Libby P. Human vascular smooth muscle cells: Target for and source of tumor necrosis factor. J Immunol 142:100, 1989.
58. Clinton SK, Libby P. Cytokines and growth factors in atherogenesis. Arch Pathol Lab Med 116:1292, 1992.
59. Häyry P, Mennander A, Räisänen-Sokolowski A, et al. Pathophysiology of vascular wall changes in chronic allograft rejection. Transplant Rev 7:1, 1993.
60. Thyberg J, Hedin U, Sjölund M, et al. Regulation of differentiated properties and proliferation of arterial smooth muscle cells. Arteriosclerosis 10:966, 1990.
61. Ip JH, Fuster V, Badimon L, et al. Syndromes of accelerated atherosclerosis: Role of vascular injury and smooth muscle cell proliferation. J Am Coll Cardiol 15:1667, 1990.
62. Reidy MA. Factors controlling smooth-muscle cell proliferation. Arch Pathol Lab Med 116:1276, 1992.
63. Ross R. Polypeptide growth factors and atherosclerosis. Trends Cardiovasc Med 1:277, 1991.
64. Ross R, Masuda J, Raines EW, et al. Localization of PDGF-B protein in macrophages in all phases of atherogenesis. Science 248:1009, 1990.
65. Lindner V, Reidy MA. Proliferation of smooth muscle cells after vascular injury is inhibited by an antibody against basic fibroblast growth factor. Proc Natl Acad Sci USA 88:3739, 1991.
66. Gordon D. Growth factors and cell proliferation in human transplant arteriosclerosis. J Heart Lung Transplant 11:S7, 1992.
67. Gordon D, Reidy MA, Benditt EP, et al. Cell proliferation in human coronary arteries. Proc Natl Acad Sci USA 87:4600, 1990.
68. Kim DN, Schmee J, Ho HT, et al. The "turning off" of excessive cell replicative activity in advanced atherosclerotic lesions of swine by a regression diet. Atherosclerosis 71:131, 1988.
69. Hansson GKL, Jonasson L, Holm J, et al. Class II MHC antigen expression in the atherosclerotic plaque: Smooth muscle cells express HLA-DR, HLA-DQ and the invariant gamma chain. Clin Exp Immunol 64:261, 1986.
70. Bieber CP, Stinson ED, Shumway NE, et al. Cardiac transplantation in man. VII. Cardiac allograft pathology. Circulation 41:753, 1970.
71. Chomette G, Auriol M, Cabrol C. Chronic rejection in human heart transplantation. J Heart Transplant 7:292, 1988.
72. Gimbrone MA Jr, Bevilacqua MP. Vascular endothelium functional modulation at the blood interface. In Simionescu N, Simionescu M (eds): Endothelial Cell Biology. New York, Plenum, 1988, p 255.
73. Kosek JC, Hurley EJ, Lower RR. Histopathology of orthotopic canine cardiac homografts. Lab Invest 19:97, 1968.
74. Alonso DR, Starek PK, Minick CR. Studies on the pathogenesis of atheroarteriosclerosis induced in rabbit cardiac allografts by the synergy of graft rejection and hypercholesterolemia. Am J Pathol 87:415, 1977.
75. Hosenpud JD, Shipley GD, Morris TE, et al. The modulation of human aortic endothelial cell ICAM-1 (CD-54) expression by serum containing high titers of anti-HLA antibodies. Transplantation 55:405, 1993.
76. Opelz G. Effect of HLA matching in heart transplantation. Transplant Proc 21:794, 1989.
77. Hess ML, Hastillo A, Mohanakumar T, et al. Accelerated atherosclerosis in cardiac transplantation: Role of cytotoxic B-cell antibodies and hyperlipidemia. Circulation 68(suppl):94, 1983.
78. Fenoglio R, Ho E, Reed E, et al. Anti-HLA antibodies and heart allograft survival. Transplant Proc 21:807, 1989.
79. Suciu-Foca N, Reed E, Marboe C, et al. The role of anti-HLA antibodies in heart transplantation. Transplantation 51:716, 1991.
80. Reed E, Hardy M, Benvenisty A, et al. Effect of anti-idiotypic antibodies to HLA on graft survival in renal allograft recipients. N Engl J Med 316:1450, 1987.
81. Reed E, Cohen DJ, Barr ML, et al. Effect of anti-HLA and anti-idiotypic antibodies on the long-term survival of heart and kidney allografts. Transplant Proc 24:2494, 1992.
82. Petrossian GA, Nichols AB, Marboe CC, et al. Relation between survival and development of coronary artery disease and anti-HLA antibodies after cardiac transplant. Circulation 80(suppl):III-122, 1989.
83. Barr ML, Berger CL, Wiedermann JG, et al. Photochemotherapy for the prevention of graft atherosclerosis in cardiac transplantation. J Heart Lung Transplant 12:S85, 1993.
84. Hammond EH, Ensley RD, Yowell RL, et al. Vascular rejection of human cardiac allografts and the role of

humoral immunity in chronic allograft rejection. Transplant Proc 23:26, 1991.

85. Ensley RD, Hammond EH, Renlund DG, et al. Clinical manifestations of vascular rejection in cardiac transplantation. Transplant Proc 23:1130, 1991.

86. Hammond EH, Wittwer CT, Greenwood J, et al. Relationship of OKT3 sensitization and vascular rejection in cardiac transplant patients receiving OKT3 rejection prophylaxis. Transplantation 50:776, 1990.

87. Hammond EH, Yowell RL, Price GD, et al. Vascular rejection and its relationship to allograft coronary artery disease. J Heart Lung Transplant 11:S111, 1992.

88. Cherry R, Nielsen H, Reed E, et al. Vascular (humoral) rejection in cardiac allograft biopsies: Relation to circulating anti-HLA antibodies. J Heart Lung Transplant 11:24, 1992.

89. Cerilli J, Brasile L, Galouzis T, et al. The vascular endothelial cell antigen system. Transplantation 39:286, 1985.

90. Paul LC, Busch GJ, Paradysz JM, et al. Definition, genetics, and possible significance of newly defined endothelial antigens in the rat. Transplantation. 36:533, 1983.

91. Cheigh JS, Chami J, Stenzel KH, et al. Renal transplantation between HLA identical siblings: Comparison with transplants from HLA semi-identical related donors. N Engl J Med 296:1030, 1977.

92. Brasile L, Zerbe T, Rabin B, et al. Identification of the antibody to vascular endothelial cells in patients undergoing cardiac transplantation. Transplantation 40:672, 1985.

93. Dunn MJ, Crisp S, Rose M, et al. Detection of anti-endothelial antibodies by Western blotting—positive correlation with coronary artery disease after cardiac transplantation. Lancet 2:1566, 1992.

94. Barr ML, Rose EA, Wiederman JG, et al. Anti-endothelial antibodies in cardiac transplantation. Submitted to J Heart Lung Transplant, 1993.

95. Iwaki Y, Terasaki P. Sensitization effect. *In* Terasaki P (ed): *Clinical Transplants.* Los Angeles, UCLA Tissue Typing Laboratory, 1986, p 257.

96. Singh G, Thompson M, Griffith B, et al. Histocompatibility in cardiac transplantation with particular reference to immunopathology of positive serologic crossmatch. Clin Immunol Immunopathol 28:56, 1983.

97. Lavee J, Kormos RL, Duquesnoy RJ, et al. Influence of panel-reactive antibody and lymphocytotoxic crossmatch on survival after heart transplantation. J Heart Lung Transplant 10:921, 1991.

98. Zerbe T, Uretsky B, Kormos R, et al. Graft atherosclerosis: Effects of cellular rejection and human lymphocyte antigen. J Heart Lung Transplant 11:S104, 1992.

99. McCloskey D, Festenstein H, Banner N, et al. The effect of HLA lymphocytotoxic antibody status and crossmatch result on cardiac transplant survival. Transplant Proc 21:804, 1989.

100. Lopez C, Simmons RL, Mauer SM, et al. Virus infections may trigger rejection in immunosuppressed renal transplant recipients. Proc Clin Dial Transplant Forum 2:107, 1972.

101. Peterson PK, Balfour HH Jr, Marker SC, et al. Cytomegalovirus disease in renal allograft recipients: A prospective study of the clinical features, risk factors and impact on renal transplantation. Medicine 59:283, 1980.

102. Light JA, Burke DS. Association of cytomegalovirus

infections with increased recipient mortality following transplantation. Transplant Proc 11:79, 1979.

103. Grattan MT, Moreno-Cabral CE, Starnes VA, et al. Cytomegalovirus infection is associated with cardiac allograft rejection and atherosclerosis. JAMA 261:3561, 1989.

104. Cameron DE, Greene PS, Alejo D, et al. Postoperative cytomegalovirus infection and older donor age predispose to coronary atherosclerosis after heart transplantation. Circulation 80 (suppl II):II-526, 1989.

105. McDonald K, Rector TS, Braunlin EA, et al. Association of coronary artery disease in cardiac transplant recipients with cytomegalovirus. Am J Cardiol 64:359, 1989.

106. Loebe M, Schüler S, Zais O, et al. Role of cytomegalovirus infection in the development of coronary artery disease in the transplanted heart. J Heart Transplant 9:707, 1990.

107. Balk AHMM, Linden M, Meeter K, et al. Is there a relationship between transplant coronary artery disease and the occurrence of CMV infection (abstract)? J Heart Lung Transplant 10:188, 1991.

108. Everett JP, Hershberger RE, Norman DJ, et al. Prolonged cytomegalovirus infection with viremia is associated with development of cardiac allograft vasculopathy. J Heart Lung Transplant 11:S133, 1992.

109. Ross R. Mechanisms of atherosclerosis—A review. Adv Nephrol 19:79, 1990.

110. Visser MR, Tracy PB, Vercellotti GM, et al. Enhanced thrombin generation and platelet binding on herpes simplex virus–infected endothelium. Proc Natl Acad Sci USA 85:8227, 1988.

111. Etingin OR, Silverstein RL, Friedman HM, et al. Viral activation of the coagulation cascade: Molecular interactions at the surface of infected endothelial cells. Cell 61:657, 1990.

112. Benditt EP. Implications of the monoclonal character of human atherosclerotic plaques. Ann NY Acad Sci 275:96, 1976.

113. Hosenpud JD, Shipley GD, Wagner CR. Cardiac allograft vasculopathy: Current concepts, recent developments, and future directions. J Heart Lung Transplant 11:9, 1992.

114. Fabricant CG, Fabricant J, et al. Virus-induced atherosclerosis. J Exp Med 148:335, 1978.

115. Hajjar DP, Nicholson AC, Hajjar KA, et al. Decreased messenger RNA transcription in herpesvirus-infected arterial cells: Effects on cholesteryl ester hydrolase. Proc Natl Acad Sci USA 86:3366, 1989.

116. von Willebrand E, Pettersson E, Ahonen J, et al. CMV infection, class II antigen expression, and human kidney allograft rejection. Transplantation 42:364, 1986.

117. van Es A, Baldwin WM, Oljans PJ, et al. Expression of HLA-DR on T lymphocytes following renal transplantation, and association with graft rejection episodes and cytomegalovirus infection. Transplantation 37:65, 1984.

118. Arnold JC, Gmelin K, Otto G, et al. Effect of cytomegalovirus infection on expression of HLA-antigens in liver allografts. Transplant Proc 23:442, 1991.

119. Sedmak DD, Roberts WH, Stephens RE, et al. Inability of cytomegalovirus infection of cultured endothelial cells to induce HLA class II antigen expression. Transplant 49:458, 1990.

120. Fujinami RS, Nelsan JA, Walker L, et al. Sequence homology and immunologic cross-reactivity of human cytomegalovirus with HLA-DR β chain: A means for graft rejection and immunosuppression. J Virol 62:100, 1988.

121. Lodge PA, Haisch CE, Huber SA, et al. Biological differences in endothelial cells depending upon organ derivation. Transplant Proc 23:216, 1991.

122. Minick CR, Fabricant CG, Fabricant J, et al. Atheroarteriosclerosis induced by infection with a herpesvirus. Am J Pathol 96:673, 1979.

123. Yamashiroya HM, Hosh L, Yang R, et al. Herpesviridae in the coronary arteries and aorta of young trauma victims. Am J Pathol 130:71, 1988.

124. Wu T-C, Hruban RH, Ambinder RF, et al. Demonstration of cytomegalovirus nucleic acids in the coronary arteries of transplanted hearts. Am J Pathol 140:739, 1992.

125. Min KW, Wickemeyer WKJ, Chandran P, et al. Fatal cytomegalovirus infection and coronary arterial thromboses after heart transplantation: A case report. J Heart Transplant 5:375, 1986.

126. Kemnitz J, Hirt SW, Haverich A, et al. Dynamik der Entwicklung der Transplantationsvaskulopathie (graft coronary disease) nach orthotoper Herztransplantation. Verh Dtsch Ges Pathol 74:476, 1990.

127. McManus B, Kendall T, Wilson J, et al. Immunoreactivity of monoclonal antibody to cytomegalovirus in coronary atherosclerosis and transplant arteriopathy. Mod Pathol 4:19A, 1991.

128. Hendrix MGR, Dormans PHJ, Kitslaar P, et al. The presence of cytomegalovirus nucleic acids in arterial walls of atherosclerotic and nonatherosclerotic patients. Am J Pathol 134:1151, 1989.

129. Hendrix MGR, Daemen M, Bruggeman CA. Cytomegalovirus nucleic acid distribution within the human vascular tree. Am J Pathol 138:563, 1991.

130. Hendrix MGR, Salimans MMM, van Boven CPA, et al. High prevalence of latently present cytomegalovirus in arterial walls of patients suffering from grade III atherosclerosis. Am J Pathol 136:23, 1990.

131. Plotkin SA, Starr SE, Friedman HM, et al. Effect of Towne live virus vaccine on cytomegalovirus disease after renal transplant. Ann Intern Med 114:525, 1991.

132. Terasaki P, Mickey MR, Iwaki Y, et al. Long-term survival of kidney grafts. Transplant Proc 21:615, 1989.

133. Kormos RL, Colson YL, Hardesty RL, et al. Immunologic and blood group compatibility in cardiac transplantation. Transplant Proc 20:741, 1988.

134. Festenstein H, Banner N, Smith J, et al. The influence of HLA matching and lymphocytotoxic antibody status in heart-lung allograft recipients receiving cyclosporin and azathioprine. Transplant Proc 1:797, 1989.

135. Shakin-Eshleman SH, Cavarocchi NC, Zmijewski CM. HLA compatibility and clinical outcome among cardiac transplant recipients. Clin Transplant 4:98, 1990.

136. Pfeffer PF, Foerster A, Froysaker T, et al. Correlation between HLA-DR mismatch and rejection episodes in cardiac transplantation. Transplant Proc 1:691, 1987.

137. Zerbe T, Arena V, Kormos R, et al. Role of major histocompatibility complex (HLA) matching in cardiac allograft rejection. Transplant Proc 1:74, 1988.

138. Laufer G, Miholic J, Laczkovics A, et al. Independent risk factors predicting acute graft rejection in cardiac transplant recipients treated by triple drug immunosuppression. J Thorac Cardiovasc Surg 98:1113, 1989.

139. Costanzo-Nordin MR. Cardiac allograft vasculopathy: Relationship with acute cellular rejection and histocompatibility. J Heart Lung Transplant 11:S90, 1992.

140. Khaghani A, Yacoub M, McCloskey D, et al. The influence of HLA matching, donor/recipient sex, and incidence of acute rejection on survival in cardiac allograft recipients receiving cyclosporin A and azathioprine. Transplant Proc 1:799, 1989.

141. Pollack MS, Ballantyne CM, Payton-Ross C, et al. HLA match and other immunological parameters in relation to survival, rejection severity, and accelerated coronary artery disease after heart transplant. Clin Transplant 4:269, 1990.

142. Narrod J, Kormos R, Armitage J, et al. Acute rejection and coronary artery disease in long-term survivors of heart transplantation. J Heart Transplant 5:418, 1989.

143. Radovancevic B, Birovljev S, Vega JD, et al. Inverse relationship between human leukocyte antigen match and development of coronary artery disease. Transplant Proc 1:1144, 1991.

144. Donaldson PT, O'Grady J, Portmann B, et al. Evidence for an immune response to HLA class I antigens in the vanishing bile duct syndrome after liver transplantation. Lancet 1:945, 1987.

145. Radovancevic B, Poindexter S, Birovljev S, et al. Risk factors for development of accelerated coronary artery disease in cardiac transplant recipients. Eur J Cardiothorac Surg 4:309, 1990.

146. Johnson MR. Transplant coronary disease: Nonimmunologic risk factors. J Heart Lung Transplant 11:S124, 1992.

147. Bilodeau M, Fitchett DH, Guerraty A, et al. Dyslipoproteinemias after heart and heart-lung transplantation: Potential relation to accelerated graft arteriosclerosis. J Heart Transplant 8:454, 1989.

148. Winters GL, Kendall TJ, Radio SJ, et al. Posttransplant obesity and hyperlipidemia: Major predictors of severity of coronary arteriopathy in failed human heart allografts. J Heart Transplant 9:364, 1990.

149. Taylor DO, Thompson JA, Hastillo A, et al. Hyperlipidemia after clinical heart transplantation. J Heart Transplant 8:209, 1989.

150. Becker DM, Chamberlain B, Swank R, et al. Relationship between corticosteroid exposure and plasma lipid levels in heart transplant recipients. Am J Med 85:632, 1988.

151. Öst L. Effects of cyclosporin on prednisolone metabolism (letter). Lancet 1:451, 1984.

152. Superko HR, Haskell WL, DiRicco CD. Lipoprotein and hepatic lipase activity and high-density lipoprotein subclasses after cardiac transplantation. Am J Cardiol 66:1131, 1990.

153. Laden AMK. Experimental atherosclerosis in rat and rabbit cardiac allografts. Arch Pathol 93:240, 1972.

154. Minick CR, Murphy GE. Experimental induction of atheroarteriosclerosis by the synergy of allergic injury to arteries and lipid-rich diet. Am J Pathol 73:265, 1973.

155. Minick CR, Alonso DR, Rankin L. Role of immunologic arterial injury in atherogenesis. Thromb Haemost 39:304, 1978.

156. Eich D, Thompson JA, Daijin K, et al. Hypercholesterolemia in long-term survivors of heart transplantation: An early marker of accelerated coronary artery disease. J Heart Lung Transplant 10:45, 1991.

157. Sharples LD, Caine N, Mullins P, et al. Risk factor analysis for the major hazards following heart transplantation—rejection, infection and coronary occlusive disease. Transplantation 52:244, 1991.

158. Olivari MT, Homans DC, Wilson RF, et al. Coronary artery disease in cardiac transplant patients receiving triple-drug immunosuppressive therapy. Circulation 80(Suppl III):III-111, 1989.

159. Gao SZ, Schroeder JS, Alderman EL, et al. Clinical and laboratory correlates of accelerated coronary artery disease in the cardiac transplant patient. Circulation 76(Suppl V):V-56, 1987.
160. Gerlach H, Esposito C, Stern DM. Modulation of endothelial hemostatic properties: An active role in the host response. Annu Rev Med 41:15, 1990.
161. Dzau VJ, Gibbons GH, Cooke JP, et al. Vascular biology and medicine in the 1990s: Scope, concepts, potentials, perspectives. Circulation 87:705, 1993.
162. Faulk WP, Labarrere CA. Vascular immunopathology and atheroma development in human allografted organs. Arch Pathol Lab Med 116:1337, 1992.
163. Hunt BJ, Segal H, Yacoub M. Hemostatic changes in heart transplant recipients and their relationship to accelerated coronary sclerosis. Transplantation 55:309, 1993.
164. Labarrere CA, Pitts D, Halbrook H, et al. Tissue plasminogen activator (tPA) in human cardiac allografts. Transplantation (in press).
165. Meilahn EN. Hemostatic factors and risk of cardiovascular disease in women. Arch Pathol Lab Med 116:1313, 1992.
166. Fuster V, Badimon L, Badimon JJ, et al. The pathogenesis of coronary artery disease and the acute coronary syndromes. N Engl J Med 326:310, 1992.
167. Davies PF, Robotewskyj A, Griem ML, et al. Hemodynamic forces and vascular cell communication in arteries. Arch Pathol Lab Med 116:1301, 1992.
168. Yeung AC, Vekshtein VI, Drantz DS, et al. The effect of atherosclerosis on the vasomotor response of coronary arteries to mental stress. N Engl J Med 325:1551, 1991.
169. Fish RD, Nabel EG, Selwyn AP, et al. Responses of coronary arteries of cardiac transplant patients to acetylcholine. J Clin Invest 81:21, 1988.
170. Yeung AC, Anderson T, Meredith I, et al. Endothelial dysfunction in the development and detection of transplant coronary artery disease. J Heart Lung Transplant 11:S69, 1992.
171. Gibbons GH. Preventive treatment of graft coronary vascular disease: The potential role for vasodilator therapy. J Heart Lung Transplant 11:S22, 1992.
172. Smith JB. Angiotensin-receptor signaling in cultured vascular smooth muscle cells. Am J Physiol 250:F759, 1986.
173. Williams LT. Signal transduction by the platelet-derived growth factor receptor. Science 243:1564, 1989.
174. Naftilan AJ, Pratt RE, Dzau VJ. Induction of platelet-derived growth factor A-chain and c-myc gene expressions by angiotensin II in cultured rat vascular smooth muscle cells. J Clin Invest 83:1419, 1989.
175. Dubin D, Pratt RE, Cooke JP, et al. Endothelin, a potent vasoconstrictor, is a vascular smooth muscle mitogen. J Vasc Med Biol 1:150, 1989.
176. Garg UC, Hassid A. Nitric oxide-generating vasodilators and 8-bromo-cyclic guanosine monophosphate inhibit mitogenesis and proliferation of cultured rat vascular smooth muscle cells. J Clin Invest 83:1774, 1989.
177. Nilsson J, Olsson AG. Prostaglandin E inhibits DNA synthesis in arterial smooth muscle cells stimulated with platelet-derived growth factor. Atherosclerosis 53:77, 1984.
178. Newby AC, Southgate KM, Assender JW. Inhibition of vascular smooth muscle proliferation by endothelium-dependent vasodilators. Herz 17:291, 1992.
179. Schroeder JS, Gao S-Z, Hunt SA, et al. Accelerated graft coronary artery disease: Diagnosis and prevention. J Heart Lung Transplant 11:S258, 1992.
180. Kobashigawa JA, Murphy FL, Stevenson LW, et al. Low-dose lovastatin safely lowers cholesterol after cardiac transplantation. Circulation 82(Suppl IV):IV-281, 1990.
181. Norman DJ, Illingsworth DR, Munson J, et al. Myolysis and acute renal failure in a heart transplant recipient receiving lovastatin (letter). N Engl J Med 318:40, 1988.
182. Ensley RD, Hunt S, Taylor DO, et al. Predictors of survival after repeat heart transplantation. J Heart Lung Transplant 11:S142, 1992.
183. Halle AA III, Wilson RF, Massin EK, et al. Clinical investigation: Coronary angioplasty in cardiac transplant patients: Results of a multicenter study. Circulation 86:458, 1992.
184. Ginsberg R, Davis K, Bristow MR, et al. Calcium antagonists suppress atherogenesis in aorta but not in the intramural coronary arteries of cholesterol-fed rabbits. Lab Invest 49:154, 1983.
185. Sugano M, Nakashima Y, Tasaki H, et al. Effects of diltiazem on suppression and regression of experimental atherosclerosis. Br J Exp Pathol 69:515, 1988.
186. Weinstein DB. The antiatherogenic potential of calcium antagonists. J Cardiovasc Pharmacol 12 (Suppl 6):S29, 1988.
187. Waters D, Lesperance J. Interventions that beneficially influence the evolution of coronary atherosclerosis. The case for calcium channel blockers. Circulation 86 (6 Suppl):III-111, 1992.
188. Block LH, Buhler FR. Atherosclerosis, cell motility, calcium and calcium channel blockers. J Cardiovasc Pharmacol 19(Suppl 2):S1, 1992.
189. Weir MR, Peppler R, Gomolka D, et al. Evidence that the antiproliferative effect of verapamil on afferent and efferent immune responses is independent of calcium channel inhibition. Transplantation 54:681, 1992.
190. Jost S, Rafflenbeul W, Deckers J, et al. Concept of antiatherosclerotic efficacy of calcium entry blockers. INTACT investigators. Eur J Epidemiol 8(Suppl 1):107, 1992.
191. Sheehan H, Vetrovec G, Graham S, et al. Calcium channel antagonists protect against the development of coronary artery disease following cardiac transplantation (abstract) J Am Coll Cardiol 17:290A, 1991.
192. Schroeder JS, Gao SZ, Alderman EL, et al. A preliminary study of diltiazem in the prevention of coronary artery disease in heart transplant recipients. N Engl J Med 328:164, 1993.
193. Feogh ML. Angiopeptin: A treatment for accelerated myointimal hyperplasia? J Heart Lung Transplant 11:S28, 1992.
194. Meiser BM, Wolf S, Devens C, et al. Continuous infusion of angiopeptin significantly reduces accelerated graft vessel disease induced by FK506 in a rat heart allograft model. Transplant Proc 24:1671, 1992.
195. Eriksen UH, Amtorp O, Bagger JP, et al. Continuous angiopeptin infusion reduces coronary restenosis following balloon angioplasty (abstract). Circulation 88:I-594, 1993.
196. Clowes AW, Reidy MA. Prevention of stenosis after vascular reconstruction: Pharmacological control of intimal hyperplasia—a review. J Vasc Surg 13:885, 1991.
197. Clowes AW, Clowes MM, Vergel SC, et al. Heparin

and cilazapril together inhibit injury induced intimal hyperplasia. Hypertension 18:1165, 1991.

198. Taylor A, Gasparro FP. Extracorporeal photochemotherapy for cutaneous T-cell lymphoma and other diseases. Semin Hematol 29:132, 1992.

199. Griepp RB, Stinson EB, Bieber CP, et al. Control of graft arteriosclerosis in human heart transplant recipients. Surgery 81:262, 1977.

200. Lurie KG, Billingham ME, Jamieson SW, et al. Patho-genesis and prevention of graft arteriosclerosis in an experimental heart transplant model. Transplantation 31:41, 1981.

201. deLorgeril M, Dureau G, Boissonnat P, et al. Platelet function and composition in heart transplant recipients compared with nontransplanted coronary patients. Arterioscler Thromb 12:222, 1992.

202. Ware JA, Heistad DD. Platelet-endothelial interactions. N Engl J Med 328:628, 1993.

8

LUNG TRANSPLANT PATHOLOGY

Susan Stewart, MD

INTRODUCTION AND MORPHOLOGY OF EXPERIMENTAL LUNG TRANSPLANTATION

Lung transplantation is now an established therapeutic procedure for end stage pulmonary vascular and parenchymal disease.[1, 2] Lungs can be transplanted singly, as a double block, or combined with the heart, depending on the primary disease and, to some extent, on donor organ availability. Eisenmenger's syndrome and some other combined cardiopulmonary diseases require replacement of the native heart and lungs, but diffuse pulmonary diseases in which the native heart is not significantly diseased can undergo bilateral or single lung replacement. The remaining native lung in single lung transplants can threaten to infect the graft in suppurative conditions, and this procedure is therefore usually confined to pulmonary fibrosis and severe emphysema.

Lung transplantation is significantly limited by donor organ availability, as there are strict selection criteria.[3] The long-term survival of the graft is limited by obliterative bronchiolitis, which can be reduced in incidence by transbronchial biopsy diagnosis of complications postoperatively.[4]

A long history of experimental lung transplantation predates successful clinical lung grafting. This work was performed mainly on dogs,[5, 6] rats,[7] and primates[8–10] in combinations of organs, as in current clinical use. Experimentally, single, bilateral, and combined heart-lung grafts have all shown similar pathologic features in the short term. Long-term survivors are seen only in primates[9] or in combined heart-lung grafts, as lower animals do not tolerate total cardiopulmonary denervation.[5, 11] In dogs, unmodified lung acute rejection causes consolidation and congestion with terminal hemorrhagic necrosis.[12] This is often accompanied by secondary infection. Microscopically, perivascular mononuclear cell infiltrates appear at days 4 to 5, progressing to alveolar infiltration. Polymorphs and necrosis are in evidence at 8 to 10 days.[13] Airways show bronchitis with mucus and inflammatory cell plugging, which eventually leads to obliterative bronchiolitis.[12] Immunosuppression modifies the histologic appearances, reducing perivascular infiltration and leaving prominent alveolar exudation.[14, 15]

Cyclosporine treatment of unmatched mongrel dogs was associated with widespread perivascular and peribronchial cuffs of lymphoid cells, more prominent than in unmodified grafts and extending into alveoli.[16] There was also a second histologic pattern confined to perivascular cuffing with normal air spaces. The latter pattern required longer immunosuppression by steroids for its reversal.[15] Increased doses of immunosuppression in baboon lung grafts decreased the intensity of the cellular infiltrates.[17] Prop and associates have detailed the histologic features of rat lung rejection using inbred strains with greater immunogenetic standardization than in dogs and primates.[18, 19] After an initial latent phase, a vascular phase of rejection comprises prominent perivascular and peribronchial mononuclear cell infiltration. This extends into the interstitium in the alveolar phase, leading to necrosis and acute inflammatory cell infiltration in the final destructive phase. The bronchial and bronchiolar changes are difficult to compare with rejection in other species owing to the prominence of rat bronchus-associated lymphoid tissue. Studies in the rat, however, suggest that post-transplantation bronchiolitis obliterans is due to rejection, with pathologic changes very similar to those in human lung grafts.[20]

Isografts in both rats and dogs show nonspecific exudate with polymorphs and macrophages but not lymphoid cells and serve as useful controls in the study of histologic appearances characteristic of rejection.[21, 22]

There is less information on chronic rejection in experimental lung allografts. Long-term appearances in primates were described by Haverich and colleagues as showing marked interstitial fibrosis and pulmonary arteriolar intimal thickening.[23] Pulmonary interstitial thickening and blunting of alveolar septa without mononuclear cell infiltrates were seen in a 144-day monkey allograft.[9] It is important to note that obliterative bronchiolitis was not seen in the presence of intimal proliferation in two long-term (5- and 7-year) primate survivors.[24]

In the case of combined grafts, Prop and associates demonstrated that the lungs are more vigorously rejected than the heart.[25] The mucosa-associated lymphoid tissue facilitates infiltration of the graft by recipient lymphocytes, providing a strong stimulus for a local immune response. This may also explain the discordance of lung and heart rejection in combined primate and human grafts.

MORPHOLOGY OF ACUTE REJECTION

The histopathologic appearances of acute lung rejection in humans have been studied in transbronchial, open biopsy, and autopsy material.[26–30] These data refer to rejection modified by immunosuppression, generally a combination of cyclosporine, azathioprine, and steroid therapy. The precise incidence of acute lung rejection is not known, but it is common in the first 3 to 6 months following transplantation. Presenting symptoms include pyrexia, breathlessness, and cough. An abnormal radiograph is seen in some cases, with new or changing infiltrates.[31] Some patients, however, may be asymptomatic. Radiographic abnor-malities are commoner in early rejection (within 1 month of operation), with ill-defined perihilar and lower zone shadowing that is generally symmetric and bilateral. Pleural effusions may be present. The chest radiograph is abnormal in the minority (23 per cent) of episodes of rejection occurring later than 1 month after transplantation.[31] During episodes of rejection there is usually a decline in pulmonary function.

The earliest histopathologic abnormality seen on transbronchial or open lung biopsy in patients undergoing acute rejection is perivascular cuffing by mononuclear cells.[28, 30] These are predominantly perivenular, although periarteriolar distribution is seen later. The cells are small lymphocytes admixed with larger, transformed-looking lymphocytes. Initially, the infiltrate is 2 to 3 cells thick and is confined to the perivascular adventitia, where there may be very mild edema. Advancing rejection involves endothelial cell hyperplasia with lymphocytic infiltration of the intima, in addition to the perivascular mononuclear cells. Eosinophils, polymorphs, and plasma cells are not conspicuous at this stage.

Increasing intensity of rejection is manifested by more widespread distribution of the infiltrates, which become more prominent and easily visible at scanning magnification (Fig. 8–1). Venules and arterioles both are cuffed, and small airways show similar periadventitial infiltration. The proportion of small, round lymphocytes decreases, with more activated lymphoid cells, eosinophils, and polymorphs present. Endotheliitis is also more frequent, with expansion of the subendothelial layer and, sometimes, reduction of the vascular lumen. Lymphocytes infiltrate through the bronchiolar walls and can be seen within the epithelium (Fig. 8–2). Larger cartilage-containing airways show lymphocytic bronchitis concomitant with this lymphocytic bronchiolitis.[32] This feature is not always seen on transbronchial biopsy samples unless specific endobronchial pieces have been taken.

Frequent cellular infiltrates around vessels and airways are associated with extension of the infiltrates into the alveolar walls and spaces as the severity of rejection increases (Fig. 8–3). At this stage the abnormalities are not likely to be missed by transbronchial sampling, and when the infiltrate extends into alveolar spaces, macrophages can become a prominent component. The interstitial involvement can remain focal or progress to confluent areas ultimately, with hemorrhage, necrosis, and

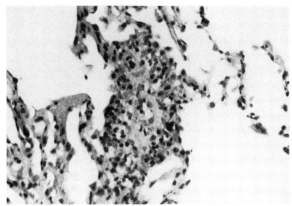

Figure 8–1. Acute pulmonary rejection (mild), showing dense perivascular infiltration around a small vessel. The infiltrate is composed of mononuclear cells with occasional polymorphs, and there is conspicuous endotheliitis. The adjacent parenchyma is unaffected. Grade A2. (Hematoxylin & eosin. High power: transbronchial biopsy)

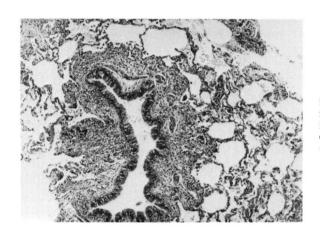

Figure 8–2. Acute lymphocytic bronchiolitis with peribronchial mononuclear cells cuffing small airways and infiltrating intact respiratory epithelium. Perivascular infiltrates were not present in this biopsy specimen. Grade B2. (Hematoxylin & eosin. Medium power: transbronchial biopsy)

Figure 8–3. Acute pulmonary rejection (moderate), showing extension of perivascular infiltrate into adjacent alveolar walls and septa and showing intra-alveolar inflammation. The peripheral areas of the biopsy are unremarkable, confirming that this is not a confluent process. Grade A3. (Hematoxylin & eosin. Low power: transbronchial biopsy)

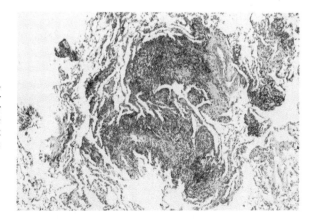

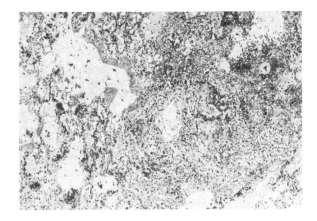

Figure 8–4. Acute pulmonary rejection of severe grade with confluent perivascular infiltrates extending into alveolar septa and spaces; hemorrhage and hyaline membrane formation are present. The central vessel shows endotheliitis. Grade A4 rejection. (Hematoxylin & eosin. Low power: autopsy section)

rarely hyaline membrane formation (Figs. 8–4 and 8–5). This stage is not commonly seen in clinical material on the present immunosuppressive regimens but may occur if immunosuppression is significantly reduced—e.g., for the treatment of lymphoproliferative disease or poor patient compliance.

Noninfiltrative cuffing of airways may similarly progress to a destructive phase, with epithelial ulceration, polymorph infiltration, and necrosis. These histologic phases of acute rejection are similar to those described in animal studies and form the basis for a classification and grading system (vide infra). It must be emphasized that all these features, although characteristic of rejection, are entirely nonspecific, and other causes of pulmonary infiltrates, particularly infectious agents, must be excluded.[28, 30] In the context of clinical lung transplantation, acute rejection often coexists with infection, but the appearances just described were seen in cases in which infection was meticulously excluded.[33]

Perivascular and peribronchiolar infiltrates are often seen together in biopsy material but may occur independently. It is generally accepted that solely perivascular infiltrates are compatible with a histologic diagnosis of acute pulmonary rejection.[26, 28, 34] The significance of peribronchiolar infiltrates or lymphocytic bronchiolitis and bronchitis in the absence of perivascular cuffing is not clear, but they may represent a form of acute rejection directed against the airways.[28] This assumes considerable importance in the context of chronic lung rejection, since the main pathologic abnormality associated with decreased graft survival is obliterative bronchiolitis and not vascular occlusive disease in the present cohorts of patients. Lymphocytic bronchiolitis may represent the progenitor lesion of obliterative bronchiolitis, requiring early recognition and treatment.[35]

MORPHOLOGY OF CHRONIC REJECTION

The long-term survival of pulmonary grafts is limited by a progressive decline in function

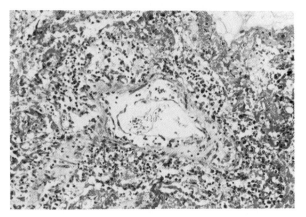

Figure 8–5. High power view of grade A4 rejection (Fig. 8–4), showing extensive endotheliitis, hemorrhage, and hyaline membranes. (Hematoxylin & eosin. High power: autopsy section)

because of obliteration of the airways.[1] Although chronic vascular changes occur similar in all respects to those in other solid organ transplants,[36] it is the progressive obliteration of bronchioles that assumes the greatest clinical importance.[37, 38] The clinical signs and symptoms of this form of chronic lung rejection include cough, copious sputum, and recurrent infections. These infections may be due to common bacterial pathogens or, in many cases, to *Aspergillus*.[30] The radiologic abnormalities include bronchiectasis and lower lobe opacities, which can be particularly well demonstrated on computed tomography. The pulmonary function progressively declines to low values of FEV_1, with little or no improvement on prolonged augmented immunosuppression.[37] These functional changes are due to obliterative bronchiolitis that appears to develop through a sequence of epithelial injury leading to submucosal scarring and finally total obliteration of bronchioles (Fig. 8–6). This fibrotic scarring process involves both membranous and respiratory bronchioles and may be eccentric or concentric, with a residual lumen in the early stages.[28] Ultimately there is total obliteration of the airway lumen by fibrous tissue, which, in the burnt out phase, is acellular. The smooth muscle layers of the bronchioles may be destroyed by extension of the fibrous tissue into the peribronchiolar interstitium, associated with mononuclear cell infiltration of all layers of the bronchiolar wall in the active phase. There may be epithelial damage with lymphocytic infiltration in addition to the fibrosis.[35] Alternatively, the epithelium may be ulcerated, with subepithelial granulation tissue growing into the lumen in a polypoid fashion prior to scarring.

During the active phase of obliterative bronchiolitis, perivascular infiltrates are noted in the adjacent parenchyma. The severity and chronicity of bronchiolar injury due to rejection may be important in the development of obliterative bronchiolitis. Nonrepetitive injury may be associated with re-epithelialization of the bronchiolar mucosa restoring the lumen to normal. Scarring can remain subtotal with only slow progression to a total obliterative phase. The active inflammatory, subtotal forms of obliterative bronchiolitis are the most likely to respond to augmented immunosuppression therapy.[37, 39, 40] The inactive total obliteration is clearly irreversible. In lung biopsies, bronchiolar scarring may be evident only on elastic tissue stains demonstrating proximity of the fibrosed structure to the pulmonary arterioles and delineating the extent of luminal narrowing by submucosal fibrosis.[28, 41] Extensive peribronchiolar fibrosis associated with destruction of the smooth muscle may result in extrinsic compression of the lumen in a constrictive form of obliterative bronchiolitis. The distribution of obliterative bronchiolitis is often patchy, particularly in the early stages, but is generally bilateral, involving all lobes extensively by the time it has caused graft failure.[29, 38]

Obliterative bronchiolitis has many possible causes in lung transplants, but in the context of the pulmonary graft it is likely to be due to rejection. Evidence for this includes the association of obliterative bronchiolitis with severe and frequent acute rejection episodes.[37, 42, 43] Persistence of acute rejection on follow-up transbronchial biopsies after augmented immunosuppression is a risk factor for the development of obliterative bronchiolitis in a lung graft.[44] A further predictor of long-term outcome is the histologic grade of acute rejection.[42, 45] High grades of rejection, however, do not always lead to the development of

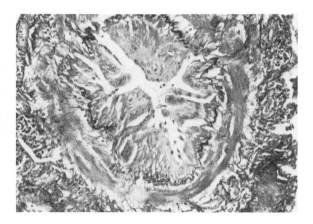

Figure 8–6. Subtotal obliterative bronchiolitis, showing marked reduction in lumen by fibrous tissue internal to bronchiolar elastica. Residual epithelium can be seen. Minimal mononuclear cell infiltration external to this bronchiole is seen, and inflammatory cells are not conspicuous in the submucosal fibrotic tissue. Obliterative bronchiolitis. Grade C1b. (Elastic van Gieson. Medium power: open biopsy)

obliterative bronchiolitis, and in some cases a clinical diagnosis of acute rejection would appear to be a better predictor of outcome.[44] When biopsy material is specifically examined for evidence of airways damage during episodes of acute rejection, there is a better correlation with the development of histologic obliterative bronchiolitis.[42] Intense and persistent rejection damage to bronchioles was associated in this study with subsequent epithelial damage and late airway fibrosis. It is necessary in all these studies to distinguish between clinical and histologic relationships. A clinical diagnosis of obliterative bronchiolitis may not be confirmed by transbronchial biopsy owing to patchiness of the process, particularly in its early phases.[46] Such biopsies, therefore, have poor negative predicter power in the investigation of this long-term graft complication.

The distal respiratory epithelium within the graft is an immune target and has been shown to express class II antigens.[47] Studies have linked the increased expression of class II major histocompatibility complex (MHC) antigens to the development of obliterative bronchiolitis.[48, 49] The induction of class II antigen expression on the bronchial epithelium is not specific to rejection and may be caused by infection, particularly viral and pneumocystic. Lymphocyte alloreactivity may also be nonspecifically upregulated following an infectious episode.[50] Animal studies have demonstrated a relationship between the extent of bronchiolar damage and degree of histocompatibility mismatch.[51] Harjula and associates found that their longest surviving lung transplant patient who did not develop obliterative bronchiolitis had the closest HLA match, compared with other heart-lung recipients.[24] Positive primed lymphocyte tests correlate with both histologic and functional obstructive airway disease in the pulmonary graft.[50] The importance of acute rejection directed at the bronchiolar epithelium in the development of obliterative bronchiolitis is confirmed by the beneficial effect of augmented immunosuppression in slowing the progression of this fibrosing condition.[32, 37, 40, 52]

Certain infectious agents have been implicated in the development of obliterative bronchiolitis in the nontransplanted population, particularly viruses, including respiratory syncytial virus, adenovirus, mycoplasma, and chlamydia.[53, 54] It is well documented that lung transplant recipients have a greatly increased susceptibility to infection by both common pathogens and opportunistic organisms,[55, 56]

and the possibility of an infectious cause for obliterative bronchiolitis must be seriously considered. Chronic persistent epithelial injury as a result of infection with inadequate healing could lead to submucosal granulation tissue and eventual total obliteration. Cytomegalovirus (CMV) has been suggested as a cause of obliterative bronchiolitis in graft recipients, since it can produce this pathologic manifestation in the nonimmunosuppressed host.[57] CMV infection has been reported to be a risk factor in some but not all lung transplant centers.[58-60] There is a higher incidence of obliterative bronchiolitis in seropositive recipients and mismatched recipients, particularly when there has been well-documented CMV pneumonitis.[59] The mechanism by which CMV increases the risk of chronic rejection is not yet elucidated. Cytokine release may lead to increased expression of class II antigens on epithelial and endothelial cells.[61, 62] Such an increase in expression of class II antigens on bronchial epithelium has been associated with obliterative bronchiolitis in human lung transplant recipients.[47] Alternatively, CMV may directly injure the graft or induce the formation of cross-reactive antibodies. The acute lung damage associated with active CMV pneumonitis may be related to activation of both macrophages and cytotoxic cells within the lung.[61]

Further evidence that obliterative bronchiolitis is a manifestation of chronic rejection is its frequent occurrence in nontransplant patients with immunologic lung disease. Obliterative bronchiolitis is well described in the collagen vascular diseases and has also been reported in bone marrow transplant recipients who have experienced graft versus host disease.[53, 63] Another suggested cause for obliterative bronchiolitis of a nonimmunologic nature includes ligation of the bronchial circulation, perhaps leading to inadequate healing after acute rejection or infection. Against this is the absence of obliterative bronchiolitis in experimental autografts. Larger cartilaginous airways do, however, show degenerative changes in the late postoperative period, which could be partly due to ischemia. The surgical procedure of transplantation also results in denervation of the graft and interruption of lymphatic drainage. The most significant effect is likely to be the loss of cough reflex leading to retention of secretions and an increased risk of pulmonary infections.[39]

Obliterative bronchiolitis in the grafted lung is commonly seen as a rather acellular fibrosing process. The accompanying mononuclear cell infiltrate is limited to the peribronchial and perivascular tissue unless the obliterative bronchiolitis is accompanied by high grade superimposed acute rejection or parenchymal infection.[30] Obliterative bronchiolitis in non-immunosuppressed patients is usually more cellular and associated with chronic interstitial pneumonitis. The latter form of obliterative bronchiolitis, however, does exist in lung transplant recipients, probably as a result of infection, and may overlap with chronic organizing pneumonia.[64, 65] In this condition, granulation tissue is present in the distal airspaces, often cellular and polypoid in configuration (Fig. 8–7). The process may be more patchily distributed than pure rejection-related bronchiolitis obliterans, and there may be foreign material and giant cells indicating likely aspiration.[64]

The large, cartilage-containing airways are affected by chronic rejection in association with the distal bronchiolitis obliterans. Bronchitis and bronchiectasis are common, with cylindric dilatation and viscid retained secretions. Acute and chronic inflammation of the airways is associated with extensive squamous metaplasia, lymphocytic infiltration of mucosa and submucosa with scarring and loss of submucosal glands.[29, 38, 66, 67] Replacement of smooth muscle by fibrous tissue is important in the dilatation of these larger airways, which can be demonstrated by specimen bronchography.[66] Individual epithelial cell necrosis is observed in association with Leu 7 positive lymphocytes in the donor tracheal and proximal bronchial epithelium.[68, 69] The obliterative fibrosing process may extend from bronchioles to involve proximal small cartilage-containing airways, thus giving the appearance of obliterative bronchitis.

Another manifestation of chronic rejection is vascular fibrointimal proliferation and sclerosis.[28, 36] The pathologic appearance of this condition is essentially similar to the proliferative vascular sclerosis of other solid organ grafts and involves both large elastic and smaller muscular vessels. As with obliterative bronchiolitis, the fibrous obliteration may be active, with marked cellularity and subendothelial and transmural infiltrates or it may be burnt out and sclerotic (Figs. 8–8 and 8–9). In the early active phases, endotheliitis with hyperplasia of the overlying endothelial cells may be present. The fibrointimal thickening often involves veins, but in these vessels the process is generally more sclerotic and acellular (Fig. 8–10). There is some correlation with obliterative bronchiolitis, but generally the airway fibrosis is both clinically and pathologically more significant than the vascular changes.[44] In combined heart-lung grafts, pulmonary vascular occlusive disease may correlate with coronary occlusive disease, but many of the heart-lung transplants monitored by transbronchial biopsies have shown chronic pulmonary rejection without evidence of coronary artery disease. This may be related to augmented immunosuppression when acute pulmonary rejection has been detected on diagnostic and surveillance biopsy material, reducing the incidence of cardiac rejection.

Chronic rejection probably results from different mechanisms to acute rejection affecting vessels, but there does seem to be a relationship between previous persistent and severe rejection and development of occlusive vascular disease. Chronic vascular rejection may develop on the basis of preservation injury and damage to the endothelium or even as a result of donor vascular pathology. A study of unused donor lungs demonstrated a high incidence of organizing thromboemboli, as well as fat and

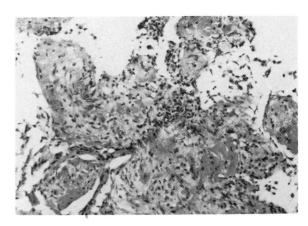

Figure 8–7. Organizing pneumonia seen on transbronchial biopsy with fibrosing granulation tissue present in distal air spaces and associated with interstitial inflammation. This is a nonspecific histologic picture and should be distinguished from obliterative bronchiolitis without distal organization. (Hematoxylin & eosin. Medium power: transbronchial biopsy)

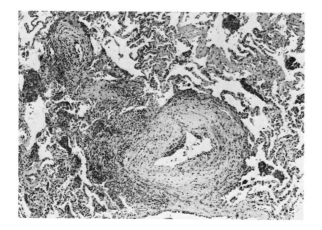

Figure 8–8. Small pulmonary artery showing vasculopathy of chronic rejection. There is a transmural infiltrate of mononuclear cells, including active endotheliitis. The vessel wall is thickened, particularly the intima. Adjacent parenchyma contained sclerotic veins and venules as well as interstitial inflammatory cells. (Hematoxylin & eosin. Medium power: open lung biopsy)

Figure 8–9. Partial occlusion of a pulmonary arteriole by fibrous cellular intimal proliferation. The adventitia is free from inflammation. Grade D vascular occlusive disease. (Hematoxylin & eosin. Medium power: open biopsy)

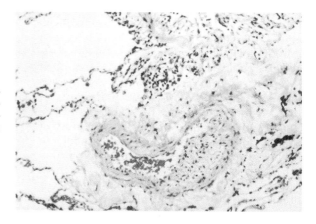

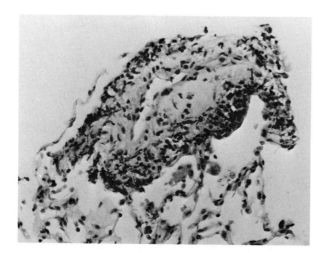

Figure 8–10. Perivascular mononuclear cell infiltrate around a vein with mild endotheliitis and hyaline intimal sclerosis. (Hematoxylin & eosin. High power: transbronchial biopsy)

bone marrow emboli that may have initiated damage onto which the features of chronic rejection are superimposed. Pulmonary occlusive disease has a patchy distribution but usually affects the vessel in a circumferential pattern of intimal proliferation. There is fragmentation of the internal elastic lamina with attenuation of the media. Lipid and cholesterol are deposited in plaques that may show cellular infiltration by lymphocytes, macrophages, and plasma cells. The significance of chronic vascular rejection of the lung is not yet certain.[42] It has been described in open biopsy and autopsy material of patients surviving longer than 3 months in the presence of normal pulmonary vascular pressure measurements.[42, 44] Only when obliterative bronchiolitis has been overcome as a long-term complication will it be possible to assess the clinical and pathologic significance of vascular occlusion in these patients. At present the chronic airways changes are the dominant factor in survival.

CLASSIFICATION AND GRADING OF LUNG REJECTION

The histologic features of acute lung rejection can be graded according to semiquantitative and semiqualitative assessments of the nature and extent of the infiltrates. A standardized nomenclature has been developed by the Lung Rejection Study Group on behalf of the International Society for Heart and Lung Transplantation.[28] This grading system has been based primarily on transbronchial biopsy specimens and is a histologic classification independent of clinical information, having excluded infection (Table 8–1). Individual transplant centers have developed their own grading systems, most of which can be incorporated within the Working Formulation. This means that data can be compared among institutions for the promotion of improved patient care. Acute rejection is graded according to the nature and frequency of perivascular mononuclear infiltrates. Four grades are recognized, corresponding to minimal, mild, moderate, and severe acute rejection. Within each grade a suffix denotes the presence (a) or absence (b) of bronchiolar inflammation, large airway inflammation (c), or the absence of bronchioles in the tissue examined (d).

Grade A1 (minimal acute rejection) comprises scattered, infrequent perivascular mononuclear infiltrates that are not obvious at scan-

Table 8–1. Working Formulation for Classification and Grading of Pulmonary Rejection

Grade A: acute rejection
  (1) Minimal acute rejection
  (2) Mild acute rejection
  (3) Moderate acute rejection
  (4) Severe acute rejection
    (a) With evidence of bronchiolar inflammation
    (b) Without evidence of bronchiolar inflammation
    (c) With large airway inflammation
    (d) No bronchioles are present

Grade B: active airway damage without scarring
  (1) Lymphocytic bronchitis
  (2) Lymphocytic bronchiolitis

Grade C: chronic airway rejection
  (1) Bronchiolitis obliterans, subtotal
  (2) Bronchiolitis obliterans, total
    (a) Active
    (b) Inactive

Grade D: chronic vascular rejection

Grade E: vasculitis

From Yousem SA, Berry GJ, Brunt EM, et al. A working formulation for the standardisation of nomenclature in the diagnosis of heart and lung rejection: Lung Rejection Study Group. J Heart Transplant 9:593, 1990.

ning magnification. The infiltrates are found particularly around venules and consist of small round lymphocytes, including transformed lymphocytes; they form a cuff of not more than three cells in thickness in the perivascular adventitia. Eosinophils may be present but scanty in this grade. *Grade A2* (mild acute rejection) shows larger, more frequent infiltrates that are readily recognized at low magnification. More activated lymphocytes are present together with macrophages and eosinophils, and there is frequently subendothelial infiltration by these mononuclear cells, resulting in endotheliitis. The perivascular interstitium may be expanded, but there is no infiltration of mononuclear cells into the adjacent alveolar septa or air spaces. Lymphocytic bronchiolitis is more common with this than in the minimal grade. *Grade A3* (moderate acute rejection) is defined by extension of the mononuclear cell infiltrate into perivascular and peribronchiolar alveolar septa and spaces. Occasional neutrophils are seen in addition to the other cellular components, and there is nearly always an associated endotheliitis. The overlying endothelium may show hyperplastic or degenerative changes. *Grade A4* (severe acute rejection) shows confluent diffuse infiltrates of perivascular interstitial and alveolar tissues. Alveolar epithelial cell damage is present, with hemorrhage, neutrophils, and sometimes hyaline membranes. Parenchymal necrosis, infarction, or necrotizing vasculitis (seen on open biopsy) may be associated with these changes.

Active airway damage without fibrous scarring is likely to be a form of cellular rejection directed at the airways.[4, 28, 35] There are no perivascular infiltrates to allow classification under acute rejection grades A1 to A4. Large and small airway inflammation without fibrous scarring or perivascular infiltrates may be the progenitor lesions for chronic airway rejection, and it may be that the identification of this separate grade helps predict those patients who will go on to develop obliterative bronchiolitis. Lymphocytic bronchitis (B1) shows mononuclear cell infiltration of mucosa and submucosa of cartilage-containing airways, with submucosal gland and epithelial injury. Squamous metaplasia may be seen. Lymphocytic bronchiolitis (B2) represents the same process involving terminal and respiratory bronchioles.

Obliterative bronchiolitis is now thought to represent chronic airway rejection of the lung graft[37, 42–45] and can be classified according to the extent of the obliteration and presence or absence of inflammatory cell infiltration. Subtotal bronchiolitis obliterans (C1) may be eccentric or concentric but retains some bronchiolar lumen. In the active phase (C1a), intra- and/or peribronchiolar mononuclear infiltrates occur with epithelial damage that is not present in the inactive (C1b) phase. Total obliteration (C2) similarly can be classified as active (a) or inactive (b).

Chronic vascular rejection is categorized separately (D), with fibrointimal thickening of arteries and veins as the characteristic abnormality. Vasculitis (E) is not usually seen on transbronchial biopsy material but has been described in open biopsies. The vessel wall shows areas of necrosis with inflammatory cell infiltration disproportionate to adjacent parenchymal inflammatory changes. This may be a form of acute rejection involving larger vessels than venules and arterioles.

This classification of acute and chronic rejection allows the pathologist to label the process by appropriate letters and numerals. Acute and chronic rejection may coexist, leading to grades such as A2a with C1a and D. Details of the grading are illustrated in the Working Formulation.[28]

The Working Formulation makes several recommendations. 1, Follow-up biopsies should be classified as ongoing, resolving, or resolved rejection when compared with a previous biopsy. 2, The grading can be applied only if a minimum number of transbronchial biopsies containing pulmonary parenchyma have been submitted. The optimum number to evaluate lung allograft rejection is uncertain,[4] but five parenchymal specimens are thought to reduce the risk of missing significant rejection to an acceptable level. 3, At least three levels should be examined with hematoxylin and eosin stains. Connective tissue stains are mandatory for the evaluation of chronic vascular and airway damage and should include an elastic stain as well as a trichrome stain. Also mandatory is a silver stain for *Pneumocystis* and fungi since the former, in particular, may closely mimic lung rejection.[70] Further stains for infectious agents, e.g. Ziehl-Neelsen, are optional, as are immunoperoxidase and in situ hybridization studies for viral pathogens, cytokines, and class II antigens. 4, Also within the recommendations are the lengthy differential diagnoses of both perivascular and interstitial mononuclear infiltrates and of submucosal airway scarring. These will be discussed in a later section. The final recommendation relates to those circumstances in which the biopsies show a mixture of rejection and infection. With experience, the pathologist may be able to indicate infection or rejection as the predominant process even though they cannot always be reliably distinguished. Re-biopsy may be the only way of correctly classifying the episode.

In practice, the grading system has been relatively straightforward to use in our institution. The rejection grades have been easily translated into simple letters and numerals for the generation of a large data base comprising details of all transbronchial biopsies performed on lung transplant recipients. It is essential that all microbiologic and serologic data are reviewed before the final classification can be made of a transbronchial biopsy as showing a particular rejection grade. This is because infection is a major problem in the histologic assessment of lung recipient biopsies, potentially limiting usefulness of such a classification.

We studied 100 consecutive transbronchial biopsy sections, analyzing histopathologic appearances in conjunction with microbiologic and serologic data.[71] These biopsies were obtained from 43 patients with clinical indications and also routine surveillance. Specimens from either the bronchoalveolar lavage (BAL) or transbronchial lung samples were sent for viral culture, including cultures for cytomegalovirus (CMV) and herpes simplex virus (HSV). Direct early antigen fluorescent focus (DEAFF) tests were performed for detection of CMV. Serologic studies and cultures were also performed to exclude *Toxoplasma*, adenovirus, influenza virus, *Mycoplasma, Legionella*, and Epstein-Barr virus (EBV) according to clinical suspicion. Microbiologic data for all specimens taken 2 days prior to and 2 days following the transbronchial biopsy were also reviewed and these included sputa, blood cultures, and throat swabs.

From these 100 biopsies, 76 were assigned a rejection grade at the time of histologic reporting. The commonest grade was mild acute rejection—that is, grade A2, and no cases of severe acute rejection were seen. In 22 of these 76 transbronchial biopsies, the caveat "exclude infection" was included in the histologic report. Analysis of the microbiologic data showed 8 of these 22 cases to have significant positive cultures. In addition, 14 of the 54 cases confidently graded as showing rejection with no histologic suspicion of infection had positive cultures or serology. Biopsy material that subsequently showed microbiologic evidence of concomitant infection did not show an excess of airways inflammation (suffix a or c). This may be because the respiratory infections diagnosed microbiologically involved upper airways proximal to those sampled in the transbronchial biopsy procedure. Rejection-related airways inflammation would appear not to be confused with airways infection in the majority of these biopsies. Rejection could not be assessed in 24 transbronchial biopsies, 2 of which were inadequate owing to lack of lung parenchyma and previous biopsy site. The remaining 22 nongradable biopsies had histologic evidence of infection that was confirmed by the appropriate culture or serology in 20 cases. The two cases initially thought to be infective but not confirmed showed features suggestive of viral pneumonitis in one case and a nonspecific pneumonitis in the other.

This study highlights the problem of infection in this group of patients. From these 100 consecutive biopsies, 54 were assigned a final grade of rejection retrospectively with no evidence of concomitant infection. This, however, does not detract from the usefulness of biopsies in diagnosing and grading rejection for the immediate management of the patient, since the cases in which infection was thought to be complicating rejection were treated with increased immunosuppression together with appropriate antimicrobial therapy. The study also highlights the usefulness of transbronchial biopsy in the diagnosis of pulmonary infections in lung transplant patients and the high specificity of the histologic appearances of infection in ungradable biopsies.[41, 71]

The use of the Working Formulation has also enabled a study of the diagnosis of chronic rejection in transbronchial biopsies. Chronic rejection was seen in 147 biopsies from a total of 961 transbronchial biopsies, only 26 of which were inadequate or inappropriate. Both chronic airways and chronic vascular rejection were present in 37 biopsies, chronic airways rejection alone in 35, and chronic vascular rejection alone in the remaining 75. The commonest C grade was C1a, subtotal active obliterative bronchiolitis. This was seen in 27 biopsies without concomitant vascular rejection and in a further 27 biopsies with vascular occlusive disease. This confirms the usefulness of transbronchial biopsy in the diagnosis of chronic rejection.[46] In the same series of biopsies, grade B rejection was noted in 18 biopsies. Four of these biopsies showed lymphocytic bronchitis and fourteen showed lymphocytic bronchiolitis, four of which were seen in conjunction with chronic airways and chronic vascular rejection. This latter association will be important to follow as increasing numbers of patients survive long enough to develop chronic graft rejection.

OPPORTUNISTIC INFECTION IN THE GRAFTED LUNG

The transplanted lung is highly susceptible to infection by both normal and opportunistic pathogens.[55, 72, 73] Some of these infections, particulary in the early postoperative period, may be donor acquired as a result of either prolonged ventilation or aspiration. Reactivation of donor latent infection may occur in the new recipient, this being of particular importance in herpes virus infections.[74] Infection is the main differential diagnosis of acute rejection and may coexist with it.[28] The Stanford and Pittsburgh groups have reported over 87 per cent of heart-lung transplant recipients experiencing infectious episodes.[55, 72] These are mainly bacterial infections of the lungs and thoracic cavity. The high rate of common bacterial and opportunistic infections in the grafted lung may be due to decreased mucociliary clearance, absent cough reflex, and augmented immunosuppression given for the treatment of acute rejection episodes. The bronchopulmonary defenses may be lowered further by the depletion of bronchus-associated lymphoid tissue (BALT).[75] This lymphoid tissue plays an important role in local pulmonary immunity and may also be a target of allograft rejection. The lung is unusual among transplanted organs in that it contains a significant amount of lymphoid tissue. Hruban and colleagues have evaluated BALT using immunoperoxidase techniques in heart-lung recipients, quantifying the number of immunoglobulin-bearing plasma cells in the lamina propria on both native trachea and donor main stem bronchus. Lung allograft rejection was associated with a marked depletion of IgA- and IgG-bearing plasma cells, which was not mirrored in the native tracheas.[75] This implies that it is not simply a manifestation of the immunosuppressive therapy. Another factor in the high incidence of infections in the transplanted lung is its direct exposure to the numerous environmental pathogens.

Cytomegalovirus is a significant viral pathogen causing both morbidity and mortality to lung transplant recipients.[58, 74] The virus may also act as a modulator of rejection.[62] CMV disease is the most common serious infection affecting this group of patients, often causing death from CMV pneumonia.[39, 58] Heart-lung transplant recipients are more susceptible to CMV pneumonia than are other solid organ recipients,[76] and there is also an association between CMV infections and other opportunistic pathogens.[77] CMV infection can be introduced by seropositive donor lungs or by positive blood products. Donor and recipient matching for CMV status reduces the incidence of primary CMV transmitted by the donor organs. Before the introduction of this matching policy, primary CMV infection from the donor usually caused a fatal pneumonitis with evidence of systemic CMV infection in other organs.[58] With the incidence of primary CMV disease in these patients having been reduced, CMV reactivation has become a more common problem. Transbronchial biopsies are often used to diagnose CMV in the grafted lung.[41] This may be during episodes of clinical illness, or the disease may be detected in follow-up or routine surveillance biopsies.

It is important to distinguish the histologic features of CMV infection (Fig. 8–11), in which CMV inclusions are identified without any evidence of associated inflammatory reaction, from CMV pneumonia in which the characteristic inclusions are associated with an active pneumonitis[26] (Fig. 8–12). The former condition may not require treatment. Lack of differentiation between CMV infection and CMV pneumonitis makes comparison of data between different centers difficult and, in particular, the relationship of CMV to other graft complications, including obliterative bronchiolitis. In our center, the following definitions are in use: CMV *pneumonia* is defined by characteristic CMV inclusions in the lung, with an active inflammatory infiltrate indicating that the virus is indeed the cause of the pneumonitis. CMV *infection* is the identification of CMV from an organ, serologic reactivation, or seroconversion. Identification of CMV includes the presence of inclusions in tissue specimens and lavage fluid. The histologic features of CMV pneumonitis in the transplanted lung are those of diffuse viral alveolitis with polymorphonuclear cell infiltrates, some of which form microabscesses, diffuse alveolar cell hyperplasia, and sometimes hyaline mem-

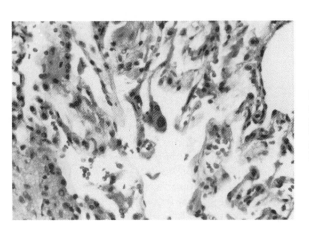

Figure 8–11. A single CMV-infected alveolar epithelial cell is present in the center of the field, with no evidence of significant inflammation in surrounding parenchyma. This indicates CMV infection rather than active CMV pneumonitis and may not be clinically significant. (Hematoxylin & eosin. High power: transbronchial biopsy)

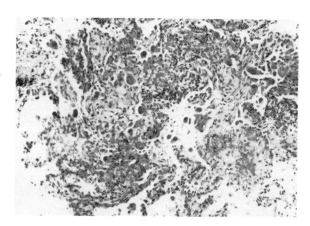

Figure 8–12. Active CMV pneumonitis with numerous intranuclear and cytoplasmic inclusions typical of cytomegalovirus. The interstitium shows inflammatory cell infiltration with both mononuclear cells and polymorphs, and there is intra-alveolar hemorrhage and fibrin. This diffuse alveolitis in which viral inclusions are related to the inflammation is easily distinguished from rejection. (Hematoxylin & eosin. Medium power: transbronchial biopsy)

branes[78] (Fig. 8–13). The characteristic inclusions are both intranuclear "owl's eye" and cytoplasmic granular inclusions, which are often obvious even on low power magnification.

In the early stages of reactivation or primary infection, the diagnosis of CMV pneumonitis may be suggested even in the absence of these characteristic inclusions by the features of viral alveolitis, perivascular edema, and neutrophil microabscesses. These features may also allow differentiation from acute lung rejection.[26] The most useful features in this regard are the perivascular edema and lack of tight perivascular cuffing by the cellular infiltrate. Also, diffusely infiltrating polymorphs or focal collections of polymorphs in the form of microabscesses are not features of acute rejection and should stimulate a search for viral changes, including inclusions. There are occasions, however, when rejection and CMV pneumonitis coexist, and treatment may have to be given for both with careful follow-up, including further transbronchial biopsies, until clinical and histologic resolution is achieved.

CMV pneumonia is known to show perivascular infiltrates similar to those of acute pulmonary rejection.[70] This has been described in a review of 42 biopsies of immunosuppressed, nontransplant patients. Three cases of CMV pneumonia showed striking perivascular infiltrates thought to be indistinguishable from those of lung rejection. Similar perivascular infiltrates were also seen in a case of combined CMV and *Pneumocystis carinii* pneumonia (PCP). The occurrence of perivascular infiltrates in CMV pneumonia has been underemphasized in pathologic descriptions of this condition in nontransplanted patients. However, it is of considerable importance when this infection occurs in a lung graft and needs to be distinguished from rejection. It is also a potential area of difficulty in distinguishing with certainty CMV infection from CMV pneumonitis. Tazelaar did not find any correlation between the tissue cellularity or the histologic pattern of pneumonia and the presence of perivascular inflammatory cell infiltrates.[70]

The histologic diagnoses of CMV infection and disease in these patients pose a challeng-

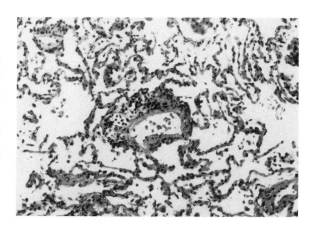

Figure 8–13. Perivascular and interstitial infiltrates consisting of mononuclear cells and significant numbers of polymorphs scattered throughout alveolar walls. Endotheliitis is not prominent. Elsewhere in this biopsy there were perivascular edema and enlarged alveolar epithelial cells, suggestive of CMV reactivation in the transplanted lung. The low power similarity to acute pulmonary rejection is striking. Serology studies confirmed CMV reactivation. (Hematoxylin & eosin. Low power: transbronchial biopsy)

ing problem because of these overlapping histologic features and the fact that pulmonary rejection has characteristic but not specific appearances (Fig. 8–13).

Further problems are encountered when the patient is already receiving antiviral therapy (ganciclovir or acyclovir). These drugs are frequently given prophylactically in the early postoperative weeks when the patient is likely to have increased immunosuppression. This prophylactic treatment reduces the clinical incidence of CMV and HSV infections in the graft and modifies the appearances of the intracellular inclusions of both these viruses. Inclusions may be recognized as viral in nature but without the characteristic CMV owl's eye appearance and with reduced intracytoplasmic inclusions. Sometimes the viral inclusions do not develop sufficiently to be recognized as such, but the cell nuclei appear rather eosinophilic and degenerate (Fig. 8–14). Also, under these conditions the inclusions of HSV and CMV may be indistinguishable.

Good clinicopathologic correlation is essential for the accurate diagnosis of transbronchial biopsies from these patients, and serologic information may be helpful. Special techniques such as immunohistochemistry and in situ hybridization may aid detection and differentiation of these viruses, improving the diagnosis of histologically confirmed infection.[79, 80] However, there are limitations to the usefulness of these techniques. The increased sensitivity of CMV detection may not solve the histologic dilemma of infection versus pneumonitis and may be disappointing in the yield of additional information. In a seropositive immunosuppressed patient, it is to be expected that occasional CMV-positive cells can be identified in tissue by these methods, and the clinical significance may be doubtful. There may be a role for these more sensitive techniques in the investigation of nonspecific pneumonitis and in the assessment of patients suffering CMV and HSV infections concomitantly.

The impact of CMV infection in heart-lung transplant recipients has been described.[58, 74] The CMV serologic status of the donor is important only if the recipient is CMV seronegative. When a seropositive donor organ was transplanted into a seronegative recipient, CMV pneumonia occurred frequently (64 per cent), with a high case fatality (57 per cent).[58] The frequency of CMV pneumonia was identical in seropositive recipients irrespective of donor serologic status. This implies that graft-associated transmission in this transplant population is of minor importance.[58] Associations were demonstrated between augmented immunosuppression for the treatment of rejection within the preceding 30 days and the development of CMV pneumonia. CMV infection and pneumonia are associated with frequent pulmonary superinfections, including bacterial pneumonia and bronchitis. This may be due to increased immunosuppression predisposing to CMV or to an immunosuppressive effect of the CMV itself. CMV pneumonia is most frequently encountered in the first 3 months post-transplant; early biopsy diagnosis and treatment by ganciclovir has improved the survival rate from this complication, reducing both morbidity and mortality. The effect on the development of obliterative bronchiolitis remains to be seen.

Herpes simplex virus (HSV) is another op-

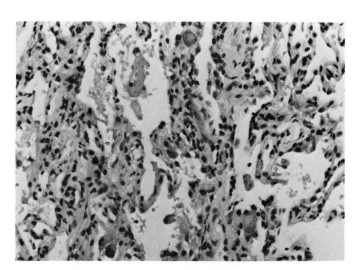

Figure 8–14. Diffuse viral alveolitis with mixed inflammatory infiltration, including conspicuous polymorphs. Alveolar epithelial cells contain viable intranuclear inclusions together with degenerate inclusions that are less hematoxyphilic. (Hematoxylin & eosin. High power: transbronchial biopsy)

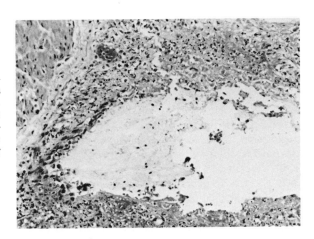

Figure 8–15. Ulcerated bronchiole with necrotic lining and luminal debris. Intranuclear viral inclusions are present (left) in the degenerate epithelial cells. Similar lesions were present in the trachea and main stem bronchi, and there was a necrotizing bronchopneumonia in which sparse herpetic inclusions were seen. (Hematoxylin & eosin. Medium power: autopsy section)

portunistic infection of the transplanted lung that often follows a period of augmented immunosuppression for rejection. In these circumstances, it may be associated with the characteristic intraoral lesions, alerting the clinician and pathologist to the possibility of an HSV pneumonia. It can be largely avoided by the use of prophylactic acyclovir. The histologic diagnosis is often more difficult than that of CMV pneumonitis. The features of HSV infection are those of bronchitis, bronchiolitis (Fig. 8–15), and bronchopneumonia, which may be distinguishable from the diffuse interstitial viral alveolitis of CMV pneumonia. The presence of necrosis and lack of cytomegaly are useful in distinguishing these two causes of viral pneumonia, but diagnostic inclusions of HSV may be very difficult to find.[77] The nuclear inclusions of HSV pneumonia are more eosinophilic than are CMV inclusions. Cytoplasmic inclusions indicate CMV. The characteristic features of HSV, however, are not as well developed in the respiratory tract as they are in the female genital tract: diagnosis may be improved by the use of immunohistochemical and DNA probe methods.[80] Herpes simplex virus infection usually occurs in the first 8 weeks of transplantation when immunosuppression is augmented. HSV may be concomitant with CMV and also with another herpes virus, EBV. One fatal case of disseminated HSV infection in our unit showed necrotizing tracheobronchitis, pneumonia, hepatitis, and esophagitis. This patient had been earlier treated for a concomitant CMV pneumonia, but there was no histologic evidence of residual CMV disease in either the grafted or nontransplanted tissues.

Pneumocystis carinii is an important opportunistic pathogen in lung transplant recipients. It has a very high frequency in some centers.[72]

The diagnosis of this infectious complication depends on histologic or cytologic assessment of material from the grafted lung. The typical histologic appearance of *Pneumocystis carinii* pneumonia (PCP) as described in AIDS patients is that of abundant intra-alveolar foamy exudate with variable interstitial inflammation.[81] Cysts are numerous and can be suspected on the hematoxylin and eosin sections by the honeycomb nature of the intra-alveolar exudate and confirmed on Grocott silver staining. In contrast, the histologic reaction in lung transplant recipients is more commonly granulomatous.[27, 30] There is interstitial inflammation, with collections of histiocytes, and well-formed epithelioid granulomas, with giant cells in some cases. Plasma cells are often strikingly numerous, and there is mild edema of the alveolar walls. Polymorphs are not a feature.

This granulomatous reaction is associated with relatively small numbers of cysts, which are usually within the granulomatous areas. They may form small clusters or occur singly and require lengthy high power screening for their diagnosis. The lack of abundant organisms within the airspaces is reflected in the paucity of pneumocysts found in the accompanying BAL samples. In some cases the organisms may be present only on the biopsy samples, and reliance on lavage cytology may lead to underdiagnosis of this complication. The small number of pneumocysts and the histologic mimicking of acute rejection make mandatory the meticulous screening of a silver stain section of all transbronchial biopsy material.[28, 70] In his study of perivascular inflammation in pulmonary infections in immunosuppressed but nontransplant patients, Tazelaar described 33 cases of *Pneumocystis* pneumonia in which 7 (21 per cent) showed perivascular mononuclear cell infiltration.[70] The infiltrates included small, round lymphocytes and macrophages with some activated lymphocytes. Eosinophils were noted, as were neutrophils. Plasma cells were found in 94 per cent of cases of *Pneumocystis* pneumonia but in only 43 per cent of cases of CMV pneumonia.

The reason for the granulomatous response to *Pneumocystis* in lung transplants is not clear. Atypical histologic reactions to *Pneumocystis* are well described[81] and are increasingly recognized in the large group of AIDS patients, especially in extrapulmonary *Pneumocystis* infections.[82] Granulomatous *Pneumocystis* does not appear to be related to the use of cyclosporine, as cardiac transplant recipients in our institution show typical intra-alveolar cysts (Table 8–2). The incidence of PCP is reduced by prophylaxis to cover periods of increased immunosuppression. It is not clear whether *Pneumocystis* represents a reactivation of latent infection in the donor lungs or new primary infection.[83] It has been noted to occur in clusters of patients at our institution.

Aspergillus infection is a significant and increasing problem in lung transplant recipients.[30] This fungus produces a range of diseases similar to those seen in nonimmunosuppressed patients.[84] *Aspergillus* may colonize the large airways of lung allografts saprophytically, and this is particularly the case when these have become bronchiectatic due to the combination of repeated infections and the development of obliterative bronchiolitis. In this type of *Aspergillus* infection, hyphae may be seen in the lavage and cultured without being present in the transbronchial biopsy. The fungus may not cause active disease under these circumstances, but its presence is a risk for more invasive disease when immunosuppression is increased or obliterative bron-

Table 8–2. Histologic Features of *Pneumocystis carinii* Pneumonia in 30 Transbronchial Biopsies from Transplant Recipients

	Lung Transplant*	Heart Transplant
Total number in group	10	12
Granuloma/ granulomatous	8	6
Intra-alveolar foam Organisms	4	9
Scanty	3	0
Intermediate	6	7
Numerous	1	5

*Eight biopsies from six heart-lung transplant patients and two biopsies from a single lung transplant patient, one transplant, one own lung.

chiolitis advances. *Aspergillus* in the large airways may become locally invasive, particularly in the region of the anastomosis where it can cause ulceration and pseudomembrane formation and is prone to invade ischemic cartilage (Fig. 8–16).[85, 86] This can be a serious complication leading to dehiscence of the anastomosis, dissemination of the fungus to other organs, or both. The fungus may be demonstrated in endobronchial biopsies or biopsies of the tracheal anastomosis, depending on the nature of the transplant. Any evidence of tissue necrosis, particularly ischemic cartilage, should prompt a search for invasion by *Aspergillus* hyphae.

In single lung transplants, in which there may be a greater ischemic problem with the bronchial anastomosis than in the well-vascularized lower tracheal anatomosis of heart-lung transplants,[87] the locally invasive *Aspergillus* disease is confined to the side of the graft. This emphasizes the importance of local defense

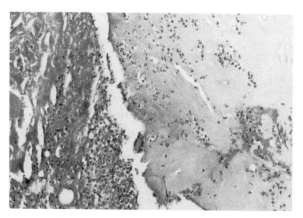

Figure 8–16. Necrotic cartilage in a bronchial biopsy specimen from an anastomotic area of a single lung transplant. Fungal hyphae were present in the acute inflammatory fibrinous exudate adjacent to the ischemic cartilage, and these were characteristic of *Aspergillus* spp on Grocott stain (not shown). This ulcerative tracheobronchial tree *Aspergillus* infection is associated with dehiscence and fungal dissemination. (Hematoxylin & eosin. Medium power: bronchial biopsy)

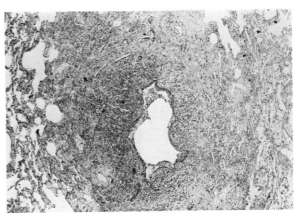

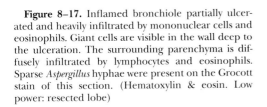

Figure 8–17. Inflamed bronchiole partially ulcerated and heavily infiltrated by mononuclear cells and eosinophils. Giant cells are visible in the wall deep to the ulceration. The surrounding parenchyma is diffusely infiltrated by lymphocytes and eosinophils. Sparse *Aspergillus* hyphae were present on the Grocott stain of this section. (Hematoxylin & eosin. Low power: resected lobe)

factors and risk factors such as ischemia. It is not a risk of immunosuppression per se. Another manifestation of large airways disease due to *Aspergillus* is tracheobronchial obstruction by a noninvading mass of fungal hyphae. This is distinguished from the previous condition by lack of tissue invasion or associated necrotic tissue, particularly cartilage. The material is usually obvious at bronchoscopy as it forms obstructing, cream-colored masses and can be lavaged as well as biopsied. This obstructive form of fungal disease may resolve completely on treatment, and it is therefore very important to recognize it as a noninvasive form.[30, 86]

Lung transplant recipients can develop bronchocentric granulomatous mycosis in the segmental and subsegmental bronchi. In this condition the fungal fragments are associated with a giant cell granulomatous response.[88] The chronic granulomatous reaction is centered on cartilage-containing airways, although it can be seen in bronchioles (Fig. 8–17). The walls of the airways may be partially destroyed

and identifiable only by the use of elastic tissue stains. There is usually central necrosis, with prominent palisading of macrophages peripherally (Fig. 8–18). The frequency of giant cells in this condition is variable. The inflammatory cell infiltrate also includes lymphocytes, neutrophils, and plasma cells, with eosinophils occurring in variable numbers. Bronchocentric granulomatous mycosis in the transplant recipient can be associated with eosinophilic pneumonia in the surrounding lung parenchyma. In some cases, particularly at autopsy, this may be the dominant histologic feature, with only small areas of granuloma formation in airways and few fungal hyphae demonstrated. Grocott stains demonstrate branching septate fungal hyphae, usually centered in the necrotic areas but with variable penetration of the granulomatous bronchial wall. This condition therefore appears to be intermediate between the saprophytic and obstructing forms seen in the larger airways and frankly invasive *Aspergillus*. It is interesting that one of our patients with bronchocentric granulomatous mycosis due to

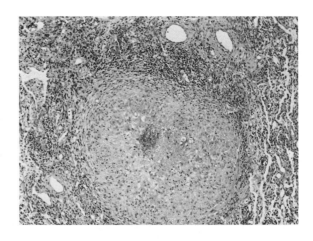

Figure 8–18. Necrotic granuloma centered on a bronchiole with mononuclear cell infiltrate external to adventitia. The eosinophilic central debris contained fungal hyphal fragments on Grocott staining. Epithelioid macrophages predominate with sparse giant cells. (Hematoxylin & eosin. Medium power: resected upper lobe of transplanted lung for severe bronchiectasis. Patient known to have *Aspergillus* in sputum)

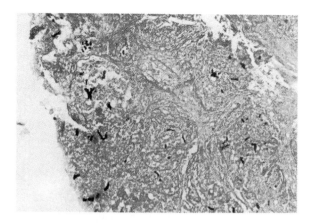

Figure 8–19. Necrotic lung parenchyma in which numerous fungal hyphae typical of *Aspergillus* are seen in a case of invasive parenchymal pulmonary aspergillosis. (Grocott's methenamine silver. Low power: transbronchial biopsy)

Aspergillus in the resected right upper lobe of a combined heart-lung graft had a strong family history of asthma and histologic features compatible with bronchial asthma in her original explanted lungs, removed for Eisenmenger's pulmonary hypertension. The immunosuppressive treatment given to lung recipients may mask the development of asthma, which is seen in association with bronchocentric granulomatosis in nonimmunosuppressed patients. Bronchocentric granulomatous mycosis does not necessarily progress to invasive *Aspergillus* disease even in these immunosuppressed patients, but the presence of viable fungus in abnormal airways inevitably poses a threat of disseminated infection when immunosuppression is significantly increased. The numbers of patients studied with this condition are as yet too small to understand the natural history of this form of fungal disease.

A common pulmonary manifestation of *Aspergillus* infection in the immunocompromised host is suppurative pneumonia with or without angioinvasion.[89] This can result in marked hemorrhage and parenchymal necrosis (Fig. 8–19). This type of invasive aspergillosis occurs in lung transplant recipients, with the same tendency to vascular invasion and dissemination to extrathoracic sites. The risk factors for the development of invasive aspergillosis in lung transplant recipients include previous episodes of persistent rejection, previous CMV pneumonia, recurrent *Pseudomonas* infections, and high sputum colony counts of *Aspergillus* greater than 2000 per ml. An FEV_1 lower than 50 per cent of that predicted is also associated with development of invasive fungal disease. Many of the patients develop new chest x-ray shadowing, which may take the form of nodules rather than diffuse infiltrates. Many of the risk factors relate to the development of oblit-

erative bronchiolitis, which is the main clinicopathologic setting of invasive *Aspergillus* in many pulmonary transplant centers. It is possible to diagnose invasive aspergillosis on transbronchial biopsy, although it is important to document necrotic parenchyma with hyphae in adjacent viable lung. With so many manifestations of *Aspergillus* disease in lung transplant patients, it is imperative to classify each episode as invasive or noninvasive disease, since this may have considerable prognostic significance (Table 8–3). Review of our data showed that histopathologic and cytologic examination of aspirates remains very important in the diagnosis of *Aspergillus* pneumonia, since clinical, radiologic, and microbiologic diagnoses are often unreliable. Unfortunately, the extent of *Aspergillus* infection may be diagnosed only at autopsy.[90]

Other opportunistic infections include those by typical and atypical mycobacteria. These are often diagnosed by a combination of transbronchial biopsy, lavage, and culture.[91] Patients with established obliterative bronchiolitis seem to be the most at risk. Any transbronchial biopsy from a lung allograft recipi-

Table 8–3. Nature of *Aspergillus* Infection in 24 Transbronchial Biopsies from 129 Lung Transplant Recipients

Tracheobronchial Aspergillosis	
Invasive	6
Saprophytic	7
BCG	6
OTBA	1
Parenchymal Aspergillosis	
Invasive	3
Cavity	1

BCG = Bronchocentric granulomatous. OTBA = Obstructive tracheobronchial aspergillosis.

ent with well-defined granulomas, granulomatous inflammation, or histiocytic infiltrates should be carefully studied for the presence of mycobacteria. Ziehl-Neelsen staining is not routine in the reporting of transplant biopsies,[28] as there is a very low incidence of mycobacterial infections in these patients. Patients transplanted for pulmonary sarcoidosis are of particular interest as they nearly always have evidence of recurrent granulomas within the graft. This can occur as early as 4 months posttransplant and necessitate the inclusion of Ziehl-Neelsen staining in all biopsies taken from patients with this primary disease. Only after meticulous exclusion of an infectious cause for the granulomas can they be ascribed to recurrent primary disease. One patient with a clinicopathologically sound diagnosis of end stage sarcoidosis that recurred in the graft finally succumbed to *Mycobacterium tuberculosis* pneumonia 3 years following transplantation. Transbronchial biopsies taken before he died showed necrosis for the first time in his granulomas, and acid-fast bacilli were easily demonstrated in the pulmonary biopsy tissue accompanying bronchial lavage.

Toxoplasmosis occurs both as a primary (donor-transmitted) and recrudescent infection in lung transplant patients. The diagnosis has been made by serology, and organisms have not been demonstrated on biopsy material from our patients.[92] Opportunistic infection due to the Epstein-Barr virus will be considered in the section on lymphoproliferative disorders. It can cause a non-neoplastic viral pneumonitis in both immunosuppressed and nonimmunosuppressed patients,[93] but there are considerable difficulties in substantiating this diagnosis in lung transplant patients in whom the histologic appearances can be confused with acute rejection.

OTHER DIFFERENTIAL DIAGNOSES OF REJECTION

Infections of the lung are by far the most common differential diagnoses of lung rejection histologically.[28, 41] However, many other conditions can mimic rejection (Table 8–4).[28] These include prominent BALT (bronchus-associated lymphoid tissue), which may be seen in the submucosa of the small airways and at the bifurcation of larger airways. The location of this often exuberant lymphoid tissue adjacent to epithelium, with limited extension into adjacent parenchyma, should enable a distinc-

Table 8–4. Differential Diagnosis of Rejection

CMV pneumonitis
Pneumocystis carinii pneumonia
EBV-associated lymphoproliferations, including
  pneumonitis
Bronchial-associated lymphoid tissue
Previous biopsy site
Recurrent primary disease, e.g., sarcoidosis, histiocytosis
  X, pulmonary fibrosis
Ischemia and preservation injury
Drug toxicity, e.g., azathioprine
Donor pathology , e.g., infection, aspiration

From Stewart S. Pathology of lung transplantation. Semin Diagn Pathol 9:210, 1992.

tion. Often this mucosa-associated lymphoid tissue shows active germinal center formation or a characteristic vascular pattern with prominent high endothelial venules. The prominence of this tissue seems to decrease in the months following transplantation and is therefore likely to be a significant differential only in the early postoperative months.[75]

Many lung transplant recipients have repeated transbronchial biopsy procedures as part of their postoperative management,[4] and occasionally the scarred parenchyma of a previous biopsy site can be included in a new diagnostic biopsy. Dense fibrosis with entrapment of lymphocytes and abundant hemosiderin accumulation is seen. The appearance can be difficult to recognize in small biopsies but has been confirmed on explanted and autopsy material, in which the subpleural, thin, wedge-shaped scarring is characteristic. The presence of a previous biopsy site renders that particular piece of parenchyma inadequate for the diagnosis of rejection, and it should not be counted toward the five transbronchial specimens required for the grading of rejection.[28]

The etiology of some of the primary pulmonary diseases for which lung transplantation is performed is uncertain, giving rise to a theoretical possibility of recurrence in the new graft.[30] In patients transplanted for sarcoidosis, noncaseating epithelioid granulomas in a typical bronchovascular distribution were seen in diagnostic transbronchial biopsies as early as the fourth month following transplantation (Fig. 8–20). Obviously, the presence of granulomas in an immunosuppressed transplant recipient must lead to the scrupulous exclusion of opportunistic infection. Having excluded other causes, we have accepted that sarcoidosis can recur in the graft. The granulomatous stage of this disease would not be confused with acute rejection but rather with infection.

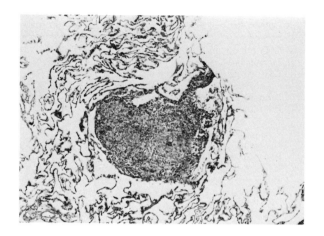

Figure 8–20. Epithelioid and giant cell noncaseating granuloma in a patient transplanted for sarcoidosis. Special stains for opportunistic organisms were all negative, allowing a diagnosis of sarcoidosis recurrent in the lung graft. Adjacent parenchyma is normal. (Hematoxylin & eosin. Medium power: transbronchial biopsy)

In the earliest forms of recurrent sarcoidosis, a lymphocytic alveolitis with perivascular mononuclear cell infiltrates is indistinguishable from acute rejection. It is imperative, therefore, to be aware of the patient's original disease before ascribing a perivascular interstitial infiltrate to rejection. Patients with idiopathic pulmonary fibrosis (IPF) of classic or desquamative patterns may also be expected to undergo recurrence, which would be very difficult indeed to distinguish from rejection or nonspecific changes in the graft. Suggestive histologic features either in biopsy or autopsy material from patients transplanted for IPF would be expected to be significantly different from the changes associated with chronic rejection. In the latter, microcystic patterns of end stage fibrosis are not a feature.[29, 66] Langerhans' cell histiocytosis (LCH) may also theoretically recur, but again there is no evidence in our own series of patients. One patient transplanted with a single lung graft for LCH has had so many complications, including numerous infections, that interpretation of her biopsy material has always been difficult, and it has never been possible absolutely to exclude recurrence of the primary disease. The risk of recurrences of all these conditions will become clearer as patients survive longer and are grafted for a wider range of pulmonary conditions.

In the early postoperative period, preservation injury due to ischemia may be noted on biopsy, ranging from focal collections of polymorphs and hyperplasia of alveolar epithelial cells to intra-alveolar fibrinous exudation. The absence of perivascular infiltrates has distinguished this from rejection. Occasionally preservation injury or severe postoperative bleeding may lead to the biopsy appearances of adult respiratory distress syndrome (ARDS) with hyaline membranes. Although the cellular infiltrates paradoxically may appear more sparse in severe acute rejection with hyaline membrane formation, these infiltrates are not a feature at all of ARDS of ischemic etiology.

Epstein-Barr virus induces lymphoproliferative disease in the lung, ranging from a viral pneumonitis to a process indistinguishable from malignant lymphoma.[93] Differential diagnosis from rejection will be considered in a later section.

The submucosal scarring of chronic rejection in the airways and lymphocytic bronchiolitis or bronchitis also have important differential diagnoses. The most frequent cause of acute and chronic inflammation of the airways is infection, including viral, bacterial, mycoplasmal, fungal, and chlamydial organisms. These have been considered in an earlier section. Lung allograft recipients are predisposed to recurrent aspiration by the loss of cough reflex, and this may cause submucosal fibrosis and inflammation (Fig. 8–21). Foreign material with an associated giant cell reaction within the airways may point to aspiration, and there may also be distal organizing pneumonia distinctive from obliterative bronchiolitis. Aspiration is only one cause of organizing pneumonia in these patients.[64, 65] Others include infection and possibly ischemic damage to the lung. The extension of the organizing granulation tissue into the distal alveolar ducts and air spaces helps distinguish the process from obliterative bronchiolitis of chronic rejection, which is more localized to the terminal and respiratory bronchioles.[64] Granulation tissue in distal air spaces is not a common feature of rejection except in persistent or partially treated cases.[65] Fibromyxoid plugs of connective tissue within terminal airways and air spaces are described by Yousem and associates

Figure 8–21. Eccentric fibrous obliteration of a bronchiole with ulceration. The occluding granulation tissue contains foreign body–type giant cells and is compatible with aspiration. The patient had recurrent laryngeal nerve palsy and developed this appearance within 3 months of transplantation. In this biopsy specimen, the orientation of the bronchiolar smooth muscle clearly defines the extent of luminal narrowing. Connective tissue stains are mandatory in order not to overlook obliterative bronchiolitis. (Hematoxylin & eosin. Medium power: transbronchial biopsy)

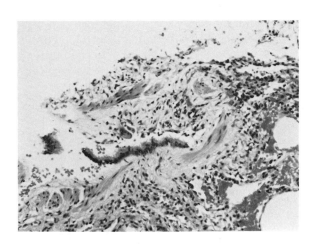

as occurring in the setting of acute lung rejection, in the healing phase of previously diagnosed diffuse alveolar damage following preservation injury, and, thirdly, in relation to infection.[65] It was documented in this study that 9 of the 11 cases of acute rejection with organizing pneumonia-like reaction resolved their granulation tissue completely. This study also shows the importance of correlating the findings with cultures and special stains for organisms.

BRONCHOALVEOLAR LAVAGE CYTOLOGY

Bronchoalveolar lavage (BAL) is a noninvasive technique to assess the inflammatory and immune response of the lung, with both clinical and research uses.[94, 95] BAL samples the surface of the lower respiratory tract; the cells obtained are assumed to be representative of those within the lung parenchyma. However, the proportion and types of cells obtained at lavage have been shown not to correspond exactly to those obtained from minced enzymatically treated lung biopsies.[96] Meticulous attention to technique is essential, as many of the lung transplants have inflamed airways with purulent or retained secretions, which may affect the differential cell count if upper and lower respiratory tract materials are mixed during the procedure. Bronchoalveolar lavage has been studied both experimentally and clinically in transplantation. The main applications in human lung transplantation are in the diagnosis of infection by culture and direct examination and also in the analysis of cell populations and their functional testing.[97] Considering its use in the diagnosis of infection, lavage is complementary to transbron-

chial biopsy and may have a higher diagnostic yield, particularly for fungi and herpes simplex virus (HSV). The high specificity for nonbacterial infectious agents and the short turnaround time for preparation and staining make this a very useful technique. The identification of herpes simplex infected cells and pneumocysts is thought always to be significant. The interpretation of aspirates containing CMV inclusions or *Aspergillus* hyphae, however, must be made in the light of clinical, radiologic, and accompanying biopsy histopathology so that colonization is not confused with active pulmonary infection. Histochemical, immunohistochemical, and in situ hybridization studies can be applied to the cytologic specimens for further elucidation of infections but are usually confirmatory rather than providing further diagnoses.

Bronchoalveolar lavage offers the opportunity to examine the nature of the immunocompetent cells infiltrating the graft.[50, 98, 99] The cellular profiles of the lavage fluid have been described in acute, resolving, and chronic rejection and also in infection. The degree of overlap among these conditions is too great to allow their differentiation. Also, there is poor correlation with the paired biopsy rejection grade.[98] The total lavage cell counts increase during episodes of illness whether due to infection or rejection in the lung. High lymphocyte counts of greater than 15 per cent were found to be supportive of a diagnosis of rejection but occurred in only 23 per cent of rejection episodes as defined on paired biopsy samples. Neutrophils are nonspecifically increased in both infection and rejection. The cellular profiles returned to those of healthy lung recipients after treatment of rejection or infection. These patients had increased numbers of alveolar macrophages, neutrophils, and lymphocytes when compared with normal, nontransplanted controls. The use of lymphocyte phenotyping has not provided additional discrimination between acute and chronic rejection and infection. CD3 and CD8 cells are increased in both types of rejection, showing a considerable overlap between these conditions and infection.[100] CD8 cells are the predominant lymphocytes in the lavage fluid, which may be due to the fact that these are the commonest lymphoid cells, both in normal and diseased respiratory epithelium.[101] The considerable difficulties in obtaining accurate cell counts and differentials in lavage fluids make it essential to standardize protocols before comparing data among various research groups.

Analysis of BAL fluid has shown that most of the donor lymphocytes within the graft are replaced by recipient cells within the first 6 weeks. Macrophages and lymphocytes of donor HLA type may persist for as long as 32 weeks after transplantation.[102] The replacement of donor by recipient lymphocytes may explain the lower incidence of rejection approximately 3 months after transplantation. Cytolytic activity of lavage fluid against donor spleen cells has been used to predict rejection episodes.[50] Spontaneous proliferation and interleukin-2 responsiveness have also been used to monitor rejection, but in some studies this has been without a biopsy "gold standard." Macrophage-lymphocyte interactions are also seen during infection, with high levels of cell-mediated lympholysis. These functional studies have the same considerable overlap as the absolute cell counts and differentials. Further studies are required to determine the role of BAL in monitoring rejection. Grafts showing established obliterative bronchiolitis have a preponderance of CD8+ cells (up to 60 per cent to 92 per cent), with these cells reactive against donor-specific class I antigens.[103, 104] This contrasts with donor-specific class II–directed reactivity associated with acute rejection in which the BAL cells are predominantly CD4 in phenotype. It remains to be seen whether any of these observations, together with studies of cytokines in the lavage fluid, become clinically useful in monitoring acute and chronic lung rejection.

LYMPHOPROLIFERATIVE DISORDERS

Lymphoproliferative post-transplant disease (LPD) is now well described in lung transplant patients.[105–107] It is associated with Epstein-Barr virus (EBV) infection and may be common in this group of patients because of the high level of immunosuppression required, compared with recipients of other solid organ grafts. Epstein-Barr virus infection can be associated with a pneumonitis that is histologically similar in many respects to acute pulmonary rejection and should be considered in its differential diagnosis. Diffuse pneumonia due to infectious mononucleosis in nontransplant patients has been described.[93] There are few detailed reports of the histopathologic features, but the characteristic abnormalities are dense lymphoplasmacytic infiltrates, predominantly perivascular, with a tendency to follow lymphatics. In patients dying nonrespiratory deaths with acute infectious mononucleosis, atypical mononuclear cells have been described in the pulmonary interstitium. Epstein-Barr virus has been detected in cases diagnosed as lymphocytic interstitial pneumonia by in situ hybridization techniques, further associating this virus with pulmonary lymphoproliferation.[108]

Lung transplant recipients have a high incidence of LPD involving the graft itself. Five of fifty-three heart lung recipients at the Pittsburgh center developed LPD, three involving the lung allograft primarily and manifesting a short interval following transplantation.[107] In transbronchial and open biopsy material the infiltrates corresponding to radiographic or CT nodules consist of sheets of lymphoid cells with varying proportions of mature and blast-like components.[30] The nodular infiltrates can be quite mature looking, with conspicuous plasma cell differentiation. A perivascular distribution similar to that of the EBV pneumonitis is often a prominent feature but with involvement of the full thickness of the vessel wall, endothelial infiltration, and fibrinoid necrosis. Coagulative necrosis is a common feature that is useful on transbronchial biopsy as a pointer to this proliferative condition. The lymphoproliferation is usually of B cell origin and can be monoclonal or polyclonal.[109] Polymorphic polyclonal proliferations point toward a florid viral pneumonitis on the background of exogenous immunosuppression.[109, 110] Monomorphic, monoclonal proliferations at the other end of the spectrum have the features of malignant non-Hodgkin's lymphoma. However, categorizing individual patients is complicated by the fact that polyclonal and monoclonal lesions can be present at the same time. Also, some patients have two or more monoclonal cellular populations. The classification of post-transplant LPD, therefore, has been problematic.[109] Lymphoproliferation must be distinguished from nonspecific reactive lymphoid hyperplasias, and this is difficult even in nodal material.[111] Frizzera and associates have recognized three categories: polymorphic, monomorphic, and minimally polymorphic. This classification does not assign significance to atypical immunoblasts and necrosis, nor does it designate any of the categories clearly as lymphoma. The presence of more than one pattern of disease in a single patient makes the application of any classification difficult.[109]

The majority of LPDs are B cell proliferations, but some T cell lymphomas have been described.[112, 113] The proportion of monoclonal B cells varies within the group of LPDs and may have prognostic significance. There is good evidence that EBV protein 2 and a latent membrane protein are present in post-transplant LPD, but it must be noted that the virus can be detected in patients without this disorder.[109] Also, not all lymphoid proliferations in transplant recipients are necessarily EBV related. The correct placement of a case of LPD on the clinicopathologic spectrum is important for treatment and prognosis. The benign polyclonal hyperplasias that resemble infectious mononucleosis often respond to acyclovir and reduction in immunosuppression.[105, 114] Overdiagnosis of LPD as a malignant lymphoma may lead to inappropriate chemotherapy with its own risks. Patients with solid tumors may be acyclovir resistant with a high mortality. Dissemination in fatal cases may involve numerous extrapulmonary sites, including the central nervous system. There is evidence that the nature of the immunosuppressive agent may be important in LPD. OKT3 monoclonal antibody has been associated with increased incidence of LPD, possibly by producing cytokines that favor the oncogenic potential of EBV.[115] The diagnosis of lymphoproliferative complications in lung transplant recipients is a particular area of difficulty for the histopathologist. Heart-lung or lung graft recipients have the highest frequency of this complication—3.8 per cent in the Pittsburgh series.[114] Differentiation from lung rejection and the frequent concomitant presence of their opportunistic infections are problematic.

REFERENCES

1. Dark J, Corris PA. The current state of lung transplantation. Thorax 44:689, 1989.

2. Theodore J, Lewiston N. Lung transplantation comes of age. N Engl J Med 332:772, 1990.
3. Kriett JM, Kaye MP. The Registrar of the International Society for Heart and Lung Transplantation: Eighth Official Report—1991. J Heart Lung Transplant 10:491, 1991.
4. Higenbottam TW, Stewart S, Penketh AR, et al. Transbronchial lung biopsy for the diagnosis of rejection in heart-lung transplant patients. Transplantation 46:532, 1988.
5. Grinnan GLB, Graham WH, Childs JW, et al. Cardiopulmonary homotransplantation. J Thorac Cardiovasc Surg 60:609, 1970.
6. Veith FJ, Koerner SK, Siegelman SS, et al. Diagnosis and reversal of rejection in experimental and clinical lung allografts. Ann Thorac Surg 16:172, 1973.
7. Prop J, Kuijpers P, Wildevuur CRH. Lung allograft rejection in the rat. I. Accelerated rejection caused by graft lymphocytes. Transplantation 40:25, 1985.
8. Castaneda AR, Arnar O, Schmidt-Habelbaum, et al. Cardiopulmonary autotransplantation in primates. J Cardiovasc Surg 37:523, 1972.
9. Reitz BA, Burton NA, Jamieson SW, et al. Heart and lung transplantation. Autotransplantation and allotransplantation in primates with extended survival. J Thorac Cardiovasc Surg 80:360, 1980.
10. Anderson WR, Coulon TF, Kiesel TM, et al. Morphologic characteristics of rejection of the baboon lung allograft. Primates Med 7:81, 1972.
11. Lower RR, Stofer RC, Hurley EJ, et al. Complete homograft replacement of the heart and both lungs. Surgery 50:842, 1961.
12. Kondo Y, Cockrell JV, Hardy JD. Histopathology of one-stage bilateral lung allograft. Ann Surg 180:753, 1974.
13. Barnes BA, Flax MH, Burke JF, et al. Experimental pulmonary homografts in the dog. 1. Morphological studies. Transplantation 1:351, 1963.
14. Veith FJ, Hagstrom JWC, Anderson SR, et al. Alveolar manifestations of rejection: An important cause of the poor results of human lung transplantation. Ann Surg 175:336, 1972.
15. Norin AJ, Emeson EE, Kamholz SL. Cyclosporin A as the initial immunosuppressive agent for canine lung transplantation: Short and long-term assessment of rejection phenomena. Transplantation 34:372, 1982.
16. Veith FJ, Norin AJ, Montefusco CM, et al. Cyclosporin A in experimental lung transplantation. Transplantation 32:474, 1981.
17. Byers JM, Sabanayagam P, Baker RR, et al. Pathologic changes in baboon lung allografts. Ann Surg 178:754, 1973.
18. Prop J, Wildevuur CRH, Nieuwenhuis P. Lung allograft rejection in the rat. III. Corresponding morphological rejection phase in various rat strain combinations. Transplantation 40:132, 1985.
19. Prop J, Tazelaar HD, Billingham ME. Rejection of combined heart-lung transplants in rats: Function and pathology. Am J Pathol 127:97, 1987.
20. Tazelaar HD, Prop J, Nieuwenhuis P, et al. Airway pathology in the transplanted rat lung. Transplantation 45:864, 1988.
21. Marck KW, Wildevuur CRH, Nieuwenhuis P. Lung transplantation in the rat: Histopathology of left lung isografts and allografts. Heart Transplant 4:263, 1985.
22. Fujimara S, Rosen V, Adomian GE, et al. Cellular characteristics of rejection response to canine lung allotransplants. J Thorac Cardiovasc Surg 65:438, 1973.
23. Haverich A, Dawkins KD, Baldwin JC, et al. Long-

term cardiac and pulmonary histology in primates following combined heart and lung transplantation. Transplantation 39:356, 1985.

24. Harjula AJL, Baldwin JC, Glanville AR, et al. Human leukocyte antigen compatibility in heart-lung transplantation. J Heart Transplant 6:162, 1987.

25. Prop J, Kuijpers K, Peterson AH, et al. Why are lung allografts more vigorously rejected than hearts? J Heart Transplant 4:433, 1985.

26. Stewart S, Higenbottam TW, Hutter JA, et al. Histopathology of transbronchial biopsies in heart-lung transplantation. Transplantation Proc XX (suppl): 764, 1988.

27. Stewart S, Cary NRB. The pathology of heart and heart-lung transplantation; An update. J Clin Pathol 44:803, 1991.

28. Yousem SA, Berry GJ, Brunt EM, et al. A Working Formulation for the standardisation of nomenclature in the diagnosis of heart and lung rejection: Lung Rejection Study Group. J Heart Transplant 9:593, 1990.

29. Tazelaar HD, Yousem SA. The pathology of combined heart-lung transplantation. An autopsy study. Hum Pathol 19:1403, 1988.

30. Stewart S. Pathology of lung transplantation. Semin Diagn Pathol 9:210, 1992.

31. Millet B, Higenbottam TW, Flower, CRD, et al. The radiographic appearances of infection and acute rejection of the lung after heart-lung transplantation. Am Rev Respir Dis 140:62, 1989.

32. Allen MD, Burke CM, McGregor CGA, et al. Steroid-responsive bronchiolitis after human heart-lung transplantation. J Thorac Cardiovasc Surg 92:449, 1986.

33. Hutter JA, Stewart S, Higenbottam TW, et al. The characteristic histological changes associated with rejection in heart-lung transplant recipients. Transplant Proc 21:435, 1989.

34. Higenbottam TW, Stewart S. Transbronchial lung biopsy in the diagnosis of rejection of the transplanted lung. In Wallwork JL (ed). Heart and Lung Transplantation. Philadelphia, WB Saunders, 1989.

35. Yousem SA, Tazelaar HD. Combined heart-lung transplantation. In Sale GE (ed). The Pathology of Organ Transplantation. Boston, Butterworths, 1990, p 153.

36. Yousem SA, Paradis IL, Dauber JH, et al. Pulmonary arteriosclerosis in long-term human heart-lung transplant recipients. Transplantation 47:564, 1989.

37. Scott JP, Higenbottam TW, Hutter JA, et al. Natural history of chronic rejection in heart-lung transplant recipients. J Heart Transplant 9:510, 1990.

38. Burke CM, Theodore J, Dawkins KD, et al. Post transplant obliterative bronchiolitis and other late lung sequelae in human heart-lung transplantation. Chest 86:824, 1984.

39. Hutter JA, Despins P, Higenbottam T, et al. Heart-lung transplantation: Better use of resources. Am J Med 85:4, 1988.

40. Granville AR, Baldwin JC, Burke CM, et al. Obliterative bronchiolitis after heart-lung transplantation: Apparent arrest by augmented immunosuppression. Ann Intern Med 107:300, 1987.

41. Higenbottam TW, Penketh AR, Stewart S, et al. The diagnosis of lung rejection and opportunistic lung infection of heart-lung transplant patients using transbronchial lung biopsy. Transplantation 46:532, 1988.

42. Yousem SA, Dauber JA, Keenan R, et al. Does histologic acute rejection in lung allografts predict the development of bronchiolitis obliterans? Transplantation 52:306, 1991.

43. Burke CM, Glanville AR, Theodore J, et al. Lung immunogenicity, rejection and obliterative bronchiolitis. Chest 92:547, 1987.

44. Scott JP, Higenbottam TW, Sharples L, et al. Risk factors of obliterative bronchiolitis in heart-lung transplant recipients. Transplantation 51:813, 1991.

45. Clelland C, Higenbottam TW, Otulana B, et al. Histologic prognostic indicators for the lung allografts of heart-lung transplants. J Heart Transplant 9:177, 1990.

46. Yousem SA, Paradis IL, Dauber JH, et al. Efficacy of transbronchial lung biopsy in the diagnosis of bronchiolitis obliterans. Transplantation 47:893, 1989.

47. Yousem SA, Curley JM, Dauber JA, et al. HLA Class II antigen expression in human heart-lung allografts. Transplantation 49:991, 1990.

48. Glanville AR, Tazelaar HD, Theodore J, et al. The distribution of MHC class I and class II antigens on bronchial epithelium. Am Rev Respir Dis 139:330, 1989.

49. Prop J, Wildevuur CRH, Nieuwenhuis P. Lung allograft rejection in the rat. II. Specific immunological properties of lung grafts. Transplantation 40:126, 1985.

50. Zeevi A, Fung JJ, Paradis IL, et al. Lymphocytes of bronchoalveolar lavage from heart-lung transplantation recipients. Heart Transplant 4:417, 1985.

51. Romaniuk A, Prop J, Peterson AH, et al. Expression of class II major histocompatibility complex antigens by bronchial epithelium in rat lung allografts. Transplantation 44:209, 1987.

52. McCarthy PM, Starnes VA, Theodore J, et al. Improved survival after heart-lung transplantation. J Thorac Cardiovasc Surg 99:54, 1990.

53. Epler GR, Colby TV. The spectrum of bronchiolitis obliterans. Chest 83:161, 1983.

54. Becroft DM. Bronchiolitis obliterans, bronchiectasis, and other sequelae of adenovirus type 21 infection in young children. J Clin Pathol 24:72, 1971.

55. Dummer SJ, Montero CG, Griffith BP, et al. Infections in heart-lung transplant recipients. Transplantation 41:325, 1986.

56. Maurer JR, Tullis E, Grossman RF, et al. Infectious complications following isolated lung transplantation. Chest 101:1056, 1992.

57. Katzenstein AL, Askin FB. Surgical Pathology of Non-Neoplastic Lung Disease. Philadelphia, WB Saunders, 1982, p 349.

58. Smyth RL, Scott JP, Borysiewicz LK, et al. Cytomegalovirus infection in heart-lung transplant recipients: Risk factors, clinical associations and response to treatment. J Infect Dis 164:1045, 1991.

59. Keenan RJ, Lega ME, Dummer S, et al. Cytomegalovirus serologic status and postoperative infection correlated with risk of developing chronic rejection after pulmonary transplantation. Transplantation 51:433, 1991.

60. Duncan AJ, Dummer JS, Paradis IL, et al. Cytomegalovirus infection and survival in lung transplant recipients. J Heart Lung Transplant 10:638, 1991.

61. Humbert M, Devergne O, Cerrina J, et al. Activation of macrophages and cytotoxic cells during cytomegalovirus pneumonia complicating lung transplants. Am Rev Respir Dis 145:1178, 1992.

62. Sissons JGP, Borysiewicz LK. Human cytomegalovirus infection. Thorax 44:241, 1989.

63. Wyatt S, Nunn J, Yin J, et al. Airways obstruction associated with graft versus host disease after bone marrow transplantation. Thorax 39:887, 1984.

64. Abernathy EC, Hruban RH, Baumgartner WA, et al. The two forms of bronchiolitis obliterans in heart-lung transplant recipients. Hum Pathol 22:1102, 1991.

65. Yousem SA, Duncan SR, Griffith BP. Interstitial and airspace granulation tissue reactions in lung transplant recipients. Am J Surg Pathol 16(9):877, 1992.

66. Yousem SA, Burke CM, Billingham ME. Pathologic pulmonary alterations in long-term human heart-lung transplantation. Hum Pathol 16:911, 1985.

67. Griffith BP, Hardesty RL, Trento A, et al. Heart-lung transplantation: Lessons learned and future hopes. Ann Thorac Surg 43:6, 1987.

68. Hruban RH, Beschorner WE, Baumgartner WA, et al. Diagnosis of lung allograft rejection by bronchial intraepithelial Leu-7 positive lymphocytes. J Thorac Cardiovasc Surg 96:939, 1988.

69. Hruban RH, Hutchins GM. The pathology of lung transplantation. *In* Baumgartner WA, Achuff SC, Reitz BA (eds). *Heart-Lung Transplantation.* Philadelphia, WB Saunders, 1990, p 372.

70. Tazelaar HD. Perivascular inflammation in pulmonary infections: Implications for the diagnosis of lung rejection. J Heart Lung Transplant 10:437, 1991.

71. Hunt JB, Stewart S, Cary N, et al. Evaluation of the International Society for Heart Transplantation grading of pulmonary rejection in 100 consecutive biopsies. Transplant Int 5(Suppl 1)S249, 1992.

72. Gryzan S, Paradis IL, Zeevi A, et al. Unexpectedly high incidence of *Pneumocystis carinii* infection after heart-lung transplantation: Implications for lung defense and allograft survival. Am Rev Respir Dis 137:1268, 1988.

73. Brookes RG, Hofflin JM, Jamieson SW, et al. Infectious complications in heart-lung recipients. Am J Med 79:412, 1985.

74. Hutter JA, Scott FP, Wreghitt T, et al. The importance of cytomegalovirus in heart-lung transplant recipients. Chest 95:627, 1989.

75. Hruban RH, Beschorner WE, Baumgartner WA, et al. Depletion of bronchus-associated lymphoid tissue with lung allograft rejection. Am J Pathol 132:6, 1988.

76. Dummer JS, White LT, Ho M, et al. Morbidity of cytomegalovirus infection heart and heart-lung transplants who received cyclosporine. J Infect Dis 152:1182, 1985.

77. Smyth RL, Higenbottam TW, Scott JP, et al. Herpes simplex virus infection in heart-lung transplant recipients. Transplantation 49:735, 1990.

78. Myerson D, Hackman RC, Nelson JA, et al. Widespread presence of histologically occult cytomegalovirus. Hum Pathol 15:430, 1984.

79. Weiss LM, Movahed LA, Berry GJ, et al. In situ hybridization studies for viral nucleic acids in heart and lung allograft biopsies. Am J Clin Pathol 93:675, 1990.

80. Niedobiteck G, Finn T, Herbst H, et al. Detection of cytomegalovirus by in-situ hybridisation and histochemistry using a monoclonal antibody CCH2. 1. Comparison of methods. J Clin Pathol 41:1005, 1988.

81. Weber WR, Askin FB, Dehner LP. Lung biopsy in *Pneumocystis carinii* pneumonia. A histological study of typical and atypical features. Am J Clin Pathol 67:11, 1977.

82. Travis WD, Pittaluga S, Lipschik GY, et al. Atypical pathologic manifestation of *Pneumocystis carinii* pneumonia in the acquired immune deficiency syndrome. Am J Surg Pathol 14:615, 1990.

83. Millard PR, Heryet AR. Observations favouring *Pneumocystis carinii* pneumonia as a primary infection: A monoclonal antibody study on paraffin sections. J Pathol 154:365, 1988.

84. Pennington JE. *Aspergillus* lung disease. Med Clin North Am 64:475, 1980.

85. Hines DW, Hauber MH, Yaremko L, et al. Pseudomembranous tracheobronchitis caused by *Aspergillus*. Am Rev Respir Dis 143:1408, 1991.

86. Kramer MR, Denning DW, Marshall SE, et al. Ulcerative tracheobronchitis after lung transplantation. Am Rev Respir Dis 144:552, 1991.

87. Schafers H-J, Haydock DA, Copper JD. The prevalence and management of bronchial anastomotic complications in lung transplantation. J Thorac Cardiovasc Surg 101:1044, 1991.

88. Tazelaar HD, Baird AM, Mill M, et al. Bronchocentric mycosis occurring in transplant recipients. Chest 96:92, 1989.

89. Denning DW, Follansbee SF, Scolaro M, et al. Pulmonary aspergillosis in the acquired immunodeficiency syndrome. N Engl J Med 324:654, 1991.

90. Boon AP, O'Brien D, Adams DH. Ten-year review of invasive aspergillosis detected at necropsy. J Clin Pathol 44:452, 1991.

91. Trulock EP, Bolman RM, Genton R. Pulmonary disease caused by *Mycobacterium chelonei* in a heart-lung transplant recipient with obliterative bronchiolitis. Am Rev Respir Dis 140:802, 1989.

92. Wreghitt TG, Hakim M, Gray JJ, et al. Toxoplasmosis in heart and lung transplant recipients. J Clin Pathol 42:194, 1989.

93. Veal CF, Carr JR, Briggs DD. Diffuse pneumonia and acute respiratory failure due to infectious mononucleosis in a middle-aged adult. Am Rev Respir Dis 141:502, 1990.

94. Hunninghake GW, Kawanami O, Ferras VJ, et al. Characteristics of the inflammatory and immune effector cells in the lung parenchyma of patients with interstitial lung disease. Am Rev Respir Dis 123:407, 1981.

95. Walters EH, Gardiner PV. Bronchoalveolar lavage as a research tool. Thorax 46:613, 1991.

96. Nibbering PH, van der Heide A, van Furth R. Macrophages in broncho-alveolar lavage fluid are not representative of macrophages in granulomas of the lungs of BCG infected mice. J Pathol 157:253, 1989.

97. Walts AE, Marcheysky AM, Morgan M. Pulmonary cytology in lung transplant recipients. Diagn Cytopathol 7:353, 1991.

98. Clelland CA, Higenbottam TW, Monk JA, et al. Bronchoalveolar lavage lymphocytes in relation to transbronchial lung biopsy in heart-lung transplants. Transplant Proc 22:1479, 1990.

99. Clelland CA, Higenbottam TW, Stewart S, et al. Bronchoalveolar lavage and transbronchial lung biopsy during acute rejection and infection in heart-lung transplant patients. Am Rev Respir Dis 147:1386, 1993.

100. Shennib H, Nguyen D, Guttmann RD, et al. Phenotypic expression of bronchoalveolar lavage cells in lung rejection and infection. Am Thorac Surg 51:630, 1991.

101. Fournier M, Lebargy F, Ladurie FLR, et al. Intraepithelial T-lymphocyte subsets in the airways of normal subjects and of patients with chronic bronchitis. Am Rev Respir Dis 140:737, 1989.

102. Paradis IL, Marrari M, Zeevi A, et al. HLA phenotype of lung lavage cells following heart-lung transplantation. Heart Transplant 4:422, 1985.

103. Reinsmoen NL, Bolman RM, Savile K, et al. Differentiation of Class I- and Class II–directed donor-specific alloreactivity in bronchoalveolar lavage lymphocytes from lung transplant recipients. Transplantation 53:181, 1992.

104. Holland VA, Cagle PT, Windsor NT, et al. Lymphocyte subset populations in bronchiolitis obliterans after heart-lung transplantation. Transplantation 50:955, 1990.

105. Rhandhawa PS, Yousem SA, Paradis IL, et al. The clinical spectrum, pathology and clonal analysis of Epstein-Barr virus associated lymphoproliferative disorders in heart-lung transplant recipients. Am J Clin Pathol 92:177, 1989.

106. Nalesnik MA, Jaffe R, Starzl TE, et al. The pathology of post-transplant lymphoproliferative disorders occurring in the setting of cyclosporine A-prednisone immunosuppression. Am J Pathol 133:1273, 1988.

107. Yousem SA, Randhawa P, Locker J, et al. Posttransplant lymphoproliferative disorders in heart-lung transplant recipients. Hum Pathol 20:361, 1989.

108. Barbera JA, Hayashi S, Hegele RG, et al. Detection of Epstein-Barr virus in lymphocytic interstitial pneumonia by in situ hybridization. Am Rev Respir Dis 145:940, 1992.

109. Swerdlow S. Post-transplant lymphoproliferative disorders: A morphologic, phenotypic and genotypic spectrum of disease. Histopathology 20:373, 1992.

110. Hanto DW. Polyclonal and monoclonal posttransplant lymphoproliferative disease (LPD). Clin Transplant 6:227, 1992.

111. Frizzera G, Hanto DW, Gajl-Peczalska KJ, et al. Polymorphic diffuse B-cell hyperplasia and lymphomas in renal transplant recipients. Cancer Res 41:4262, 1981.

112. Berg LC, Copenhaver CM, Morrison VA, et al. B-cell lymphoproliferative disorders in solid organ transplant patients: Detection of Epstein-Barr virus by in situ hybridization. Hum Pathol 23:159, 1992.

113. Ih-Jen S, Kai-Hsin L, Chi-Jong C, et al. Epstein-Barr virus–associated peripheral T-cell lymphoma of activated CD8 phenotype. Cancer 66:2557, 1990.

114. Nalesnik MA, Locker J, Jaffe R, et al. Experience with posttransplant lymphoproliferative disorders in solid organ transplant recipients. Clin Transplant 6:249, 1992.

115. Goldman M, Gerard C, Abramowicz D, et al. Induction of interleukin-6 and interleukin-10 by the OKT3 monoclonal antibody: Possible relevance to posttransplant lymphoproliferative disorders. Clin Transplant 6:265, 1992.

9

DIFFERENTIAL DIAGNOSIS OF RENAL ALLOGRAFT BIOPSIES

SHANE M. MEEHAN, MD, and ROBERT B. COLVIN, MD

Renal biopsy remains the definitive diagnostic test for allograft rejection and the various lesions that affect the renal allograft (Table 9–1). The differential diagnosis of rejection and cyclosporine toxicity is not distinguishable by clinical criteria alone.[1–4] Biopsy provides clinically unsuspected diagnostic information in 38 per cent to 42 per cent of cases. Antirejection therapy with its attendant morbidity was avoided in 40 per cent to 47 per cent of cases because of the biopsy results.[5–7] Although acute rejection is known to be patchy, a needle biopsy of the cortex gives a representative picture of the pathologic process in most instances.[6–8] A biopsy sample containing only medulla will miss the diagnosis in 42 per cent and underestimate the severity in 50 per cent of cases.[9] Therefore, a biopsy without any cortical tissue must be deemed inadequate and the clinician informed for consideration of rebiopsy. It is also important to have sufficient clinical information for optimal biopsy interpretation (Table 9–2).

Technique. The tissue is divided at the bedside for light, immunofluorescence, and electron microscopy. We recommend taking the ends of the needle core for electron microscopy, followed by splitting the remaining tissue longitudinally. The presence of cortex can be confirmed by looking for glomeruli with a dissecting microscope. The longitudinal halves are each submitted for immunofluorescence and paraffin section, respectively. The paraffin-embedded tissue is sectioned at 2 and 4 microns and stained with hematoxylin and eosin and with periodic acid–Schiff reagent. We routinely stain for IgG, IgM, IgA, C3, fibrinogen, and albumin by immunofluorescence. The diagnosis can usually be rendered on light microscopic examination alone. Electron microscopy is necessary if glomerular disease is suspected.

Donor Biopsy. It is useful to obtain a biopsy of the transplanted kidney immediately after

Table 9–1. Diagnostic Classification of Renal Allograft Biopsies

1. Allograft rejection
   A. Antibody mediated
      Hyperacute allograft rejection
      Necrotizing arteritis (accelerated rejection)
      Thrombotic vasculopathy
   B. T cell mediated
      Acute cellular allograft rejection
      (i) Tubulointerstitial
      (ii) Vascular
      (iii) Glomerular (acute allograft glomerulopathy)
   C. Pathogenesis unknown
      Chronic allograft rejection
      (i) Tubulointerstitial
      (ii) Vascular
      (iii) Glomerular (chronic allograft glomerulopathy)
2. Drug toxicity
   Cyclosporine nephrotoxicity
   FK506 nephrotoxicity
   Acute allergic interstitial nephritis
3. Ischemic injury
   Acute tubular necrosis
   Perfusion injury
   Major vessel occlusion
4. Obstruction and reflux
5. Infection
   Bacterial, fungal, viral
6. Recurrent primary disease
7. Post-transplant lymphoproliferative disease

Table 9–2. Clinical Information Relevant to Renal Allograft Biopsy Interpretation

Donor
  Source (living related or unrelated; cadaver)
  HLA match
Graft
  Ischemic time
  Donor biopsy
  Initial function
Recipient
  Primary renal disease
  Days post-transplant
  Previous rejection episodes
  Symptoms
  Signs
    Creatinine and rate of rise
    Proteinuria
    Renal scan
Therapy
  Cyclosporine dose, route, levels (peak, trough)
  Drugs interactive with cyclosporine
  Monoclonal antibodies
  Nephrotoxic drugs
Other Complicating Problems
  Urinary obstruction
  Renal artery or venous stenosis
  Infection
  Hypertension
  Dehydration

revascularization to assess the state of the donor kidney (especially chronic vascular disease and acute tubular necrosis). Tubular damage can be quantified in terms of the amount of tubular dilatation or desquamation. The presence of significant tubular damage is useful in management of the patient, since such patients may require alteration in their cyclosporine dosages until their creatinine level is below 3 mg/dl. Kidneys exposed to prolonged cold ischemia time may show a perfusion-induced glomerulopathy that spontaneously resolves. This glomerulopathy is manifested by infiltration of glomerular capillary loops by neutrophils and occlusion of capillary loops by endothelial cells, giving the glomerulus a swollen and bloodless appearance. Another change occasionally noted in donor biopsies is the presence of patchy cortical necrosis, a finding that may portend significant delay in re-establishment of renal function. Furthermore, primary glomerular disease is detected occasionally by immunofluorescence in less than 5 per cent of the cases.[10]

DIFFERENTIAL DIAGNOSIS

Whenever an allograft biopsy is examined, the differential diagnosis should include rejec-

tion, infection, drug toxicity, ischemia, obstruction, recurrent and de novo renal disease, and post-transplant lymphoproliferative disease (Table 9–1). The timing of the biopsy alters the probability of these diagnoses. A biopsy taken in the first few hours for nonfunction will show acute tubular ischemic necrosis (ATN), preservation injury, or, in rare instances, hyperacute rejection. In the early post-transplant period (less than 2 months), lesions that enter the differential diagnosis of a rising serum creatinine level are, in approximate decreasing order of frequency:

Acute cellular rejection (tubulointerstitial, vascular, and/or glomerular)
Acute cyclosporine nephrotoxicity (including hemolytic-uremic syndrome)
Acute tubular necrosis
Drug-induced allergic interstitial nephritis
Recurrent glomerular disease
Extrarenal complications such as ureteral leakage or obstruction, renal vein thrombosis, and renal artery injury/thrombosis
Viral interstitial nephritis
Accelerated (humoral) vascular rejection
Recurrent glomerular disease
Acute pyelonephritis

Processes to be considered in patients with renal dysfunction in the late post-transplant period (more than 2 months) include the following:

Chronic allograft rejection
Chronic cyclosporine nephrotoxicity
Acute cellular rejection
De novo glomerular disease
Recurrent glomerular disease
Viral interstitial nephritis
Acute pyelonephritis
Reflux nephropathy
Renovascular disease
Post-transplant lymphoproliferative disease

Table 9–3. Vascular Lesions of Allografts

Endothelium and Intima
  Endothelialitis/endarteritis
  Endothelial injury and intravascular coagulation
  Thrombotic microangiopathy
  Edema and myxoid change
  Proliferation
  Hyalinosis
Media
  Myocyte vacuolization
  Myocyte degeneration/necrosis
  Necrosis
  Hyalinosis

The general approach to an allograft is like that to any other renal biopsy: the vessels, tubules, interstitium, and glomeruli are each inspected in turn for clues to the morphologic and etiologic diagnosis. This chapter is organized according to the differential diagnosis of the patterns seen in each of these components in renal allograft biopsies. Vascular lesions are considered first, since they are the most crucial in the differential diagnosis.

VASCULAR LESIONS (Table 9–3)

Hyperacute Rejection

Hyperacute allograft rejection is an antibody-mediated response to donor alloantigens occurring in the immediate post-transplant period and up to 72 hours thereafter. Antibody is deposited along the endothelium of capillaries, arterioles, and small arteries, with activation of complement and the clotting cascade, resulting in thrombosis, ischemia, and tissue damage. The glomeruli, peritubular capillaries, and small arteries show neutrophils and microthrombi (Fig. 9–1). Biopsy specimens in the first hour show neutrophil margination in capillaries, platelet accumulation, and fibrin

deposition, with extensive occlusion of the microvasculature.[11] The interstitium is edematous and has rare mononuclear cells. Over a few hours there are progressive losses of endothelium, interstitial hemorrhage, and tubular damage. Within 12 to 24 hours there is cortical infarction culminating in complete cortical necrosis, necessitating graft nephrectomy; invariably, there is graft loss. Immunofluorescence in the earliest stages reveals IgG and C3 in the glomerular and peritubular capillary walls and fibrin in the vessel lumina.[11] The deposits are scanty or absent in specimens examined after the first few hours, probably because of endothelial loss, rapid degradation of antibody, or both. In current clinical practice, this phenomenon is very rare.

Necrotizing Arteritis (Accelerated Rejection)

This form of rejection, also termed *accelerated rejection* or *vascular rejection*, usually occurs between 72 hours and 6 weeks and is thought to be due to antidonor antibody.[6, 12] The characteristic lesions show necrosis of myocytes, destruction of the elastica, and accumulation of eosinophilic material (fibrinoid) in the arterial

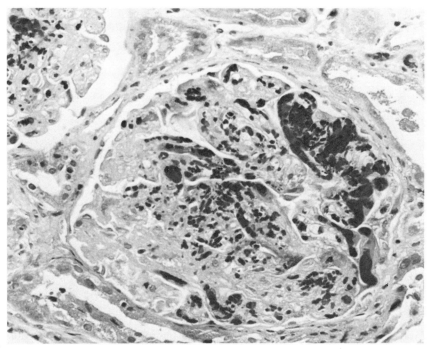

Figure 9–1. Hyperacute rejection. Glomerulus with endothelial swelling, capillary lumen obliteration, thrombi, and scattered neutrophils. (× 313)

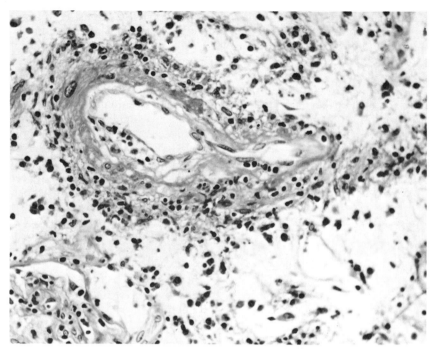

Figure 9–2. Accelerated rejection. Necrotizing arteritis with fibrinoid necrosis of the media and a mural and perivascular infiltrate of lymphocytes and neutrophils are present. This artery has a more intense mononuclear infiltrate than is usual in accelerated rejection. (× 313)

and arteriolar intima and media (Fig. 9–2). There is accompanying thrombosis with a peri-vascular neutrophilic infiltrate, and there may be leukocytoclasis; hence the lesions may resemble those of polyarteritis nodosa. Immunofluorescence shows fibrin, C3, IgG, and IgM in the areas of fibrinoid necrosis. This vascular lesion develops in presensitized individuals (by blood transfusion, previous transplant, and pregnancy), and it usually occurs in the first 6 weeks. Patients have anti-ABO or anti-HLA class I antibodies.[13–15] Why these patients have a delayed onset of rejection is not known. The prognosis is ominous, with a 1-year graft survival of 29 per cent.[5, 12] Rarely, the lesion is seen as a terminal stage of severe acute cellular rejection.

Acute Cellular Rejection

Acute cellular rejection is a T cell–mediated reaction to donor-specific antigens. It has an acute course, typically associated with an acute deterioration in graft function, fever, swelling, and tenderness of the graft, and an increased serum creatinine level. The process classically arises 1 to 4 weeks post-transplant but can oc-

cur at any time. There are three pathologic patterns: (1) tubulointerstitial infiltrate of lymphocytes and macrophages with tubulitis, (2) arterial subendothelial mononuclear cell infiltration (endothelialitis), and (3) acute allograft glomerulopathy. These may occur separately or together in any combination.

Endothelialitis is the sine qua non of acute cellular rejection. This lesion, also termed *intimal arteritis, arterial endovasculitis,* and *endarteritis,* distinguishes active cellular rejection from all other causes of graft failure. The diagnosis of acute rejection can be made in its absence, but only by exclusion of other causes. *Vascular rejection* is a confusing term in the literature that is used for two separate lesions, necrotizing arteritis or endothelialitis.

Endothelialitis is characterized by infiltration of the arterial intima by mononuclear cells, with undermining of the endothelium (Fig. 9–3). The earliest change is margination of mononuclear cells in medium and small arteries, with endothelial swelling. The endothelium is then undermined by the inflammatory cells and appears separated from the underlying intima. The intima is edematous, with scattered lymphocytes (CD4+ and CD8+) and macrophages.[16] As the mononuclear cell

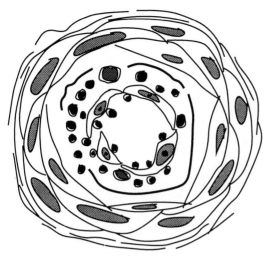

Figure 9–3. Diagrammatic representation of typical endothelialitis with adherent lymphocytes, reactive endothelial cells, and intimal inflammatory cells undermining the endothelium.

population increases, the intima expands (Fig. 9–4). Meanwhile, the endothelium is sloughed and individual endothelial cells have intense cytoplasmic basophilia and prominent nucleoli. Focal endothelial cell necrosis is also seen. There may be fibrin deposits in sloughed areas. Infarction and glomerular ischemia are rare consequences.

As the lesion progresses, it encroaches on the vessel lumen; the mononuclear cells infiltrate centrifugally to the media; and patchy necrosis with fibrin deposition may be seen.[12] Medial necrosis is rare in acute cellular rejection, and one must consider the diagnosis of accelerated (humoral) rejection when there is necrotizing arteritis. Endothelialitis is not present in all vessels in a given biopsy and is known to be a patchy process. It is estimated to be present in only 50 per cent of biopsies of acute cellular rejection.[2] We have found it in about 60 per cent of cases.

CD8 + lymphocytes predominate in the intima with lesser amounts of macrophages.[16, 17] Immunofluorescence reveals trace amounts of fibrin but no antibody;[12] C3d and C4d can also be detected.[18] The target antigens appear to be heterogeneous MHC class I and II antigens and non-MHC antigens. Class I antigens are abundant on renal arterial, venous, and capillary endothelium. After transplantation, their expression is not as evident,[19, 20] possibly owing to capillary damage.[21] In acute cellular rejection, class II antigens and adhesion molecules ICAM-1 and VCAM-1 are expressed on the en-

dothelium of larger arteries; these express little or none of these antigens under normal circumstances.[22, 23]

The responsiveness of this lesion to steroid therapy is not clear; some reports cite steroid resistance, whereas others claim the lesion is responsive.[22, 24] The steroid-resistant cases may be responsive to OKT3 or FK506.[25–27] One study suggests that although vascular lesions are reversible with OKT3 therapy, graft loss may be greater than in patients with acute cellular rejection lacking vascular involvement.[27]

Acute Vascular Cyclosporine Toxicity

A variety of renal lesions are caused by cyclosporin A, with varied time courses and reversibility. Acute nephrotoxicity is characterized by acute tubular injury or microangiopathy typical of hemolytic-uremic syndrome. Chronic toxicity shows arterial medial hyalinization, myocyte degeneration, mucoid intimal thickening, "striped" interstitial fibrosis, and tubular atrophy (discussed later).

The acute vascular lesion is morphologically identical to thrombotic microangiopathy (vasculopathy), which is the term given to the vascular changes seen in the hemolytic-uremic syndrome, thrombotic thrombocytopenic purpura, malignant hypertension, and scleroderma crisis. A similar pattern of vascular injury was observed in some recipients not on cyclosporine, probably as a manifestation (albeit rare) of allograft rejection.[28] Renal transplant patients whose primary renal disease was hemolytic-uremic syndrome may develop this vasculopathy as a recurrence of their primary renal disease.

The earliest discernible change is arteriolar endothelial swelling and edema of the intima. Later, the vessel wall has fibrin deposits and fragmented red cells (Figs. 9–5 and 9–6). The fibrin deposits are sometimes referred to as fibrinoid necrosis; however, there is no medial necrosis or leukocytoclasis. Endothelial proliferation can be dramatic with the appearance of glomeruloid bodies. Later, there is proliferation of myointimal cells with luminal narrowing. These intimal changes are thought to resolve by fibrosis. Immunofluorescence shows fibrin in the vessel walls and lumen, with granular C3 and IgM. Fibrin thrombi in the arterioles may extend into the glomerular tuft. Aneurysmal dilation of the thrombosed afferent arteriole is a distinctive finding (Fig. 9–7). The glomeruli may have capillary loop thick-

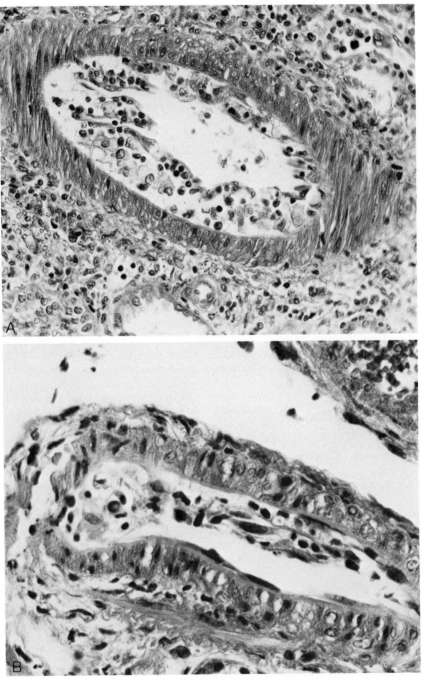

Figure 9–4. Endothelialitis in acute cellular rejection. The endothelium of an arcuate artery *(A)* and branch *(B)* is undermined by an infiltrate of lymphocytes and macrophages. *(A,* × 313; *B,* × 500)

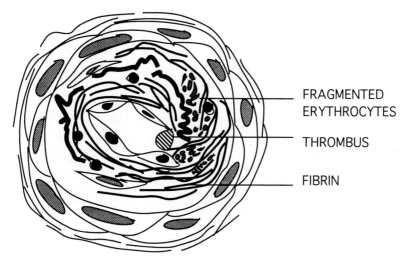

FRAGMENTED
ERYTHROCYTES

THROMBUS

FIBRIN

Figure 9–5. Diagrammatic representation of thrombotic microangiopathy involving a small artery.

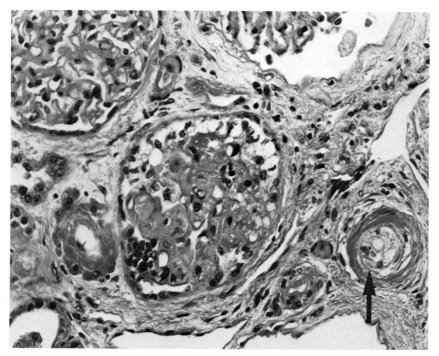

Figure 9–6. Thrombotic microangiopathy with afferent arteriole containing fragmented red cells and fibrin deposits (arrow). ($\times$ 313)

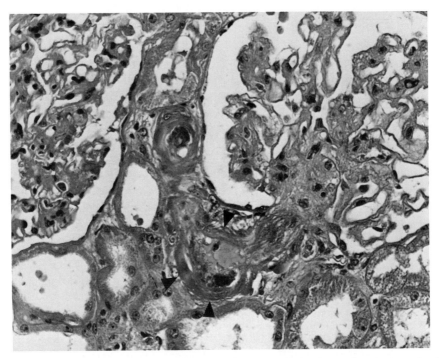

Figure 9-7. Aneurysmally dilated, thrombosed afferent arteriole in thrombotic microangiopathy (arrowheads). ($\times$ 313)

ening as a result of endothelial separation from the basement membrane, giving rise to a double contour on PAS or silver staining. The mesangium may have mesangiolysis or a fibrillary appearance. Fragmented red cells may be present in the mesangium and in Bowman's space. The interstitial infiltrate is variable and not helpful in the differential diagnosis.

Similar renal vascular lesions can be seen in nontransplanted kidneys in patients treated with cyclosporine for other reasons.[29, 30] Cyclosporine causes direct endothelial damage in vitro.[31] It initially stimulates prostacyclin synthesis by endothelium, later causing exhaustion (see below).[31, 32] There is augmentation of thromboplastin and macrophage factor VII synthesis in response to endotoxin.[33] Some patients have increased serum factor VIII and antithrombin-III.[34] Intravascular coagulation therefore may be promoted in response to endothelial damage by factors in the allograft not yet defined. The prognosis of thrombotic microangiopathy is poor, with 75 per cent graft loss in one series.[35]

Chronic Rejection

Chronic allograft rejection is a process characterized pathologically by vascular myointi-mal hyperplasia, interstitial fibrosis, tubular atrophy, and chronic allograft glomerulopathy in varied combinations. The clinical features are gradual deterioration of graft function and proteinuria usually more than 6 months post-transplant. The process is presumably immunologically mediated, although the pathogenesis has not been proved.

Intimal proliferation is the most common manifestation of chronic rejection, which probably evolves from acute vascular rejection with or without antibodies; the lesions may be present without clinical episodes of acute rejection and without loss of function. The number of early acute rejection episodes is correlated with the development of chronic rejection.[36] Intimal proliferation is typically seen more than 6 months post-transplantation but has appeared as early as 4 weeks. The implications of chronic rejection are grave, with progressive deterioration and irreversible graft failure being the rule. The clinical picture is often complicated by hypertension. The mean time from diagnosis of chronic rejection to graft failure is 1.9 years.[37]

The lesions are present in the interlobar, arcuate, and interlobular arteries down to the small arteries. As in acute cellular vascular rejection, the process is patchy. On light microscopy there is concentric intimal thickening and luminal narrowing mainly affecting medium-sized muscular arteries (over 50 μm).[38] The intima contains a cellular spindle cell proliferation with scattered mononuclear cells (Figs. 9–8 and 9–9). T lymphocytes are predominant.[38] Variable amounts of foamy histiocytes are present, especially along the elastica. The intimal stroma takes up little stain with hematoxylin and eosin. The internal elastic lamina is often focally ruptured and on occasion is reduplicated. The media may be thick, thin, or fibrotic. The smooth muscle cells may be vacuolated, adjacent to disruptions in the elastic lamina. Vacuolation like this may also be seen in cyclosporine toxicity, but the intimal changes are usually distinctive enough to enable differentiation. Additional findings include tubular atrophy, patchy to diffuse interstitial fibrosis, and tubulointerstitial inflammation. The glomeruli have increased mesangial matrix with segmental basement membrane duplication. Ischemic basement membrane wrinkling may be seen in advanced lesions.

The vascular lesion is histologically similar to that of atherosclerosis and may represent an accelerated form of the process in response to immunologic endothelial injury.[22, 37, 38] Growth factor release from intimal macrophages or platelets is thought to stimulate myointimal cells, resulting in myocyte migration from the media and proliferation, accumulation of foamy histiocytes, and an increase in intimal proteoglycans, analogous to atherosclerosis arising over a period of weeks to months. Cigarette smoking at the time of transplantation is independently correlated with the development of chronic rejection.[37]

Intimal hyalinosis appears as eccentric eosinophilic subendothelial deposits, often with extension into the media. The differential diagnosis is cyclosporine toxicity, hypertensive arteriolopathy, diabetes mellitus, and chronic rejection. In cyclosporine toxicity, florid hyalin deposits may extend from the media into the intima (see later). In chronic rejection there is large vessel involvement also. One must rely on ancillary morphologic features to make the differential diagnosis. Arteriolar hyalin may be seen in kidneys as an early manifestation of recurrent diabetes in the graft after the first year.[39] However, efferent and afferent arteriolar hyalinosis can be seen in allografts from patients without diabetes and is therefore not a specific marker of disease recurrence.[40] Glomerular changes (mesangial expansion and basement membrane thickening) are frequent and reliable signs of recurrent diabetic disease, being present in almost 100 per cent of patients at 2 years post-transplantation.[41]

Chronic Cyclosporine Toxicity

Medial hyalinosis is a relatively specific manifestation of chronic cyclosporine toxicity.[34, 42] This form of hyalinosis primarily affects the media of cortical afferent arterioles and small arteries with less than two layers of smooth muscle.[34] The hyalin is eosinophilic and segmentally distributed in nodules or knobs (Figs. 9–10 and 9–11), or in what has been referred to as a necklace or cloverleaf pattern.[34] The deposits may cause luminal narrowing. There is myocyte damage with flattening and cytoplasmic vacuolation. In both hypertensive and diabetic arteriolopathy, the hyalin tends to be predominantly subendothelial but may extend into the media. Medial hyalinosis arises after the second month post-transplant.[34] Rare reports have found hyalinosis at 35 days post-transplant[43, 44] in patients given high dose cyclosporine; some report the presence of the lesion in the first week.[45] The accompanying edematous or mucoid intimal thickening of small arteries may cause severe vascular luminal narrowing (see Fig. 9–14). This may arise anywhere from 5 weeks to 2 years post-transplant[44] and should be distinguished from the intimal proliferation of thrombotic microangiopathy and chronic rejection; these entities have relatively greater intimal cellular proliferation.

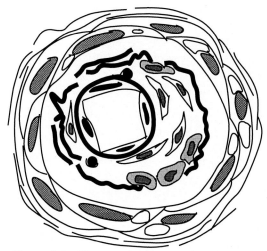

Figure 9–8. Diagram showing vascular changes of chronic rejection, with intimal proliferative changes, luminal narrowing, disruption, and duplication of the elastica. (× 313)

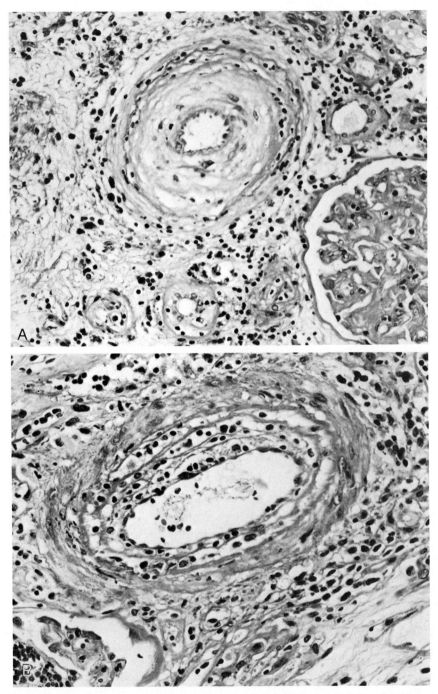

Figure 9–9. A, Chronic rejection with intimal thickening, myointimal proliferation, and fibrosis of the media. (× 290) B, Similar to A, with intimal and medial mononuclear cell infiltrate. (× 313)

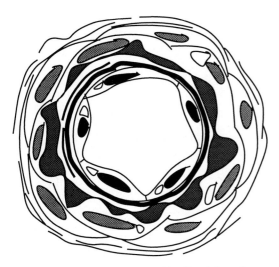

Figure 9–10. Diagram of medial hyalinosis in cyclosporine toxicity, with endothelial and smooth muscle vacuolization. ($\times$ 313)

Immunofluorescence reveals IgM, C3, C1q, and occasionally fibrin deposits in the vessel walls.[34] On electron microscopy there is smooth muscle damage with moth-eaten-appearing myofibrils, disappearance or clumping of fusiform densities, apoptosis, and compression atrophy of smooth muscle cells.[12, 46] The

insudation is finely granular and amorphous, with a mass effect compressing and replacing smooth muscle and separating collagen bundles. The internal elastic lamina is thickened, laminated, and sometimes convoluted.[34, 46] Intimal hyalin can also be seen.[44, 46] It is interesting that both endothelial and smooth muscle cells can have extensive cytoplasmic vacuolation, single cell necrosis, and conspicuous lysosomes, as seen in acute cyclosporine-induced renal tubular epithelial damage.

The electron microscopic finding of extracellular nodular deposits replacing smooth muscle cells is helpful in the differential diagnosis of cyclosporine hyalinosis from diabetic or hypertensive arteriolopathy, in which focal nodular deposits are inside intact smooth muscle cells. This is helpful only in the early stages of these disorders. In more advanced lesions the distinction may be impossible. In addition to the arteriolopathy, one sees "striped" interstitial fibrosis and tubular atrophy.

The presence of arteriolar medial hyalin, myocyte degeneration and focal necrosis, intravascular coagulation, and mucoid intimal thickening of small arteries defines cyclosporine-associated vasculopathy.[34, 42] Glomerular and arteriolar thrombi are seen in about 3 per cent of biopsies of patients on cyclosporine.[47]

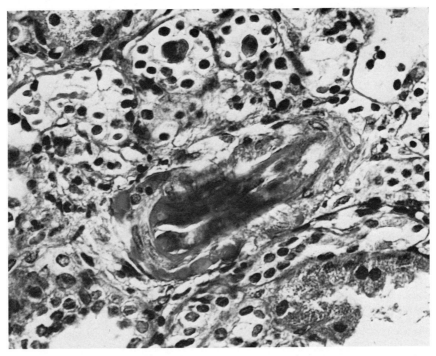

Figure 9–11. Chronic cyclosporine vasculopathy. Small artery with medial hyalin in a necklace pattern (arrow) and large amounts of intimal hyalin. (Reticulin stain $\times$ 500)

Although the vascular lesion is associated with interstitial scarring and tubular atrophy, renal function may be little affected despite histologic changes.[48] The spectrum of vascular and interstitial changes, called vascular-interstitial cyclosporine toxicity by some, is seen in 15 per cent of cases treated with cyclosporine.[34]

Cyclosporine vasculopathy may be progressive or may regress if therapy is discontinued or if the dose is reduced.[42] Regression of the arteriolopathy may be seen as early as 3 months after cessation of therapy or reduction of dosage and consists of remodeling of the vascular wall, recovery of luminal patency, and diminution of the acute changes. Patients with persistent lesions have greater cumulative doses of cyclosporine and greater severity of vascular mural changes than those showing regression. The reversibility of lesions, even in patients maintained on reduced doses of cyclosporine, has important implications for patient management, particularly in view of the fact that cessation of cyclosporine introduces a high risk of rejection.

TUBULOINTERSTITIAL LESIONS

Tubulointerstitial lesions are the commonest lesions seen in renal transplant biopsies and probably create the greatest diagnostic difficulty in isolation. The differential diagnosis includes the entities in Tables 9–4 and 9–5. Normal host adaptation to an allograft is associated with tubulointerstitial infiltration.[48–50] In the normal donor the infiltrate occupies about 2 per cent of the area of the cortex.[50] In biopsies of normally functioning grafts in the first 3 weeks, about 10 per cent of the cortex is occupied by mononuclear cells. This figure drops to approximately 6 per cent by the third month. The infiltrate stays at this level for the

Table 9–4. Tubulointerstitial Lesions

Diffuse Mononuclear Cell Infiltrate
Acute cellular rejection
Acute on chronic cellular rejection
Acute interstitial nephritis due to drug allergy
Post-transplant lymphoproliferative diseases
Focal Mild Mononuclear Cell Infiltrate
Cyclosporine nephrotoxicity
FK506 nephrotoxicity
Ischemic tubular injury (acute tubular necrosis, ATN)
Subcapsular cortical ischemia
Viral infection
Pyelonephritis

Table 9–5. Tubular Lesions in Allografts

Tubulitis
Vacuolization
Tubular necrosis
Apoptosis
Loss of brush border
Regenerative changes
Casts
Cellular debris
Leukocytes
Erythrocytes
Pigment
Proteinaceous
Calcification
Tubular atrophy

remainder of the first year and slowly tapers to 2 per cent at between 3 and 8 years.[50] However, diffuse interstitial lymphocytic infiltrates can be seen in long-term stable grafts.[48] Tubulitis is rare in these circumstances. Staining with lymphocyte monoclonal antibodies and point counting give a 95 per cent probability of stable graft function, with an interstitial leukocyte infiltration of less than 14 per cent in patients treated with azathioprine and prednisolone. The probability is similar with an interstitial infiltrate of less than 8 per cent in cyclosporine-treated patients and with an infiltrate of less than 16 per cent in triple therapy.[51] The infiltrate is diffuse in 77 per cent of the cases of acute cellular rejection and focal in 23 per cent.[2, 52] Diffuse cortical interstitial infiltrates occupying more than 18 per cent to 21 per cent of the area of the biopsy can be considered to represent acute cellular rejection until proved otherwise.[45]

Acute Cellular Rejection

Acute cellular tubulointerstitial rejection (ACR) is characterized by interstitial edema, an extensive infiltrate of mononuclear cells in the interstitium, and infiltration of tubular epithelium (Fig. 9–12), often termed _tubulitis_. Tubulitis is usually multifocal, and there are lymphocytes and macrophages in the tubular epithelium and tubular casts made up of mononuclear cells. It can be seen in 77 per cent of acute rejection episodes and is said to involve distal tubules to a greater extent than proximal tubules.[53] The small nuclei of lymphocytes must be distinguished from apoptotic tubular cell nuclei.

The earliest lesion observed by light microscopy is a perivascular infiltrate around the ar-

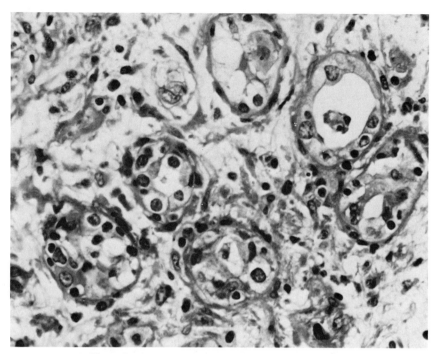

Figure 9–12. Tubulitis in acute cellular rejection. (× 500)

cuate vessels and an accompanying scattered interstitial infiltrate of mononuclear cells. The infiltrate intensifies acutely to become a polymorphous dense cellular lesion involving the cortex and outer medulla. On light microscopy one can distinguish small lymphocytes, larger lymphoblasts with abundant pyroninophilic cytoplasm, and prominent nucleoli, macrophages, and occasional granulocytes. The lymphoid cells may have mitotic figures (Fig. 9–13). If the acute changes are superimposed on a background of chronic rejection (i.e., vascular intimal proliferation, interstitial fibrosis, tubular atrophy, and glomerulopathy), then a diagnosis of acute on chronic cellular rejection can be made.

Either T cells or macrophages are the predominant cell type, probably varying with the timing of the biopsy, the severity of rejection,[54, 55] and the immunosuppressive therapy used.[5, 56, 57] Typically, T cells comprise just over 50 per cent of the cells and macrophages, 25 per cent to 40 per cent. The remainder are neutrophils, basophils, and eosinophils. Up to 33 per cent of the lymphoid population in ACR are lymphoblasts. Expression of Ki67, the IL-2 receptor (CD25), the transferrin receptor, CD38, and MHC class II antigen is evidence of lymphoid activation. These antigens are not expressed by resting T cells.[58] In one study, 6.3

per cent of CD45+ cells expressed Ki67, 4.1 per cent expressed CD25, and 6.9 per cent had detectable transferrin receptor.[58] The proportion of CD4+ and CD8+ cells varies,[50, 54, 58–61] usually with CD8+ predominance. CD4+ T cells may predominate early in ACR. As the lesion evolves, CD4+ cells are concentrated around vessels and the diffuse interstitial infiltrate is dominated by CD8+ cells.[12, 60]

The rejection episodes generally respond to high dose steroids, anti–T cell antibody or antilymphocyte globulin within 24 hours. The interstitial infiltrate rarely disappears completely but decreases to about 7 per cent of the area of the biopsy in patients on cyclosporine.[51] Additionally, the lymphoid cells are less activated in appearance and lose staining with activation markers, CD25, and antitransferrin.[58] Mononuclear cells may remain in the tubules longer than in the interstitium.

Prognostic Significance of the Infiltrate. The intensity of the mononuclear infiltration has no correlation with reversal of rejection.[50, 54] Two studies found that cases with greater amounts of CD8+ than CD4+ cells in the interstitial infiltrate had a somewhat worse prognosis.[54, 62] The latter study suggests that a diffuse cortical infiltrate of CD8+ T cells increases the relative risk of graft failure by more than 40 times. T lymphocytes infiltrating glo-

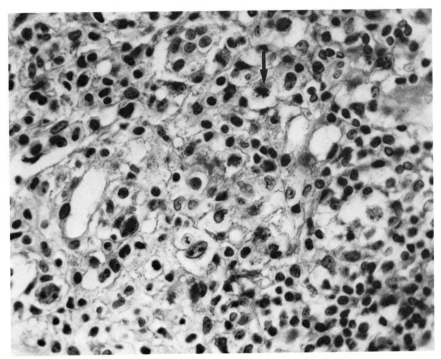

Figure 9–13. Mononuclear cell infiltrate in acute cellular rejection, with abundant activated cells and mitosis (arrow). ($\times$ 500)

meruli have been associated with a worsened prognosis.[54] Another report tentatively suggests that there are increased populations of CD8+/CD57+ T cells in rejecting allografts resistant to therapy with steroids and OKT3.[63] Two studies reported an association between eosinophils and prognosis. Grafts having irreversible ACR have higher percentages of eosinophils than those with reversible rejection (21.4 versus 3.8).[64] In a small study, biopsy samples with more than 2 per cent eosinophils were associated with graft loss in 86 per cent of cases, whereas 37 per cent of grafts with less than 2 per cent eosinophils were lost.[65] Eosinophil levels in the peripheral blood are not reliable indicators of irreversible rejection.

High numbers of macrophages in the infiltrate in early graft rejection have also been associated with refractory rejection,[66] as seen by staining with monoclonal antibody RFD7. In contrast, cases with a predominance of interstitial lymphocytes were associated with reversible rejection. Interstitial hemorrhage and necrosis are associated with poor graft survival.[67]

Acute Tubular Necrosis

Acute tubular necrosis (ATN) is a common cause of delayed primary graft function due to ischemia in graft harvesting and transplantation. Recovery from pure ATN is usually rapid, with return of complete function in days to weeks depending on the extent of tubular damage. The problem is often complicated by acute rejection in the anuric period. The reasons for this are obscure, but it is possible that tubular damage releases alloantigen and that there is increased MHC expression by graft cells.

The pathologic features of ATN in renal allografts are similar to those in the nonallograft kidney, although some morphologic distinctions have been claimed. Significant scalloping of the luminal border of proximal and distal convoluted tubules, ragged dissolution of renal tubular epithelial cells with sloughing of such cells into the tubular lumen, patchy cast formation, and occasional denudation of entire tubules characterize the lesion. In allograft ATN, the tubules are less flattened, have less severe loss of brush border on staining with PAS, and more overt tubular cell necrosis and apoptosis.[68] In addition, there are more peritubular calcium oxalate crystals, fewer cell casts, and a greater mononuclear cell infiltrate in the interstitium[68, 69] in the transplanted kidney. In well-preserved sections there may be obvious vacuolation of proximal tubular cells (Fig. 9–14), similar to that in cyclosporine nephrotoxicity (see later).

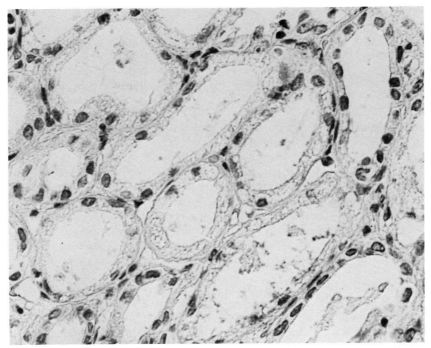

Figure 9–14. Acute ischemic tubular injury with coarse vacuolization of tubular epithelium. Compare with Figure 9–15. (× 500)

Several features confound the distinction between ATN and ACR. Interstitial edema can be marked in either ischemic injury or ACR. Limited tubulitis can be seen in ischemic injury; it is not a good discriminant of ACR, unless it is extensive. Tubular damage is usually evident in ACR. However, in ischemic tubular injury the interstitial infiltrate is rarely as intense, activated lymphoid cells are less prominent, and mitoses in the infiltrating cells are rare to undetectable. In ATN, significant accumulation of lymphocytes and occasional neutrophils can be seen at the corticomedullary junction, and the vasa recti can contain large numbers of such inflammatory cells. Interstitial hemorrhage is not a feature of ATN.

If extensive interstitial hemorrhage is encountered, renal vein thrombosis should be suspected. If cortical necrosis is present in the absence of renal hemorrhage, a compromise of the renal arteries should be suspected. ATN can also occur from obstruction. In such a case, one should look for the presence of dilation of tubules with inspissated casts and occasional rupture of tubules with interstitial inflammation (a PAS stain is helpful in detecting the extratubular cast protein). These are the features of reflux nephropathy, which can coexist with findings of ATN.

Evaluation of the biopsy in association with that taken at the time of transplantation will be very helpful. Subcapsular cortical ischemia may occasionally cause diagnostic difficulty, especially in the first 2 weeks post-transplant. The outer cortex is partially dependent on capsular vessels that are lost at transplantation. The ischemic zone extends for a depth of up to 1 mm of the outer cortex and can show tubulointerstitial inflammation and tubular necrosis. However, if an adequately deep biopsy is obtained, the zonal nature of the process should be apparent.

Acute Cyclosporine Toxicity

There are few pathognomonic lesions of acute cyclosporine nephrotoxicity. The diagnosis is made in concert with the clinical findings, including cyclosporine dosage and peak and trough serum levels. Patients treated with more than 15 mg/kg per day of cyclosporine are likely to suffer from acute cyclosporine nephrotoxicity.[70] However, a normal, or even subtherapeutic, level does not exclude cyclosporine toxicity, since patients vary considerably in their sensitivity to its effects. Patients who are given cyclosporine in the face of significant ATN or a persistently elevated serum creatinine level are more likely to develop acute cyclosporine nephrotoxicity.[70] Similarly, patients treated with cyclosporine who take other drugs that either decrease the hepatic clearance of this drug or increase the blood levels are also at risk.

The pathologic manifestations of cyclosporine nephrotoxicity are often nonspecific. The change most clearly associated with acute cyclosporine nephrotoxicity is the vasculopathy described earlier under vascular lesions (i.e., individual myocyte degeneration without inflammation); hemolytic uremic syndrome (HUS) occurs rarely, but the lesions are not distinguishable from idiopathic HUS. The incidence of arteriopathy has declined as the dosage of cyclosporine has declined, but it still occurs, and in our experience represents a significant fraction of the cases of toxicity that are biopsied.

Other changes that are associated with acute cyclosporine nephrotoxicity but are *not specific* include microcalcification of tubules, increasing severity of ATN as compared with the biopsy at the time of implantation, increased interstitial fibrosis over the biopsy at the time of implantation, and isometric vacuolization of renal tubular epithelial cells.[71] Since none of these changes are specific, they can be used only to implicate cyclosporine nephrotoxicity in the appropriate clinical setting. The differential diagnosis of tubular vacuolization includes nephrotoxicity (cyclosporine or FK506), acute tubular necrosis, osmotic diuretics (mannitol or dextran), and intravenous radiocontrast media. The most common cause in allografts is cyclosporine toxicity. Vacuolization was frequently seen early in the cyclosporine era when higher doses were used and can be rapidly induced in rats.[34]

In acute cyclosporine toxicity both proximal and distal tubules are affected, the features being more pronounced in the proximal tubules (Fig. 9–15).[34] The straight portion of the proximal tubule is more often affected than the convoluted part. The vacuoles are about one fifth of the diameter of the nucleus and are isometric. They may be single or confluent. The vacuoles seen in cyclosporine toxicity are indistinguishable from those caused by FK506.[25] The vacuoles of ischemic tubular injury tend to be larger, coarser, and irregular in size and shape (Fig. 9–14). Additionally, there tends to be more tubular cell necrosis, tubular dilation, and loss of brush border in tubular injury due to ischemia. Features of ACR are seen concomitantly with tubular vacuolar changes in 64 per cent of patients with cyclosporine toxicity and 79 per cent of patients with toxicity due to FK506.[25] Signs of chronic toxicity may also be present (striped

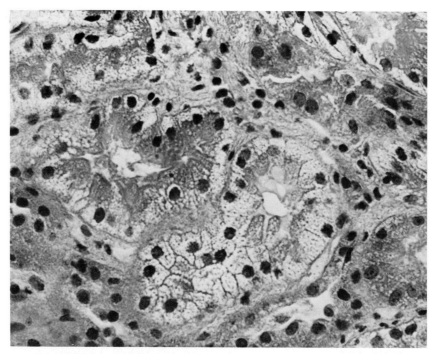

Figure 9–15. Proximal tubular vacuolization in acute cyclosporine toxicity. ($\times$ 500)

interstitial fibrosis and vascular hyalinosis). The vacuoles are reversible within 10 days of stopping cyclosporine and are dose dependent. The reversibility of these lesions with FK506 has not been determined. Ultrastructurally, the vacuoles of cyclosporine toxicity are dilated rough endoplasmic reticulum, lysosomes, and pinocytotic vesicles. These features are absent in vacuoles caused by osmotic diuresis.[34]

Other features seen by electron microscopy in patients with cyclosporine toxicity are giant mitochondria, enlarged multiple lysosomes, and microcalcifications in the tubular epithelium.[34] These features may be seen singly or in combination. Unlike the vacuolation, the giant mitochondria are more frequently found in the convoluted (S1 and S2) segments of the proximal tubule and are not found in the same cell. They are irregularly distributed and difficult to find, even in cases of severe toxicity. Thus they are largely unhelpful diagnostically.

Calcifications in tubular epithelium and basement membrane are most likely due to drug injury and appear to be dystrophic in nature. It appears that renal calcium flux is a dynamic process, and repeat biopsy may demonstrate resolution of calcium deposits over several days.[25] In calcification associated with ischemic injury, seen as deposition of calcium oxalate crystals, the crystals tend to be larger and coarser than those seen in drug toxicity. The uremic state with associated higher blood oxalate levels contributes to this process.

Patchy interstitial inflammation can also be seen. This should not necessarily be regarded as evidence of acute tubulointerstitial rejection unless the inflammation is associated with edema and tubulitis (see acute tubulointerstitial rejection). A small amount of interstitial infiltrate, particularly if it occurs in nodular aggregates or is associated with interstitial scar tissue, should not be considered evidence of acute tubulointerstitial rejection. It has been noted that most transplanted kidneys will show an increase in the numbers of interstitial lymphocytes even in the absence of clinically significant rejection. This is probably a manifestation of low-grade allograft rejection or perhaps corresponds to the infiltrate seen in "tolerant" animals.

The differentiation of cyclosporine toxicity from ACR is sometimes difficult. The absolute distinction often cannot be made since the two conditions coexist. The problem then becomes one of judgment of the relative contribution of each to allograft dysfunction. Interstitial infiltrates are common in both and are suggestive of nephrotoxicity only when minimal.[2, 3, 72, 73] Diffuse mononuclear cell infiltrates can be seen in cyclosporine toxicity, albeit less commonly than focal infiltrates. The lack of tubulitis and activated lymphocytes argues strongly against ACR. Interstitial edema,[73] tubulitis,[2] and peritubular capillary congestion[2, 3] with mononuclear cells have little diagnostic value. Anticyclosporine antibodies can be used on paraffin-embedded material. It has been claimed that fine granular tubular and interstitial staining, combined with a sparse CD8+ infiltrate, can be useful in making the diagnosis of cyclosporine toxicity.[74]

The pathogenesis of acute cyclosporine toxicity is related to arterial vasoconstriction caused by arachidonic acid metabolites.[31, 32, 75] In cyclosporine-treated animals, thromboxane A_2 production is increased.[32] This substance has profound vasoconstrictive effects. The renal blood flow is decreased and the glomerular filtration rate reduced, resulting in a diminished regenerative capacity of renal epithelium and prolongation of post-transplant ATN. In addition, the decrease in perfusion of the nephrons leads to activation of the renin-angiotensin system and causes fluid retention and hypertension. All these acute changes are reversible with cessation of therapy. Calcium antagonists have been used to ameliorate the vasoconstricting effects of cyclosporine, but these have not produced significant long-term benefit. Cyclosporine increases endothelial prostacyclin synthesis, which may be a negative feedback mechanism against the overproduction of thromboxane A_2.[31, 32, 75] Endothelial cells damaged by cyclosporine are further injured by the known ability of cyclosporine to produce platelet aggregation. All these features potentiate the ability of cyclosporine to produce vascular thrombosis.[76, 77]

Lymphoproliferative Disease

A diffuse mononuclear cell interstitial infiltrate in a renal transplant biopsy raises the differential of post-transplant lymphoproliferative diseases (PTLD). These range from benign lymphoid proliferations with mononucleosis-like symptoms to monoclonal proliferations behaving like non-Hodgkin's lymphoma. The proliferations are commonly of B cell origin and may be monoclonal or polyclonal. The vast majority have detectable Epstein-Barr virus (EBV) DNA and EBV nuclear proteins and tend to regress if immunosuppressive therapy is withdrawn.[78–80] The lesions occur in 1 per cent to 2.5 per cent of renal transplant recipients in extranodal sites, particularly the central nervous system, gastrointestinal tract, skin, and bone.[78, 80, 81] They may be unifocal or multifocal and can involve the transplant as an initial manifestation. In one series, there was initial involvement of the allograft kidney in two cases.[78] The patients presented with declining renal function and fever, at 1.5 and 2.2 months post-transplant, mimicking ACR. In one of these cases the disease presented at an advanced stage.

In general, the infiltrates in PTLD can be subclassified as polymorphous and monomorphous.[78–80, 82] Polymorphous infiltrates are composed of diffusely infiltrative lymphoid populations, containing varied proportions of small lymphocytes, small and large cleaved and noncleaved lymphocytes, immunoblasts, plasmacytoid lymphocytes, and mature plasma cells (Fig. 9–16). A minority of cases are made up of uniform populations of lymphoid cells, so-called monomorphic PTLD, most commonly small or large noncleaved lymphocytes. There is a relative paucity of macrophages, unlike the case in ACR.[78] The majority stain for B cell markers; T cell phenotypes are extremely rare.

Many cases are immunoglobulin negative but have a detectable immunoglobulin gene rearrangement or have monoclonality detectable by EBV DNA analysis.[83]

Acute Allergic Interstitial Nephritis

Acute interstitial nephritis caused by drug allergy also comes into the differential diagnosis of tubulointerstitial processes in a renal transplant biopsy. Tubulitis, indistinguishable from that seen in rejection, can be seen in drug allergy. The most helpful features in making the distinction are a greater preponderance of CD4+ lymphocytes in the infiltrate and more numerous eosinophils in allergic interstitial nephritis. However, ACR can contain numerous eosinophils,[64, 65] especially in severe rejection. In this setting, only the presence of endothelialitis can prove that rejection is present.[12]

Acute Pyelonephritis

Acute pyelonephritis is another tubulointerstitial infiltrative process to consider. There are minor differences between pyelonephritis

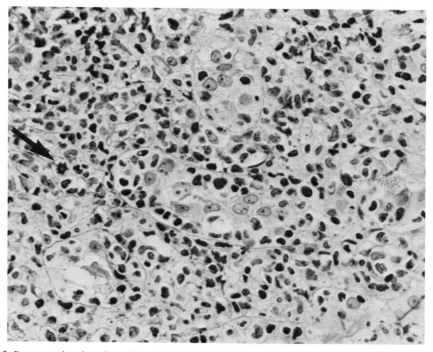

Figure 9–16. Post-transplant lymphoproliferative disease with polymorphous atypical lymphoid infiltrate, intraepithelial lymphoid cells simulating tubulitis, and mitosis (arrow). (× 500) (Courtesy of Dr. Samy S. Iskandar, Bowman Gray School of Medicine).

in an allograft and that in a nontransplanted kidney. In the setting of immunosuppression, the threshold for significant inflammation ought to be lower than usual. The number of neutrophils, both in the interstitium and infiltrating tubular epithelium, and neutrophil cast formation are less intense than one expects for the degree of tissue damage. Neutrophils may be abundant in the interstitium, with direct extension into Bowman's capsule. However, neutrophils, even in casts, can be seen in ACR. An abundance of mononuclear cells, tubulitis, and especially endothelialitis indicate ACR. Involvement of cortical tubules with relative sparing of medullary tubules and collecting ducts suggests rejection. Stains for microorganisms are rarely helpful.

The most significant viral infection in renal transplants is cytomegalovirus, although there are only occasional reports of interstitial nephritis in transplant kidneys that may be due to this organism.[85, 86] The infiltrate is focal, lymphocytic, and histiocytic, with a granulomatous appearance surrounding the tubules. Epithelial cells with typical nuclear and cytoplasmic inclusions are seen occasionally.[86] Acute cellular rejection is frequently a concomitant feature.[86, 87] CMV early and intermediate-early antigens may be detected in the infiltrating mononuclear cells.[87]

Interstitial Fibrosis

Interstitial fibrosis is an ominous sign in the renal allograft and may herald progressive graft failure. However, there have been reports of diffuse fibrosis in the presence of normal, stable graft function in patients on cyclosporine.[48] Clinically, there is insidious decline in graft function with symptoms arising with the onset of renal failure. The differential diagnoses are listed in Table 9–6.

Chronic cyclosporine toxicity gives rise to so-called "striped" interstitial fibrosis (Fig. 9–17): radial, linear cortical bands of fibrosis perpendicular to the capsule. Frequently there are associated vascular lesions, as described earlier, and the pattern is believed to arise because of chronic ischemia in watershed zones. Atrophic tubules, which accompany the fibrosis, have a diminished outer diameter, with basement membrane wrinkling and thickening and flattening of tubular epithelial cells. The pattern is not simply atrophy, however, since increased cytoplasmic basophilia and enlarged vesicular nuclei with prominent nucleoli can

Table 9–6. Causes of Interstitial Fibrosis

Donor disease (e.g, benign nephrosclerosis)
Chronic rejection
Hypertension
Renal artery stenosis
Arterial thrombosis
Obstructive uropathy
Nephrotoxicity
  Cyclosporine
  FK506
  Aminoglycosides
Scar from previous acute rejection
Subcapsular scar (surgical trauma)
Residual from acute tubular necrosis
Biopsy site

be found, indicative of a reactive process. Tubular loss can be extensive and is usually accompanied by glomerular obsolescence.

Unfortunately, this pattern is rarely distinctive by itself in a renal allograft. Among the other possibilities for interstitial fibrosis and tubular atrophy are renal artery stenosis, in which the tubules are small and simplified, often without intervening fibrosis, and benign nephrosclerosis, in which the scars are concentrated in the outer cortex. Vascular lesions help distinguish chronic rejection, cyclosporine toxicity, and hypertension. If intimal fibrosis and glomerular lesions of chronic rejection are absent, then chronic cyclosporine toxicity should be favored.

GLOMERULAR LESIONS

Glomeruli are relatively spared in typical acute cellular rejection.[84] However, studies with leukocyte markers have indicated that minor numbers of T cells and macrophages can be found in glomerular capillary loops in otherwise typical rejection,[88] and electron microscopy can reveal segmental endothelial injury. When these lesions are diffuse and well developed, the term *acute allograft glomerulopathy* is appropriate[17] (Table 9–7).

Acute Allograft Glomerulopathy

Acute allograft glomerulopathy is a form of cell-mediated rejection characterized by endothelial swelling, capillary luminal obliteration, PAS-positive mesangial webs, accumulation of T cells, and mesangiolysis.[17, 89] This typically arises 1 to 3 months post-transplant and is heralded by an acute loss of function, with azo-

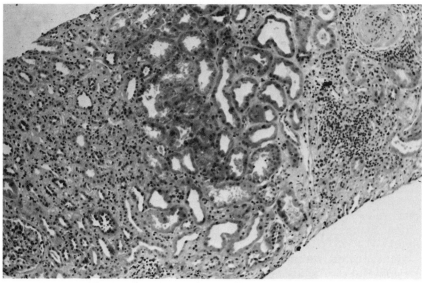

Figure 9–17. Biopsy specimen showing striped interstitial fibrosis in chronic cyclosporine toxicity. ($\times$ 79)

Table 9–7. Glomerular Lesions

Endothelial Swelling and Thrombi
    Preservation injury
    Hyperacute rejection
    Acute transplant glomerulopathy
    Hemolytic-uremic syndrome
    Acute cyclosporine toxicity
    OKT3 toxicity
    Disseminated intravascular coagulation
Hypercellularity
    Mesangial cells
        Chronic transplant glomerulopathy
        Recurrent/de novo glomerulonephritis
    Leukocytes
        Acute transplant glomerulopathy (mononuclear
          cells)
        Hyperacute rejection (neutrophils)
        Renal vein thrombosis (neutrophils, monocytes)
Necrosis
    Hyperacute rejection
    Recurrent idiopathic crescentic glomerulonephritis
    Hemolytic uremic syndrome
Glomerulosclerosis
    Chronic transplant glomerulopathy
    Focal segmental glomerulosclerosis
    Diabetes mellitus
    Hypertensive nephrosclerosis
    Cyclosporine toxicity
    Reflux nephropathy
Glomerular Basement Membrane
    Thickening
        Diabetes mellitus
        Membranous glomerulonephropathy
        Compensatory hypertrophy
    Duplication
        Acute transplant glomerulopathy (webbing)
        Membranoproliferative glomerulonephritis
        Chronic allograft glomerulopathy (tram-track)
    Wrinkling
        Ischemic collapse/vascular disease

temia and proteinuria. Acute allograft glomerulopathy is present in about 4 per cent of renal transplant biopsies.[12]

Morphologically, the earliest recognizable feature is diffuse glomerular endothelial cell swelling, progressing to capillary luminal occlusion. There is glomerular hypercellularity with endocapillary proliferation and infiltration by mononuclear cells (Fig. 9–18). There are substantially greater numbers of T lymphocytes in the glomeruli in acute glomerulopathy compared with acute cellular vascular rejection alone.[17] The glomerular inflammatory infiltrate consists predominantly of T lymphocytes of the CD3+ and CD8+ phenotype, as well as monocytes. The mesangium contains PAS-positive material, and the basement membrane may have a double contour. The most distinctive feature is a webbing pattern on PAS stain[89] (Fig. 9–18B). These lesions have been collectively referred to as "pseudoglomerulitis," and they may be global or segmental. Some have described evolving lesions from minimal endothelial swelling with capillary lumen obliteration and glomerular enlargement to focal mild hypercellularity, matrix increase, and basement membrane reduplication.[90]

Immunofluorescence reveals scant IgM and C3 deposits in the mesangium, with some deposits in the intima and media of arteries. Fibrinogen deposits are seen in capillary walls and mesangium. Electron microscopy discloses separation of the endothelium from the basement membrane, with flocculent material in the subendothelial space. Later there is split-

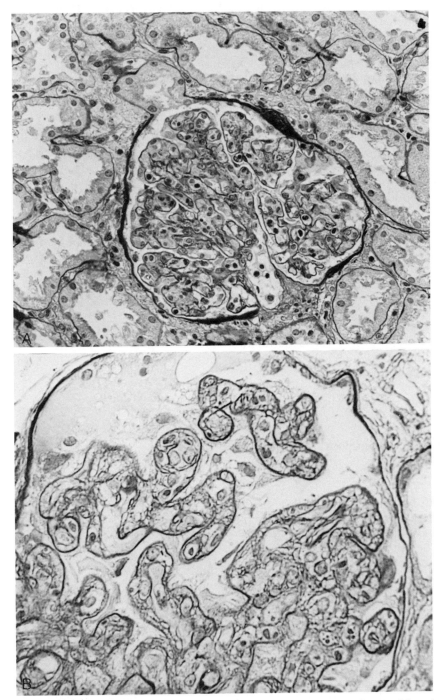

Figure 9–18. *A,* Acute allograft glomerulopathy with endothelial swelling, capillary lumen obliteration, and focal lymphocytic infiltrate. (× 313) *B,* Webbing, mesangiolysis, and basement duplication are seen on periodic acid–Schiff stains. (× 500)

ting of the basement membrane as the separated endothelium makes new basement membrane material. The intermembranous space contains cell debris and mesangial cell processes (mesangial interposition).

Acute glomerulopathy is associated with vascular injury in up to 92 per cent of cases,[12] but the interstitium may have little or no infiltrate. The interstitial infiltrate has a significantly greater amount of CD8+ cells and CD57+ cells than in the usual acute cellular rejection. The high frequency of associated lesions of ACR suggests that the process is a manifestation of rejection at the level of the endothelium, probably triggered by viral infection or other causes; the first well-documented series was in patients with cytomegaloviremia. The number of CD8+ T cells in the glomeruli is correlated with a poor prognosis, even when the lesions are not fully developed.[17, 88] The lesion is associated with a high rate of graft loss in the first year; in a combined series, there was a 67 per cent graft loss in 6 months after diagnosis.[12]

The differential diagnosis includes hemolytic-uremic syndrome and membranoproliferative glomerulonephritis. In the latter there are subendothelial, subepithelial, and mesangial electron-dense deposits. The hemolytic-uremic syndrome has distinctive vascular and glomerular changes, as described earlier.

Chronic Allograft Glomerulopathy

Chronic allograft glomerulopathy is clinically characterized by proteinuria, usually greater than 1 gram/24 hours, and a progressive decline in allograft function. The proteinuria is progressive, and patients may become nephrotic. The process usually begins after the third post-transplant month[12] but may begin earlier. The lesion develops in patients without previous glomerular disease and is thought to be a response to rejection, therapy, or infection. A few documented cases have progressed from acute glomerulopathy to chronic glomerulopathy.[90] It is rare in grafts from HLA-identical siblings.[91] Progressive graft failure commonly ensues; in one series, 77 per cent had failed at 10 years.[90]

The glomerular lesion is often focal and segmental. Glomerulosclerosis may vary from segmental to global in the same biopsy material. The glomeruli are hypercellular, with an increase in mesangial matrix, thickened capillary loops, segmental scars, and synechium formation between scarred lobules and parietal Bowman's capsule. Basement membrane duplication is apparent on PAS or methenamine silver staining (Fig. 9–19). The extent of duplication varies from moderate segmental to diffuse marked.[90] Electron microscopy shows foot process effacement and loss of endothelial fenestrations.[12] Subendothelial rarefactions are also prominent, and these contain various amounts of flocculent material, granular debris, vesicles, and ribbons.[92] The basement membrane is thickened and duplicated with mesangial cell interposition. Mesangiolysis is a frequent finding. There are no deposits on electron microscopy. Immunofluorescence reveals a typically segmental, granular IgG or IgM and C3 in the mesangium and capillary walls. Sometimes fibrin is also seen. There is no correlation between the severity of the glomerular changes and the immunofluorescent pattern. The differential diagnosis includes membranoproliferative glomerulonephritis, type I, which usually may be distinguished by diffuse hypercellularity with abundant subendothelial and mesangial electron-dense deposits. The recovery phase of the hemolytic-uremic syndrome also has prominent basement membrane duplication.

Cyclosporine Toxicity

Cyclosporine toxicity can also cause glomerular lesions as part of the hemolytic-uremic syndrome, or as an isolated finding.[34] The lesions can be found in 3 per cent of patients treated with cyclosporine. Twenty-five per cent to fifty per cent of the patients with thrombi have associated cyclosporine arteriolopathy. In one series, cyclosporine glomerulopathy was identified in biopsies taken at between 6 and 53 months, always in association with vasculopathy.[93] Patients present with a decline in graft function, hypertension and proteinuria, sometimes with hematuria. Histologically, there are glomerular capillary platelet/fibrin thrombi, visceral epithelial capping, exudations, rare crescent formation, and even thrombotic microangiopathy in severe cases. The lesions are focal and segmental in distribution and are not specific by light, immunofluorescent, or electron microscopy.

Recurrent Glomerulonephritis

Recurrent glomerulonephritis denotes glomerulonephritis in the graft that is morpho-

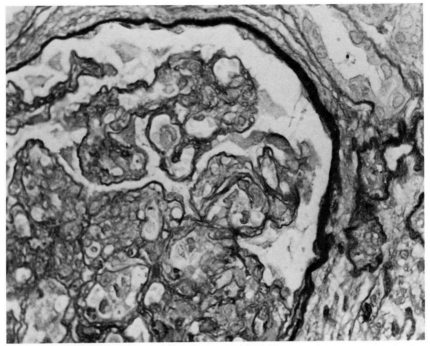

Figure 9–19. Chronic allograft glomerulopathy, with basement membrane duplication and increased mesangial matrix. (Periodic acid–Schiff, × 500)

logically identical to the original disease by light, immunofluorescent, and electron microscopy, arising from persistence of the original pathogenetic process in the recipient.[84] Recurrent glomerulonephritis is not uncommon, especially with increased long-term graft survival. The diagnosis can be established only if the previous diagnosis is documented by light, immunofluorescent, and electron microscopy, ideally by biopsy at an early stage, and is matched by the findings in the transplant biopsy, and if the donor kidney is known to be normal at transplantation. Glomerular lesions are often not clinically significant in the first 2 years after transplantation. The lesions most likely to recur are dense deposit disease (90 per cent),[94, 95] hemolytic-uremic syndrome (41 per cent),[96] IgA nephropathy (38 per cent),[95] Henoch-Schönlein purpura (10 per cent to 15 per cent),[97] and focal segmental glomerulosclerosis (20 per cent to 30 per cent).[41, 98]

De Novo Glomerulonephritis

This is, by definition, morphologically distinct from the original disease and from transplant glomerulopathy and is not present in the graft at the time of transplantation. Many cases may be coincidental, but two entities are worthy of mention as they arise specifically in the context of the transplanted allograft. These are membranous glomerulonephritis and anti-glomerular basement membrane (anti-GBM) disease arising in patients with Alport's syndrome.

More than 130 cases of de novo membranous glomerulonephritis (MGN) have been reported. The incidence is uncertain; figures from 1.2 per cent to 9.3 per cent have been cited in the literature.[99, 100] Clinically, the lesion presents anywhere from 2 to 58 months post-transplant (mean, 26 months), usually with proteinuria. There is no known relationship to HLA status. The lesion occurs equally in cadaveric and living related allografts. Few cases have been HBsAg positive; staining of the biopsy for HBsAg was negative in these reports.[101]

Microscopically, most lesions are stage I or II and diffuse at presentation (Fig. 9–20). Electron microscopy shows that the subepithelial deposits are atypical compared with those seen in idiopathic MGN in native kidneys. Additional lesions seen with light microscopy include a mononuclear cell interstitial infiltrate, transplant glomerulopathy in 33 per cent of cases, and vascular rejection in 50 per cent of

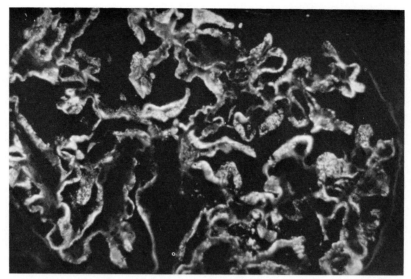

Figure 9–20. Membranous glomerulopathy, de novo, with granular IgG along the basement membrane. (Immunofluorescence, × 500)

cases.[101] The differential diagnosis includes the usual form of chronic transplant glomerulopathy, which may be distinguished by the paucity or complete absence of immune deposits on electron microscopy. The graft survival appears not to be compromised by this lesion. Patients with nephrotic-range proteinuria and creatinine levels greater than 1.3 mg/dl almost always develop graft failure, however.[12]

Anti-GBM nephritis can arise in allografts transplanted into patients with Alport's syndrome. A subset of Alport's patients lack an epitope on the noncollagenous domain of type IV collagen. The recipient can develop antibodies to this epitope in as little as 2 weeks post-transplant, which will bind to normal basement membrane. Linear IgG deposits along the GBM are detectable in 15 per cent of patients with Alport's syndrome. Circulating serum antibodies are detectable by Western blot in 50 per cent of these.[102] The linear IgG deposits are frequently transient and asymptomatic. Approximately 20 per cent of the patients with these deposits develop proteinuria, hematuria, or both. A significant portion of these patients develop graft failure.[103]

Reflux Nephropathy

Reflux nephropathy, an obstructive condition of the ureter or ureteral-vesical junction may appear at any time post-transplant. Like other types of chronic pyelonephritis, it is characterized by obstruction of tubules, with cast formation, interstitial inflammation (which is noninvasive), and interstitial fibrosis. If the process is long-standing, the tubules may be atrophic. Thus, the process may resemble chronic rejection or chronic cyclosporine nephrotoxicity. In acute cases resembling acute pyelonephritis, leukocytes or leukocyte casts in tubules may be found. In such cases, focal proliferative vasculopathy and focal global glomerulosclerosis may be found. This condition may therefore be confused with recurrent focal segmental glomerulosclerosis, which may also show tubular dilation and cast formation. In such cases, a pretransplant history is very helpful. Also, a history of proteinuria will be useful; patients with focal glomerulosclerosis will have significant proteinuria.

Renovascular Disease

Abnormalities of the renal artery anastomosis may lead to renal ischemia and renal compromise. The features seen in the biopsy may resemble those of chronic rejection. The only useful differential feature is the presence of juxtaglomerular apparatus proliferation in the absence of features of chronic rejection. If these findings are noted, the clinician should be alerted to look for renal artery disease.

REFERENCES

1. Kiss D, Landman J, Mihatsch M, et al. Risks and benefits of graft biopsy in renal transplantation under cyclosporin-A. Clin Nephrol 38:132, 1992.

2. Sibley RK, Rynasiewicz J, Ferguson RM, et al. Morphology of cyclosporine nephrotoxicity and acute rejection in patients immunosuppressed with cyclosporine and prednisone. Surgery 94:225, 1983.
3. Taube DH, Neild GH, Williams DG, et al. Differentiation between allograft rejection and cyclosporin nephrotoxicity in renal transplant recipients. Lancet 2:171, 1985.
4. Yagisawa T, Takahashi K, Toma H. One hundred eighty graft biopsies in cyclosporine treated kidney transplants. Transplant Proc 20:772, 1988.
5. Waltzer WC, Miller F, Arnold A, et al. Immunohistologic analysis of human renal allograft dysfunction. Transplantation 43:100, 1987.
6. Matas AJ, Sibley R, Mauer M, et al. A retrospective study of biopsies performed during putative rejection episodes. Transplantation 22:420, 1983.
7. Matas AJ, Tellis VA, Sablay L, et al. The value of needle renal allograft biopsy. III. A prospective study. Surgery 98:922, 1985.
8. Pardo-Mindan F, Guillen R, Virto R, et al. Kidney allograft biopsy: A valuable tool in assessing the diagnosis of acute rejection. Clin Nephrol 24:37, 1985.
9. Bonsib SM, Reznicek MJ, Wright FH. Renal medulla in the diagnosis of acute cellular rejection. Transplantation 48:690, 1989.
10. Curschellas E, Landmann J, Durig M, et al. Morphologic findings in "zero-hour" biopsies of renal transplants. Clin Nephrol 36:215, 1991.
11. Ito S, Camussi G, Tetta C, et al. Hyperacute renal allograft rejection in the rabbit. Lab Invest 51:148, 1984.
12. Colvin R. Renal allografts. *In* Colvin R, Bhan A, McCluskey R (eds). *Diagnostic Immunopathology.* New York, Raven Press, 1988, p 151.
13. Halloran PF, Schlaut J, Solez K, Srinivasa NS. The significance of the anti-class I response. II. Clinical and pathologic features of renal transplants with anti-class I-like antibody. Transplantation 53:550, 1992.
14. Scornik JC, LeFor WM, Cicciarelli JC, et al. Hyperacute and acute kidney graft rejection due to antibodies against B cells. Transplantation 54:61, 1992.
15. Paul L, Class F, van Es L, et al. Accelerated rejection of a renal allograft associated with pretransplantation antibodies directed against donor antigens on endothelium and monocytes. N Engl J Med 300:1258, 1979.
16. Alpers CE, Gordon D, Gown AM. Immunophenotype of vascular rejection in renal transplants. Mod Pathol 3:198, 1990.
17. Tuazon TV, Schneeberger EE, Bhan AK, et al. Mononuclear cells in acute allograft glomerulopathy. Am J Pathol 129:119, 1987.
18. Feucht H, Felber E, Gokel M. Vascular deposition of complement-split products in kidney allografts with cell-mediated rejection. Clin Exp Immunol 86:464, 1991.
19. von Willebrand E, Pettersson E, Ahonen J, Hayry P. CMV infection, Class II antigen expression, and human kidney allograft rejection. Transplantation 42:364, 1986.
20. Bishop GA, Waugh JA, Landers DV, et al. Microvascular destruction in renal transplant rejection. Transplantation 48:408, 1989.
21. Leszczynski D, Maszczynska M, Halttunen J, Hayry P. Renal target structures in acute allograft rejection: A histochemical study. Kidney Int 31:1311, 1987.
22. Colvin RB. The pathogenesis of vascular rejection. Transplant Proc 23:2052, 1991.
23. Fuggle SV, Sanderson JB, Gray DW, et al. Variation in expression of endothelial adhesion molecules in pretransplant and transplanted kidneys—correlation with intragraft events. Transplantation 55:117, 1993.
24. Kreis H. Antilymphocyte globulins in kidney transplantation. Kidney Int 42:188, 1992.
25. Randhawa PS, Shapiro R, Jordan ML, et al. The histopathological changes associated with allograft rejection and drug toxicity in renal transplant recipients maintained on FK506. Clinical significance and comparison with cyclosporine. Am J Surg Pathol 17:60, 1993.
26. Delaney VB, Campbell WG, Nasr SA, et al. Efficacy of OKT3 monoclonal antibody therapy in steroid-resistant, predominantly vascular acute rejection. Transplantation 47:817, 1988.
27. Schroeder TJ, Weiss MA, Smith RD, et al. The efficacy of OKT3 in vascular rejection. Transplantation 51:312, 1991.
28. Schwarz A, Krause PH, Offermann G, Keller F. Recurrent and de novo renal disease after kidney transplantation with or without cyclosporine A. Am J Kidney Dis 17:524, 1991.
29. Nizze H, Mihatsch M, Zollinger H, et al. Cyclosporine-associated nephropathy in patients with heart and bone marrow transplants. Clin Nephrol 30:248, 1988.
30. Myers B, Newton L. Cyclosporine-induced chronic nephropathy: An obliterative microvascular renal injury. J Am Soc Nephrol 2:S45, 1991.
31. Zoja C, Furci L, Ghilardi F, et al. Cyclosporin induced endothelial cell injury. Lab Invest 55:455, 1986.
32. Voss BL, Hamilton KK, Samara SEN, McKee PA. Cyclosporine suppression of endothelial prostacyclin generation. Transplantation 45:793, 1988.
33. Harlan J, Harker L, Reidy M, et al. Lipopolysaccharide-mediated bovine endothelial cell injury in vitro. Lab Invest 48:269, 1983.
34. Mihatsch M, Thiel G, Ryffel B. Histopathology of cyclosporine nephrotoxicity. Histopathology 20:759, 1988.
35. Keown PA, Stiller CR, Wallace AC. Nephrotoxicity of cyclosporin A. *In* Burdick JF, Solez K, Williams GM (eds). *Kidney Transplant Rejection: Diagnosis and Treatment.* New York, Marcel Dekker, 1992, p 637.
36. Basadonna G, Matas A, Gillingham K, et al. Early versus late acute renal allograft rejection: Impact on chronic rejection. Transplantation 55:993, 1993.
37. Kasiske BL, Kalil RS, Lee HS, Rao KV. Histopathologic findings associated with a chronic, progressive decline in renal allograft function. Kidney Int 40:514, 1991.
38. Demetris A, Zerbe T, Banner B. Morphology of solid organ allograft arteriopathy: Identification of proliferating intimal cell populations. Transplant Proc 21:3667, 1989.
39. Mauer SM, Barbosa J, Vernier RL, et al. Development of diabetic vascular lesions in normal kidneys transplanted into patients with diabetes mellitus. Cell Immunol 29:1, 1976.
40. Porter KA, Dossetor JB, Marchioro TL, et al. Human renal transplants. I. Glomerular changes. Lab Invest 16:153, 1967.
41. Ramos E. Recurrent diseases in the renal allograft. J Am Soc Nephrol 2:109, 1991.
42. Morozumi K, Thiel G, Albert FW, et al. Studies on morphological outcome of cyclosporine-associated arteriolopathy after discontinuation of cyclosporine in renal allografts. Clin Nephrol 38:1, 1992.
43. Larsen S, Brun C, Duun S, et al. Early arteriolopathy following "high-dose" cyclosporine in kidney transplantation. APMIS Suppl 4:66, 1988.

44. Rossmann P, Jirka J, Chadimova M, et al. Arteriosclerosis of the human renal allograft: Morphology, origin, life history and relationship to cyclosporine therapy. Virchows Arch A Pathol Anat 418:129, 1991.

45. Neild G, Taube D, Hartley R, et al. Morphological differentiation between rejection and cyclosporin nephrotoxicity in renal allografts. J Clin Pathol 39:152, 1986.

46. Yamaguchi Y, Teraoka S, Yagisawa T, et al. Ultrastructural study of cyclosporine-associated arteriolopathy in renal allografts. Transplant Proc 21:1517, 1989.

47. Landmann J, Mihatsch M, Ratschek M, Thiel G. Cyclosporine A and intravascular coagulation. Transplant Proc 19:1817, 1987.

48. Isoniemi HM, Krogerus L, von Willebrand E, et al. Histopathological findings in well-functioning, long-term renal allografts. Kidney Int 41:155, 1992.

49. Burdick JF, Beschorner WE, Smith WJ, et al. Characteristics of early routine renal allograft biopsies. Transplantation 38:679, 1984.

50. McWhinnie DL, Thompson JF, Taylor HM, et al. Morphometric analysis of cellular infiltration assessed by monoclonal antibody labeling in sequential human renal allograft biopsies. Transplantation 2:352, 1986.

51. McWhinnie D, Azevedo L, Carter N, et al. Diagnosis of renal allograft rejection by analysis of infiltrating cell profiles: An assessment of cyclosporine, azathioprine/prednisolone, and triple therapy. Transplant Proc 19:1633, 1987.

52. d'Ardenne A, Dunnill M, Thompson J, et al. Cyclosporin and renal graft histology. J Clin Pathol 39:145, 1986.

53. Nasady T, Ormos J, Stiller D, et al. Tubular ultrastructure in rejected human renal allografts. Ultrastruct Pathol 12:195, 1988.

54. Bishop GA, Hall BM, Duggin GG, et al. Immunopathology of renal allograft rejection analyzed with monoclonal antibodies to mononuclear cell markers. Kidney Int 29:708, 1986.

55. Dooper IM, Bogman MJ, Hoitsma AJ, et al. Detection of interstitial increase in macrophages, characteristic of acute interstitial rejection, in routinely processed renal allograft biopsies using the monoclonal antibody KP1. Transplant Int 5:209, 1992.

56. Waltzer W, Miller F, Arnold A, et al. Immunologic analysis of cellular infiltrates during human renal allograft dysfunction. Transplant Proc 20:111, 1988.

57. von Willebrand E, Hayry P. Composition and in vitro cytotoxicity of cellular infiltrates in rejecting human kidney allografts. Cell Immunol 41:358, 1978.

58. Seron D, Alexopoulos E, Raftery MJ, et al. Diagnosis of rejection in renal allograft biopsies using the presence of activated and proliferating cells. J Exp Med 166:1132, 1989.

59. Hancock W, Thomson N, Atkins R. Composition of interstitial cellular infiltrate identified by monoclonal antibodies in renal biopsies of rejecting human renal allografts. Transplantation 35:458, 1983.

60. Sako H, Nakane O, Nishihara K, et al. Immunohistochemical study of the cells infiltrating human renal allografts by the ABC and the IGSS method using monoclonal antibodies. Transplantation 44:202, 1987.

61. Guettier C, Nochy D, Hinglais N, et al. Distinct phenotypic composition of diffuse interstitial and perivascular focal infiltrates in renal allografts: A morphometric analysis of cellular infiltration under conventional immunosuppressive therapy and under cyclosporine A. Clin Nephrol 30:97, 1988.

62. Sanfilippo F, Kolbeck PC, Vaughn WK, Bollinger RR. Renal allograft cell infiltrates associated with irreversible rejection. Transplantation 40:679, 1985.

63. Malinowski K, Waltzer W, Jao S, et al. Homing of CD8+/CD57+ T lymphocytes into acutely rejected renal allografts. Transplantation 54:1013, 1992.

64. Kormendi F, Amend W. The importance of eosinophil cells in kidney allograft rejection. Transplantation 45:537, 1988.

65. Weir MR, Hall CM, Shen SY, et al. The prognostic value of the eosinophil in acute renal allograft rejection. Transplantation 41:709, 1986.

66. Raftery M, Seron D, Hartley B, et al. Immunohistological analysis of the early renal allograft biopsy. Transplant Proc 21:280, 1989.

67. Herbertson BM, Evans DB, Calne RY, Banerjee AK. Percutaneous needle biopsies of renal allografts: The relationship between morphological changes present in the biopsies and subsequent allograft function. Histopathology 1:161, 1977.

68. Olsen S, Burdick J, Keown P, et al. Primary acute renal failure ("acute tubular necrosis") in the transplanted kidney: Morphology and pathogenesis. Medicine 68:173, 1989.

69. Solez K, Racusen L, Burdick J, et al. Transplant "acute tubular necrosis" in cyclosporine treated patients. Kidney Int 37:495, 1990.

70. Mihatsch MJ, Thiel G, Ryffel B. Cyclosporin nephrotoxicity. A tubulo-interstitial and vascular disease. *In* Betani T, Remuzzi G, Garattini S (ed.). *Drugs and the Kidney*. New York, Raven Press, 1986, p 153.

71. Ruiz P, Kolbeck PC, Sroggs MW, Sanfilippo F. Associations between cyclosporine therapy and interstitial fibrosis in renal allograft biopsies. Transplantation 45:91, 1988.

72. Ryffel B, Siegel H, Thiel G, Mihatsch MJ. Experimental cyclosporine nephrotoxicity. *In* Burdick JF, Williams GM, Solez K (eds). *Kidney Transplant Rejection: Diagnosis and Treatment*. New York, Marcel Dekker, 1992, p 601.

73. Farnsworth A, Hall BM, Ng A, et al. Renal biopsy morphology in renal transplantation. Am J Surg Pathol 8:243, 1984.

74. Kolbeck PC, Wolfe JA, Burchette J, Sanfilippo F. Immunopathologic patterns of cyclosporine deposition associated with nephrotoxicity in renal allograft biopsies. Transplantation 3:218, 1987.

75. Coffman T, Carr DR, Yarger W, Klotman P. Evidence that renal prostaglandin and thromboxane production is stimulated in chronic cyclosporine nephrotoxicity. Transplantation 43:282, 1987.

76. First MR, Smith RD, Weiss MA, et al. Cyclosporine-associated glomerular and arteriolar thrombosis following renal transplantation. Transplant Proc 21:1567, 1989.

77. Gruber SA, Chavers B, Payne W, et al. Thrombosis/lack of increase with cyclosporine immunosuppression. Transplantation 47:475, 1989.

78. Nalesnik M, Jaffe R, Starzi T, et al. The pathology of posttransplant lymphoproliferative disorders occurring in the setting of cyclosporine A–prednisone immunosuppression. Am J Pathol 133:173, 1988.

79. Craig F, Gulley M, Banks P. Post-transplantation lymphoproliferative disorders. Am J Clin Path 99:265, 1993.

80. Ferry J, Jacobson J, Conti D, et al. Lymphoproliferative disorders and hematologic malignancies following organ transplantation. Mod Pathol 2:583, 1989.

81. Hanto D, Frizzera G, Gajl-Peczalska K, Simmons R.

Epstein-Barr virus, immunodeficiency, and B cell lymphoproliferation. Transplantation 39:461, 1985.

82. Swerdlow S. Post-transplant lymphoproliferative disorders: A morphologic, phenotypic and genotypic spectrum of disease. Histopathology 20:373, 1992.

83. Locker J, Nalesnik M. Molecular genetic analysis of lymphoid tumors arising after organ transplantation. Am J Pathol 135:977, 1989.

84. Cameron JS. Glomerulonephritis in renal transplants. Transplantation 34:237, 1982.

85. Platt JL, Sibley RK, Michael AF. Interstitial nephritis associated with cytomegalovirus infection. Kidney Int 28:550, 1985.

86. Battegay E, Mihatsch M, Mazzucchelli L, et al. Cytomegalovirus and kidney. Clin Nephrol 30:239, 1988.

87. Pflaumer S, Sedmak D, Tesi R, Ferguson R. The significance of immunohistochemically detected cytomegalovirus in renal allograft biopsies (abstract). Am J Clin Pathol 99:331, 1993.

88. Hiki Y, Leong AY, Mathew TH, et al. Typing of intraglomerular mononuclear cells associated with transplant glomerular rejection. Clin Nephrol 6:244, 1986.

89. Richardson WP, Colvin RB, Cheeseman SH, et al. Glomerulopathy associated with cytomegalovirus viremia in renal allografts. N Engl J Med 305:57, 1981.

90. Maryniak R, First RM, Weiss MA. Transplant glomerulopathy: Evolution of morphologically distinct changes. Transplantation 41:262, 1985.

91. Rowlands DT Jr, Burkholder PM, et al. Renal allografts in HL-A matched recipients: Light, immunofluorescence and electron microscopic studies. Am J Pathol 61:177, 1970.

92. Olsen S, Bohman SO, Petersen VP. Ultrastructure of the glomerular basement membrane in long-term renal allografts with transplant glomerular disease. Lab Invest 30:176, 1974.

93. Morozumi K, Yoshida A, Suganuma T, et al. Morphological analysis of glomerular lesions in renal transplants immunosuppressed with cyclosporine A (CYA): Has CYA induced a new transplant glomerular lesion? Transplant Proc 21:282, 1989.

94. Cameron JS. Recurrent primary disease and de novo nephritis following renal transplantation. Pediatr Nephrol 5:412, 1991.

95. Morzycka M, Croker BP, et al. Evaluation of recurrent glomerulonephritis in kidney allografts. Am J Med 72:588, 1982.

96. Hebert D, Kim EM, Sibley RK, Mauer MS. Post-transplantation outcome of patients with hemolytic-uremic syndrome: Update. Pediatr Nephrol 5:162, 1991.

97. Nast CC, Ward HJ, Koyle MA, Cohen AH. Recurrent Henoch-Schönlein purpura following renal transplantation. Am J Kidney Dis 9:39, 1987.

98. Verani RR, Hawkins EP. Recurrent focal segmental glomerulosclerosis; A pathological study of the early lesion. Am J Nephrol 6:263, 1986.

99. Antignac C, Hinglais N, Gubler MC, et al. De novo membranous glomerulonephritis in renal allografts in children. Clin Nephrol 30:1, 1988.

100. Charpentier B, Levy M. Étude cooperative des glomerulonephrites extra-membraneuses de novo sur allogreffe rénale humaine: Rapport de 19 nouveaux cas sur 1550 transplantes rénaux du groupe de transplantation de l'Ile de France. Nephrology 3:158, 1982.

101. Truong L, Gelfand J, D'Agati V, et al. De novo membranous glomerulonephropathy in renal allografts: A report of ten cases and review of the literature. Am J Kidney Dis 14:131, 1989.

102. Savige J, Mavrova L, Kincaid-Smith P. Inhibitable anti-GBM antibody activity after renal transplantation in Alport's syndrome. Transplantation 48:704, 1989.

103. Shah B, First M, Mendoza N, et al. Risk of glomerulonephritis induced by anti-glomerular basement membrane antibody after renal transplantation. Nephron 50:34, 1988.

10

LIVER TRANSPLANT PATHOLOGY

ROBERT L. FLINNER, MD, and ELIZABETH H. HAMMOND, MD

In the patient with a liver allograft, a number of events may occur that could lead to loss of the allograft and death of the patient. These include technical problems with the anastomoses, immunologic rejection of the graft, and infection involving either the graft itself or other areas such as the lungs. Examination of a liver biopsy is extremely important in evaluating problems in these patients, and a biopsy should be done before deciding on a treatment course. Furthermore, routine protocol biopsies at weekly intervals are useful in patients who are having no problems. This will often identify important changes before they become clinically evident. Day 0 biopsies are useful in evaluating the quality of the graft at the time of implantation. If all goes well, the protocol biopsies may be discontinued after 1 month, but later biopsies should be done if any problem occurs. Biopsy findings should always be correlated with the clinical findings. The major diagnostic uses are listed in Table 10–1.

TECHNICAL PROBLEMS WITH ANASTOMOSES

A major technical problem may occur with the vascular anastomoses.[1–3] The hepatic artery may become occluded in up to 3 per cent of adult liver transplants and up to 12 per cent of pediatric liver transplants. A very high mortality rate is associated with this complication (73 per cent).[1] In these cases there is either massive infarction or multiple smaller areas of in-

farction with resulting sepsis. Chronic ischemia may result from gradual vascular stenosis. This will show the changes of chronic rejection with central ballooning, hepatic cell loss, and regeneration. Portal vein obstruction may present as portal hypertension. With portal vein obstruction there is ischemic change in the hepatic cells, with centrilobular hepatocellular atrophy, sinusoidal dilatation, and hepatocellular dropout. Stenosis of suprahepatic vena cava[4, 5] leads to Budd-Chiari syndrome. There is central congestion and atrophy of parenchymal cells. It may be impossible to differentiate this from portal vein obstruction or congestive heart failure; radiologic studies are necessary to make this distinction. Leakage is the most common technical problem with the bile duct

Table 10–1. Diagnostic Uses of Liver Biopsies in Liver Transplantation

Clinical problems with vascular and bile duct anastomoses
Evaluation of day 0 (zero) biopsy
Preservation injury
Monitoring for rejection:
  Hyperacute
  Acute
  Chronic
Drug toxicity and hypersensitivity
Recurrence of primary disease
Diagnosis of infection:
  Viral
  Fungal
  Bacterial
Lymphoproliferative disorder
Graft versus host disease

anastomoses.[3] This has no direct effect on liver function but may lead to sepsis that subsequently may alter hepatic function.

If there is obstruction of the bile duct, liver function tests will be abnormal but will not differ significantly from those seen in rejection. Cyclosporine absorption may be impaired in the presence of obstruction, which will lead to low cyclosporine blood levels that may predispose the patient to rejection. Histologically, the findings are not always clear-cut and may be a problem in differentiating obstruction from rejection.[6]

EVALUATION OF DAY 0 BIOPSIES

A biopsy of the transplanted liver at the time of transplantation is recommended. This provides a baseline for subsequent evaluations of biopsies and may discover abnormalities that will aid in understanding subsequent problems with the allograft. In most cases the liver will appear histologically normal. Occasionally subcapsular or central areas of necrosis or dissociation of parenchymal cells will be seen (Fig. 10–1). Uncommonly, there is some swelling of centrilobular cells (Fig. 10–2).

A common feature detected in these biopsies is termed *surgical hepatitis*. This process is characterized by clusters of polymorphonuclear leukocytes (PMNs) in sinusoids with no associated hepatocellular injury (Fig. 10–3).

Surgical hepatitis is considered to be caused by the prolonged handling of the liver, the effects of surgical retractors, and other technical events.[2] However, there is a possibility that this change may represent a humoral immune response in a previously sensitized host. This possibility has never been rigorously evaluated.

The most important finding in a day 0 biopsy is the presence of fatty change. A severe fatty change may result in primary nonfunction of the graft.[7, 8] Severe fatty change is diagnosed when greater than two thirds of the parenchymal cells contain large fat droplets. Fatty change is considered moderate when one third to two thirds of cells are affected; mild fatty change involves fewer than one third of parenchymal cells. Fatty change is often associated with impaired liver function during the first 3 days following transplantation. Clinically, this change is associated with elevated serum glutamic-oxaloacetic transaminase (SGOT), decreased bile flow, and prolonged prothrombin time. The amount of functional impairment correlates with the severity of the fatty change. The fatty change may also result in the liver being more sensitive to subsequent preservation injury.[9] After several days, the fatty liver may recover from the functional impairment.[10] Nevertheless, transplanted livers with fatty change, especially of severe degree, are more likely to fail compared with nonfatty livers.[9] Livers with only mild fatty change have no associated poor outcome and such livers

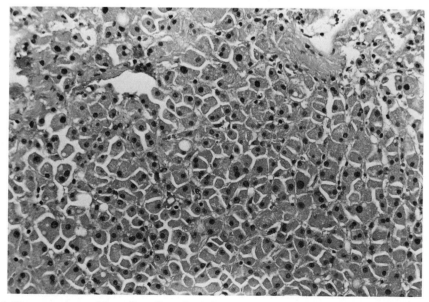

Figure 10–1. Biopsy specimen of liver allograft on day 0. Dissociation of parenchymal cells is seen. This may be in part an artifact. (Hematoxylin & eosin, × 250)

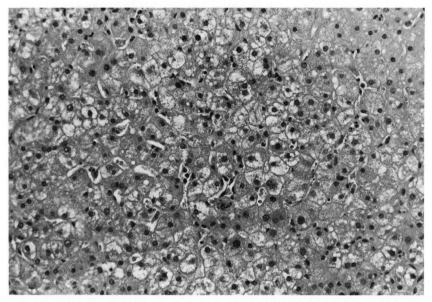

Figure 10–2. Day 0 biopsy specimen of liver allograft showing cytoplasmic swelling of parenchymal cells. (Hematoxylin & eosin, × 250)

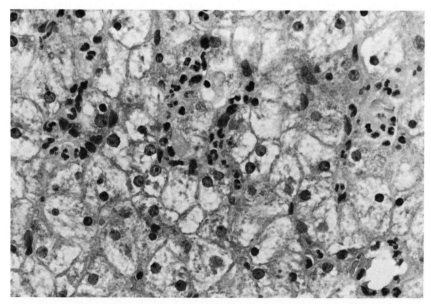

Figure 10–3. Surgical hepatitis in a day 0 biopsy specimen. There are neutrophils in sinusoids with no cell necrosis. (Hematoxylin & eosin, × 400)

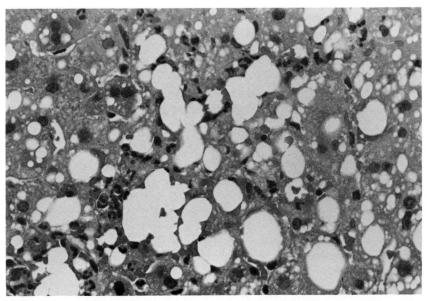

Figure 10–4. Severe fatty change in a day 0 biopsy specimen of liver allograft. Note the irregularly shaped, coalesced fat droplets in sinusoids. There is also fat in hepatic cells. (Hematoxylin & eosin, × 400)

are acceptable for transplantation. On the other hand, livers with severe fatty change should not be used for transplantation. Livers with moderate fatty change are less desirable but may be used since many will have a successful outcome.[9] In evaluating a liver for fatty change, those severely affected can usually be identified on gross examination: there is hepatomegaly, a rounded liver edge, and a yellow color. It has been recommended that frozen section examination be done on livers suspected of having significant fatty change prior to transplantation.[11]

The high risk of primary nonfunction of the liver with severe fatty change may be due to rupture of fat-filled cells with release of large fat droplets into sinusoids (Fig. 10–4). This may cause obstruction and disruption of the microcirculation.[7] The rupture of these cells may be enhanced by solidification of the triglycerides by the cold temperature used to preserve the liver prior to transplantation. It has also been postulated that release of the triglycerides and fatty acids activates phospholipases and lipid peroxidases. The resultant free radicals may cause cell damage.[8]

Hydropic changes (ballooning degeneration) in the day 0 biopsy may occur and may be associated with primary nonfunction of the graft.[8] The injured cells are unable to pump the inward-diffusing sodium and water from the cells; this is probably related to membrane injury and decreased adenosine triphosphate

(ATP) activity because of injured mitochondria.[8] Occasionally the day 0 biopsy will contain evidence of chronic active hepatitis or chronic persistent hepatitis. In the few cases studied in which subsequent biopsies were available, most showed a disappearance of the inflammatory infiltrates, presumably due to the effect of the immunosuppressive drugs (personal observation). However, these cases are at high risk for recurrence of the hepatitis.

PRESERVATION INJURY

Preservation injury occurs in about one third of patients and is associated with cholestatic jaundice. The histologic change that has been termed preservation injury is *not* seen in the day 0 biopsy and is first noted at 5 to 7 days post-transplant. This injury is characterized by marked cytoplasmic swelling of central parenchymal cells (Figs. 10–5 and 10–6).[12] In more severe examples, midzonal and periportal cells may also be affected (Fig. 10–7). The cells have a finely vacuolated, clear cytoplasm, with the organelles displaced to the pericanalicular zone of the cytoplasm. There usually is faint bile staining in the affected area, with bile plugs in canaliculi. This change has also been termed *balloon degeneration*, which is a good descriptive term.

A distinction must be made between the early ballooning change of preservation injury and ballooning occurring in a day 0 biopsy.

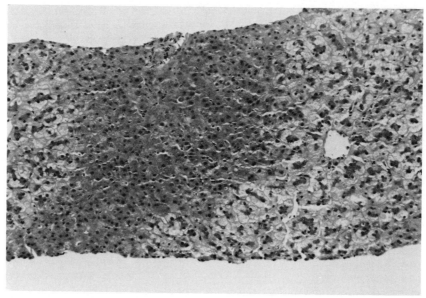

Figure 10–5. Preservation injury of liver allograft at 1 week post-transplant. Central and midzonal swelling of parenchymal cells is seen. (Hematoxylin & eosin, × 100) Compare with Figure 10–21.

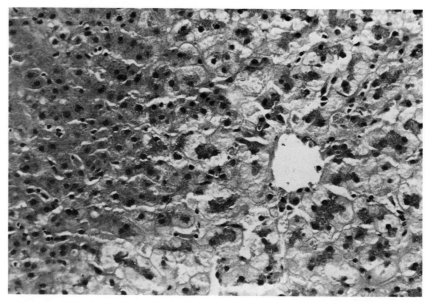

Figure 10–6. Central zone from Figure 10–5 showing preservation injury. There is cytoplasmic swelling with displacement of organelles to the pericanalicular zone of the parenchymal cells. (Hematoxylin & eosin, × 250)

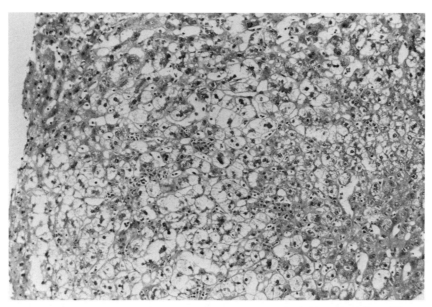

Figure 10–7. Severe preservation injury involving all zones of the lobules, 1 week post-transplant. (Hematoxylin & eosin, × 100)

Swelling or balloon changes in the day 0 biopsy do not show the striking displacement of cytoplasmic organelles, and there is no associated cholestasis. A distinction must also be made between preservation injury and the balloon change associated with rejection vasculopathy. If the ballooning appears for the first time in the third week or later, this change is not preservation injury and suggests that either vasculopathy or a mechanical problem with the hepatic artery is developing.

The ballooning change in preservation injury differs histologically from the ballooning degeneration noted in chronic rejection. In chronic rejection, the striking displacement of the organelles is not as evident. In preservation injury, there is no cell dropout or inflammatory response as would be seen in chronic rejection. In preservation injury, there is no alteration of the hepatic architecture, whereas chronic rejection shows disruption of the hepatic cords in central areas. The change in preservation injury is completely reversible and has usually resolved within 2 to 3 weeks post-transplant (Fig. 10–8).

Although preservation injury is rather striking histologically and would suggest significant injury to the cells, the presence of mitoses in the affected cells and the lack of parenchymal cell necrosis indicate that the injury is not of a serious nature. The cellular appearance suggests that there has been membrane damage probably related to early ischemia. This membrane injury may interfere with the pumping action of the membrane to remove sodium and water from the cell. There is evidence that preservation injury may predispose patients to a higher incidence of acute cellular rejection.[13] It has been postulated that ischemic injury to endothelial cells in the liver may expose hepatic antigens to the host and that inflammatory cells may be attracted to these areas, thus enhancing the possibility of a rejection episode. There is no evidence of either chronic or humoral rejection to account for this change. It does not appear to be related to cyclosporine levels. Events leading to greater ischemic time may exaggerate this change, but it has been seen in livers from stable donors with fewer than 6 hours of cold ischemia.[12]

HEPATIC INFARCTION

Hepatic infarcts are uncommon owing to the presence of a rich dual circulation in the liver (Fig. 10–9). The most common cause of hepatic infarction in transplanted livers is thrombosis of one of the major vessels to the liver. Infarction may also occur in the absence of vascular occlusion, and this is usually explained by hypoperfusion due to hypotension and shock.[14] Hypoperfusion in the graft may occur because of low output failure in the donor or because of a prolonged interval between harvest and revascularization of the

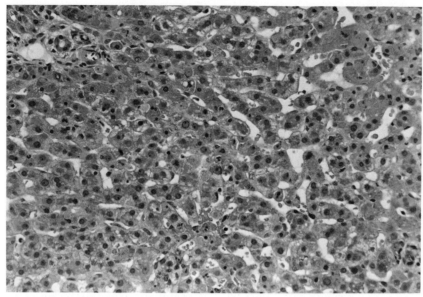

Figure 10–8. Resolved preservation injury at 3 weeks post-transplant. The changes at 1 week post-transplant are seen in Figures 10–5 and 10–6. (Hematoxylin & eosin, × 250)

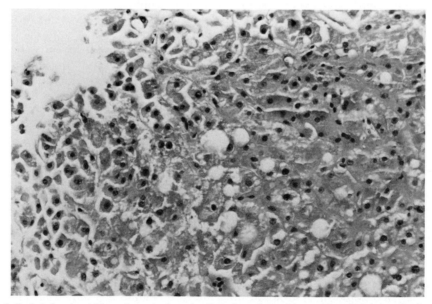

Figure 10–9. Early infarction of hepatic parenchymal cells at 1 week post-biopsy. Note shrinkage of cells with pyknotic nuclei. (Hematoxylin & eosin, × 250)

graft. Some infarcts may occur because of disproportionate size between the graft and the abdominal space, resulting in localized pressure points. In such cases there may be rather extensive areas of subcapsular infarction without vascular occlusion. If these areas of subcapsular necrosis are sampled in needle biopsies, the findings could be quite misleading and suggest massive necrosis of the liver. Correlating the needle biopsy findings with the patient's clinical condition and the laboratory data should clarify this problem.

IMMUNOLOGICALLY MEDIATED TRANSPLANT REJECTION

In the transplanted liver, recognition by the host of foreign HLA antigens is often rather intense during the first several weeks posttransplant. It has been postulated that this recognition of foreign antigens later subsides, in part owing to replacement of the donor endothelium and Kupffer cells by host cells.[15] This in effect may "shield" the antigen-containing liver cells from recognition by the host. In addition, cells from the graft migrate to other sites in the body and in successful transplants develop a state of chimerism.[16] This is thought to contribute greatly to decreasing acute rejection and promoting graft tolerance. The degree of donor cell recognition may be enhanced by preservation injury to the host cells

and modified by the degree of antigen match between the allograft and the donor.[13] Because of the early, intense host response to foreign antigen, immunosuppression must be greater early in the course whereas later this suppression may be reduced.

Rejection of the allograft may take one of several forms, including hyperacute rejection, acute cellular rejection, and chronic rejection.

Hyperacute Rejection

It is not known how frequently this occurs, but many or most cases designated as primary graft failure include instances of hyperacute rejection. In these cases the liver fails to function normally from the time of transplantation.[17] Within a period of several days there may be extensive infarction of the hepatic parenchyma associated with portal polymorphonuclear leukocyte infiltrate and necrotizing arteritis. Large arteries may show intimal fibroblastic proliferation with an infiltrate of neutrophils (Fig. 10–10) or accumulation of foamy macrophages and neutrophils beneath the intima (Fig. 10–11). Hyperacute rejection is mediated by preformed antidonor antibodies.[18, 19] Such rejection is more common in patients with high levels of circulating panel-reactive antibodies (more than 25 per cent) pretransplant and in patients with positive T or B cell cross-matches in which the antibody

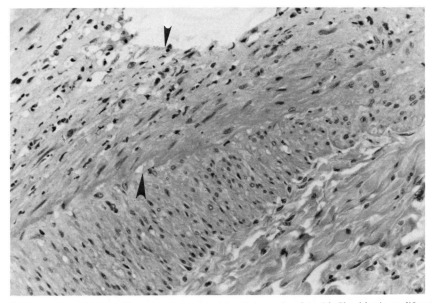

Figure 10–10. Hyperacute rejection. There is a large arterial wall (arrowheads) with fibroblastic proliferation of intima and neutrophilic infiltrate. (Hematoxylin & eosin, × 250)

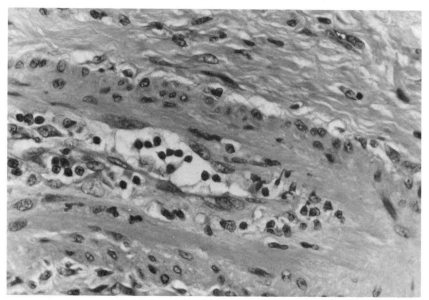

Figure 10–11. Hyperacute rejection. A large artery shows accumulation of macrophages, lymphocytes, and neutrophils beneath enlarged endothelial cells. (Hematoxylin & eosin, × 250)

is IgG.[18] Such antibodies can be demonstrated in blood vessel walls by immunofluorescence microscopy in frozen sections of unfixed biopsies. Immunoglobulin G (IgG) or IgM is colocalized with complement components. Antibody can also be seen in sinusoids in these situations, associated with Kupffer cells. Such patients have been successfully treated with high dose steroids in combination with prostaglandin E_1.[20]

Acute Cellular Rejection

Acute cellular rejection is first seen 5 to 7 days post-transplantation. At least one acute rejection episode occurs in up to 75 per cent of liver transplant patients.[2, 21] If there is no early rejection episode, it is unlikely that late rejection will occur. For the first episode of acute rejection to occur several months or a year following transplantation is most unusual and should raise the question of other processes such as hepatitis. Three histologic findings are necessary to make the diagnosis of acute cellular rejection:[2, 10]

1. There is a mixed cellular infiltrate in the portal triads that may be focal or involve only a few triads. Lymphocytes predominate, but there are also neutrophils and eosinophils (Fig. 10–12). The presence of eosinophils is an important criterion for the diagnosis of re-

jection; the absence of eosinophils suggests that rejection is not present and that the infiltrate represents another process. On the other hand, eosinophils are commonly seen in drug reactions affecting the liver.

2. Bile duct damage is seen, which may be focal or widespread. Lymphocytes and neutrophils are infiltrating the bile duct epithelium (Figs. 10–13 and 10–14). The nuclei of ducts show enlargement and pleomorphism, with overlapping of nuclei in some areas and loss of nuclei in other areas. There may be cytoplasmic vacuoles. Bile duct damage must be evaluated only in the true bile ducts in the portal triad, since proliferating ductules often show atypical epithelial changes associated with inflammatory infiltrates (Figs. 10–15 and 10–16). Bile duct damage identical to that of rejection changes may occur in viral hepatitis, drug reactions, and primary biliary cirrhosis. In cases having an intense inflammatory infiltrate in the portal triads, bile ducts may be obscured and difficult to evaluate. Trichrome stain will accentuate the bile duct. When bile ducts cannot be identified in the inflammatory infiltrates, staining of ductal epithelium with immunoperoxidase techniques using keratin antibodies may be very helpful.

3. Venous endothelialitis is the most specific finding in diagnosing acute cellular rejection. This is often a focal change and is the first finding to disappear following treatment for rejection. The endothelialitis affects both

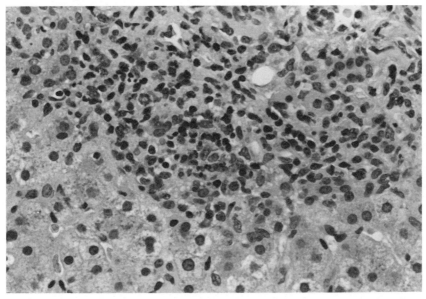

Figure 10–12. Acute cellular rejection in a liver allograft. A mixed cellular infiltrate in a portal triad is noted. Some of the cells are eosinophils. (Hematoxylin & eosin, × 400)

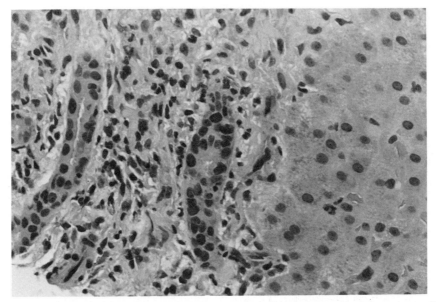

Figure 10–13. Acute cellular rejection in a liver allograft. Two bile ducts are infiltrated by inflammatory cells, with atypia of bile duct epithelium. (Hematoxylin & eosin, × 400)

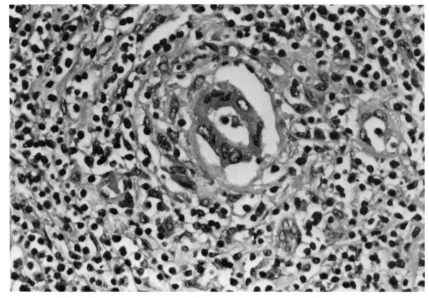

Figure 10–14. Acute cellular rejection. There is a damaged bile duct with nuclear atypia and infiltration by lymphocytes. (Hematoxylin & eosin, × 450)

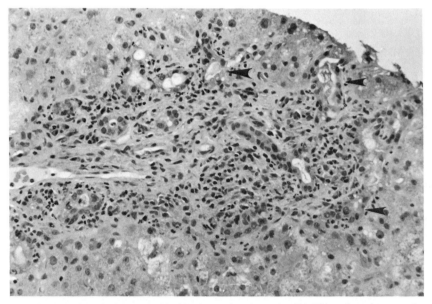

Figure 10–15. Proliferating bile ducts associated with obstruction (arrowheads). These ducts have atypia and inflammation but do not indicate rejection since they are not the true bile duct. (Hematoxylin & eosin, × 250)

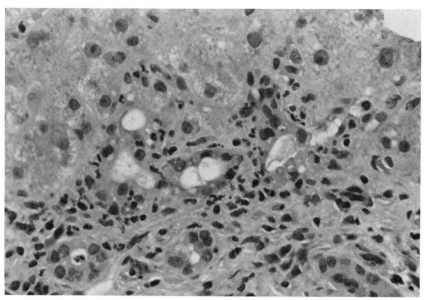

Figure 10–16. The proliferating bile ducts shown in Figure 10–15. Note neutrophils associated with these ducts; this is not evidence of rejection. (Hematoxylin & eosin, × 400)

the portal vein within the triad and central veins (Figs. 10–17 and 10–18). At times it is difficult to evaluate the presence of endothelialitis in the portal veins because of the intensity of the portal inflammatory infiltrate. Venous endothelialitis is characterized by attachment of lymphocytes to the endothelial cells. This cellular adherence is associated with damage to the endothelial cells, enlargement of endothelial nuclei, and lifting of the endothelium from the basement membrane. It is necessary to identify attachment of the lymphocytes to the endothelial cells; the mere presence of unattached lymphocytes within the vessels is not significant. The attachment may be characterized by cytoplasmic processes of the lympho-

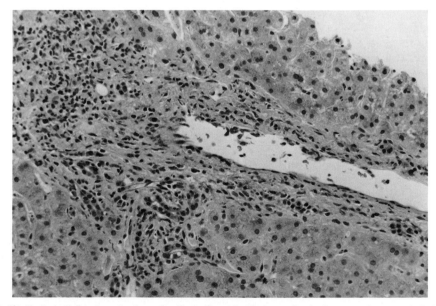

Figure 10–17. Endothelialitis in rejection of a liver allograft. The portal vein has prominent endothelial cells with lymphocytes attached to the endothelium. (Hematoxylin & eosin, × 250)

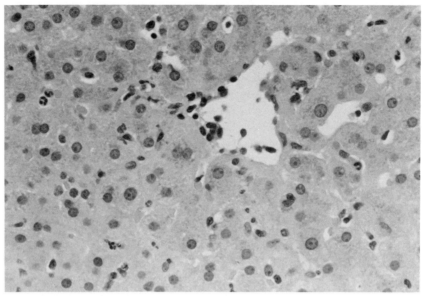

Figure 10–18. Endothelialitis in rejection of a liver allograft. Lymphocytes are attached to the endothelium of a central vein. (Hematoxylin & eosin, × 450)

cytes touching the endothelial cells or by "tenting" of the endothelial cell cytoplasm, which then touches the lymphocytes. There may also be subendothelial aggregates of lymphocytes that lift the endothelial cell from the basement membrane.

4. A nonspecific finding is canalicular cholestasis, which is common in the transplanted liver and is of no diagnostic help in recognizing cellular rejection (Fig. 10–19). One may also see ballooning of hepatic cells and focal hepatic necrosis with acidophilic bodies. These findings are nondiagnostic for rejection. Central ballooning due to preservation injury may be seen in the first several weeks post-transplant. This is a reversible change and is not

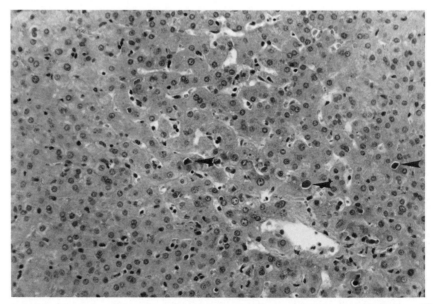

Figure 10–19. Canalicular cholestasis in a liver allograft (arrowheads), a common nonspecific finding. (Hematoxylin & eosin, × 250)

diagnostic of rejection. However, a ballooning change may predispose to a greater likelihood of cellular rejection.

Grading of Acute Rejection

A grade indicating the intensity of rejection should be used in reporting the findings.[2] Grading is based on the amount of cellular infiltrate and the percentage of bile ducts showing damage. Snover and colleagues have divided acute rejection into four categories (Table 10–2).[2, 6] In cases that have not received additional immunosuppressive therapy for rejection, endothelialitis should be present, and this is diagnostic of rejection. According to Snover's criteria, cases with *mild acute rejection* have endothelialitis and mixed cellular infiltrate in portal triads, with less than 50 per cent of the bile ducts showing damage. If an inflammatory infiltrate is seen without endothelialitis, the biopsy is diagnosed as *consistent with but not diagnostic of rejection. Moderate acute rejection* has a mixed portal infiltrate with greater than 50 per cent of bile ducts showing damage with or without endothelialitis. With this degree of bile duct damage, endothelialitis is not necessary for the diagnosis although it is helpful.

In *severe acute rejection,* there are additional findings of central balloon cell degeneration, with confluent dropout of hepatocytes and multinucleated giant cells in central areas. This change is most likely related to arteritis or endarteritis of larger vessels (transplant vasculopathy). Changes in the vessels themselves are usually not seen in biopsy material, since they occur in vessels larger than those biopsied. Another finding that is graded as severe rejection is the vanishing bile duct syndrome (VBDS). In this condition none of the portal triads contain bile ducts. There may be lesser degrees of bile duct loss, with some triads still containing a bile duct. This has been termed *paucity of bile ducts,* or *ductopenia.* The changes of severe acute rejection are potentially reversible but identify patients that are at great risk for progressing to irreversible rejection and loss of the allograft.

Adequacy of Biopsy

Since the changes that are diagnostic of cellular rejection occur mainly in the portal triads, it is necessary to have an adequate number of triads for evaluation. At least three or four portal triads should be present in the biopsy sample, since milder degrees of rejection may be spotty in distribution and may not affect every triad. One should be cautious about trying to diagnose rejection on a small biopsy sample containing only one or two triads. Such cases may show no change in the triads although the patient is experiencing cellular rejection. A comment that the biopsy material is suboptimal for evaluation should be made.

Response to Therapy

There may be total resolution of all the histologic findings within a week following treatment. Often there is evidence of histologic improvement but with residual findings of rejection. The first finding to disappear following treatment is endothelialitis. The bile duct damage may persist for several weeks following resolution of the rejection episode. These changes may persist and are not sufficient for diagnosing ongoing rejection. It is not unusual to see an occasional bile duct infiltrated by small numbers of lymphocytes and showing some cytologic atypia of the bile duct epithelium. In the absence of a mixed cellular infil-

Table 10–2. Grading of Cellular Rejection

	Mixed Cellular Infiltrate	Bile Duct Damage	Endothelialitis	Confluent Loss of Central Cells	Decrease/Loss of Bile Ducts
Consistent with/suggestive of rejection/can't rule out rejection	+	+ <50%	−	−	−
Mild rejection	+	+ <50%	+	−	−
Moderate rejection	+	+ >50%	±	−	−
Severe rejection a. Arteriopathy b. VBDS*	± −	± ±	± −	+ ±	± +

*Vanishing bile duct syndrome.

trate and endothelialitis, this should not be diagnosed as ongoing rejection. The minimal bile duct change may indicate that minimal rejection is occurring, but it is not sufficient to require additional therapy. Portal infiltrates also resolve, and especially the lymphocytes decrease in number during OKT3 treatment. However, neutrophils and eosinophils may persist and be prominent. These may infiltrate bile ducts, a finding that suggests large duct obstruction.

Chronic Rejection

Clinically, chronic rejection is associated with progressive liver failure. Chronic rejection occurs in about 10 per cent of liver transplants.[22] It implies irreversible changes leading to graft failure. This is due to rejection that was not recognized and treated or was not controlled by the immunosuppressive therapy. Chronic rejection has been more specifically defined by using both clinical and pathologic parameters.[23] Clinically, chronic rejection is a process characterized by significant serum elevations of liver enzymes and bilirubin, lasting longer than 2 months, and not responding to immunosuppressive therapy.

Other processes may produce a clinico-pathologic picture resembling chronic rejection, including chronic hepatitis, drug toxicity, hepatic artery thrombosis, and possibly recurrence of the primary disease.[24]

Pathologically, for discussion purposes, it is useful to divide chronic rejection into two distinct categories: (1) rejection vasculopathy with confluent dropout of centrilobular parenchymal cells, and (2) loss of portal bile ducts. Although these two processes may occur independently of each other, they frequently are found together, either concurrently or with one process preceding the other.[22, 24]

Rejection Vasculopathy (Obliterative Endarteritis). This is seen only in larger arteries in the liver (greater than 300 microns in diameter)[25] and is not usually found in a needle biopsy. The patients have a more rapid downhill course than that seen in pure ductopenic rejection. Many of these patients will also have severe bile duct injury or loss. Histologically, the artery has an accumulation of lipid-filled macrophages, or there may be extensive subendothelial fibrosis with narrowing and occlusion (Fig. 10–20). Grossly, the affected vessel may be yellow because of the large amounts of lipid. Small numbers of foam cells may be found in portal and hepatic vein branches.[26]

As a result of the obliterative change, central ischemic changes occur in the hepatic cells. This is characterized by a ballooning type of degeneration of parenchymal cells with confluent dropout of cells (Fig. 10–21). The balloon cell change differs from that seen in preservation injury: the cells tend to have large amounts of bile pigment within them, do not show aggregation of the organelles, and are often multinucleated. Furthermore, the cen-

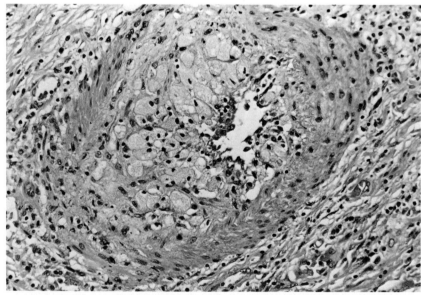

Figure 10–20. Rejection vasculopathy. Foamy cells are accumulating in the endothelial layer and obliterating the lumen. (Hematoxylin & eosin, × 250)

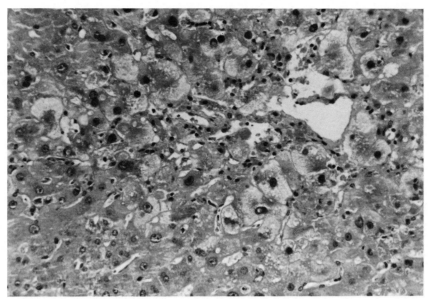

Figure 10–21. Chronic rejection. Ballooning and dropout of centrilobular cells are seen. (Hematoxylin & eosin, × 400)

tral areas show considerable disruption of the architecture with loss of many cells and with an inflammatory infiltrate consisting of lymphocytes and macrophages (Fig. 10–22). Many of the macrophages contain bile and lipochrome pigment. In the central area, in addition to cell loss, there is fibrosis and evidence of collapse of the architecture. Central loss of cells may involve all of zone 3 of the lobule and result in a "punched out" appearance in this area[24] (Fig. 10–23). The lesion is not always obvious on routine hematoxylin & eosin sections.

Clues to the diagnosis are central congestion of sinusoids (Fig. 10–24), multinucleated hepatic cells, and occasionally extramedullary hematopoiesis. A reticulin stain highlights the central collapse of the reticulin framework (Fig. 10–25). The central loss of cells may first occur from several weeks to many months

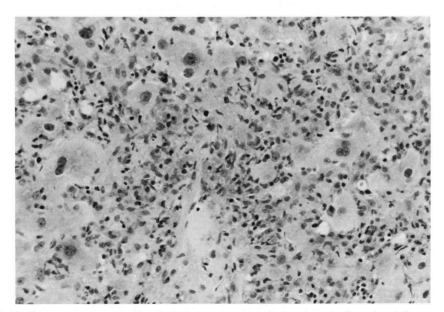

Figure 10–22. Chronic rejection. Centrilobular ballooning, multinucleation, loss of cells, and an inflammatory infiltrate are seen. (Hematoxylin & eosin, × 400)

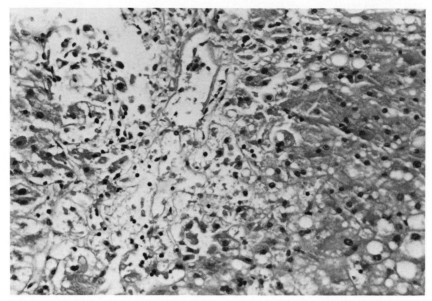

Figure 10–23. Chronic rejection. There is central loss of cells, with a "punched-out" appearance. (Hematoxylin & eosin, × 400)

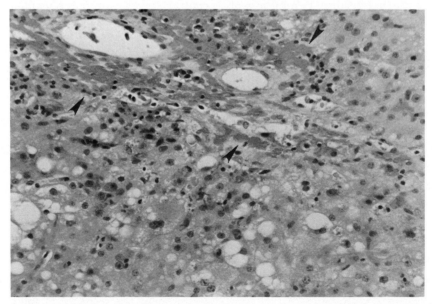

Figure 10–24. Chronic rejection. Central loss of cells is accompanied with congestion of sinusoids (arrowheads). (Hematoxylin and eosin, × 400)

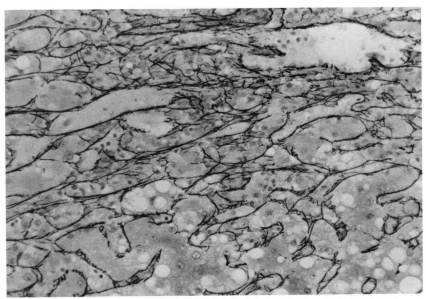

Figure 10–25. Chronic rejection. Collapse of the reticulin, indicating where hepatocytes have dropped out is noted. (Reticulin stain, × 400)

post-transplant. In a small percentage of cases, the central loss will be transient on serial biopsies and not associated with a poor prognosis.[24] However, most cases show a persistence of this change and have an associated poor prognosis with ductopenia and ultimate failure of the allograft. Rejection vasculopathy involving larger arteries is often suspected of being the underlying cause of the central cell loss, but such vascular lesions are not always present.[24] Thus, it appears that rejection vasculopathy is not the sole cause.

An alternative proposed cause is central vein damage from endothelialitis, leading to venous outflow obstruction and ischemia.[24] Usually there have been previous episodes of cellular rejection, and it appears that chronic rejection evolves from episodes of acute cellular rejection that may or may not have responded to therapy.[23] Some of the changes may suggest early cirrhotic change[23] (Fig. 10–26). True cirrhosis with reorganization of the architecture and regenerative nodules is unusual, although it may occur (Fig. 10–27).

Loss of Portal Bile Ducts. Acute cellular rejection may produce severe bile duct damage, resulting in loss of these ducts.[23, 27] If a majority or all of the bile ducts are lost, this will usually be associated with irreversible changes leading to allograft loss, the vanishing bile duct syndrome (VBDS). The terms *ductopenic rejection* and *paucity of bile ducts* are used if there is a significant decrease in ducts but some ducts

are still present. To evaluate the status of the ducts, the specimen must contain adequate numbers of portal areas. It has been recommended that at least 20 portal areas be examined; several consecutive biopsies may be required to achieve this.[25]

In the normal liver, 80 per cent to 100 per cent of portal triads will be found to contain a bile duct (Fig. 10–28). Large portal triads with bile ducts may occasionally appear in a biopsy but should not be counted in the evaluation since ducts larger than 50 microns are not affected by this process[25] (Fig. 10–29). Later, even these larger ducts may disappear. If less than 50 per cent of triads contain ducts, then the biopsy is considered to be ductopenic; if less than 25 per cent of triads contain bile ducts, irreversible rejection with vanishing bile duct syndrome is likely. Some cases will have complete absences of ducts. In triads that have no bile duct, the inflammation will have subsided and the area has a burnt-out, scarred appearance[28] (Figs. 10–30 and 10–31). Proliferating ductules are usually not present. If there is an intense portal inflammatory infiltrate, the bile duct may be obscured and thus not counted. Immunperoxidase stain for keratin may identify the otherwise obscure duct.

Other findings associated with the ductopenia are intense central cholestasis and central loss of parenchymal cells. Central loss of parenchymal cells may be associated with transplant vasculopathy; many but not all cases

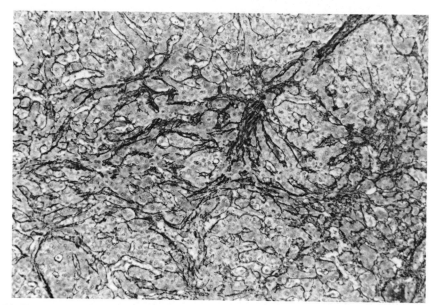

Figure 10–26. Chronic rejection, with precirrhotic fibrosis highlighted by condensation of the reticulin. (Reticulin stain, × 100)

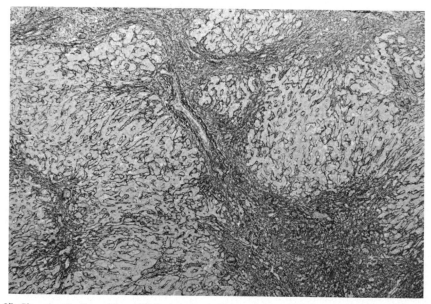

Figure 10–27. Chronic rejection with established cirrhosis. Regenerative nodules are outlined by fibrous bands. (Reticulin stain, × 30)

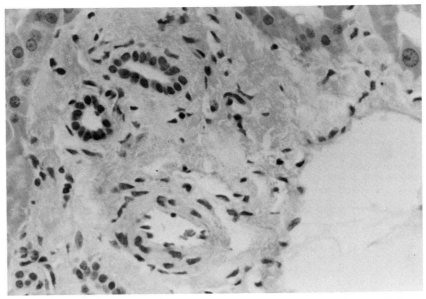

Figure 10–28. A normal portal triad. Note the two bile ducts adjacent to an artery. (Hematoxylin & eosin, × 400)

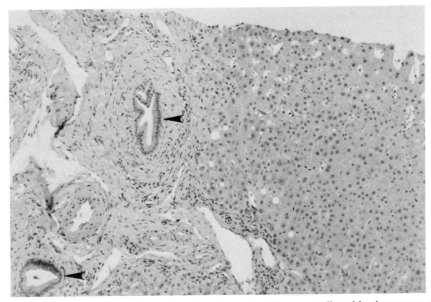

Figure 10–29. Vanishing bile duct syndrome. Large ducts (arrowheads) are not affected by the process. (Hematoxylin & eosin, × 100)

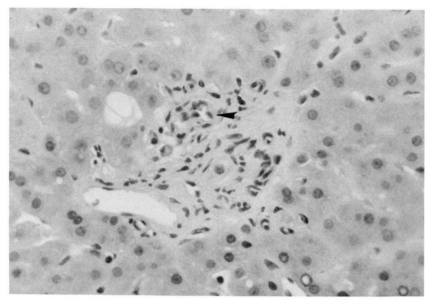

Figure 10–30. Vanishing bile duct syndrome. The portal triad has an artery (arrowhead) but no accompanying bile duct. The triad has a scarred appearance, and there is no inflammation. (Hematoxylin & eosin, × 400)

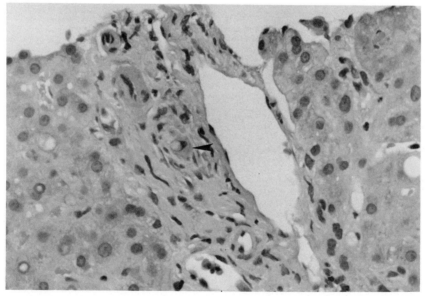

Figure 10–31. Vanishing bile duct syndrome. A remnant of a bile duct is noted, with one cell remaining (arrowhead). (Hematoxylin & eosin, × 400)

of ductopenia will have transplant vasculopathy.[28] The vasculopathy may be partially responsible for the bile duct loss, since the bile ducts derive their blood supply entirely from the hepatic artery. However, the occurrence of ductopenia is almost always preceded by a lymphocytic attack on the bile ducts, suggesting that cellular rejection is the usual mechanism of duct loss.

The vanishing bile duct syndrome and ductopenic rejection occur in about 10 per cent of liver transplants and are associated with irreversible progression to allograft loss.[25] There is often a more prolonged, relatively benign clinical course in these patients, compared with those with rejection vasculopathy. The process may occur as early as the second week post-transplantation, which has been termed the *acute vanishing bile duct syndrome,* or it may occur several months post-transplantation and is thus termed *chronic vanishing bile duct syndrome.*[25, 28] Rare cases of VBDS occurring as much as 3 years post-transplantation have been recorded.[27] Some cases of ductopenia will show fluctuating degrees of bile duct loss on serial biopsies, with the variation extending from normal to low levels. Severe cholestasis may occur, and the patient may progress to liver failure and death unless retransplanted.

More recently, it has become evident that the VBDS is not always irreversible and that up to 20 per cent of cases will show reconstitution of the bile ducts, with either improvement or remission of the cholestatic jaundice.[24, 28, 29] Those cases with complete loss of ducts may be more likely to be irreversible than those with a decreased number of ducts. However, graft loss may occur with ductopenia, and recovery of ducts may occur in cases that have had total loss of ducts. Furthermore, several cases have been reported in which clinical and biochemical recovery occurred but with persistence of ductopenia.[28]

In making a diagnosis of irreversible rejection based on absence or paucity of bile ducts, several other factors must be considered. The observed ductopenia must be present in more than one biopsy. Because of the variable clinical course of VBDS, it is recommended that patients with ductopenia who are clinically stable not be retransplanted unless there is further deterioration of their status.[29] Some of these patients will be observed to regain their bile ducts and have associated improvement of the clinical status. Whether some cases of chronic rejection can be reversed by more aggressive treatment is not known. It is likely that the vascular lesions are irreversible, whereas bile duct loss is potentially reversible. In a patient who has lost an allograft because of VBDS, there is a high likelihood of VBDS occurring in the retransplanted liver (91 per cent of cases in one series).[30]

Immunopathologic Findings in Liver Allografts

Liver allografts studied immunopathologically have shown findings that can be correlated with rejection. Acute rejection of liver allografts is associated with increased expression of major histocompatibility complex (MHC) I and II by the bile ducts and vascular endothelial cells.[31] Such cells are also induced to express the vascular intercellular adhesion molecule ICAM-1, which has been identified in such allograft biopsies immunocytochemically.[32] Likely mediators of this induction are the cytokines tumor necrosis factor (TNF), interleukin-1 (IL-1), and interferon-gamma (IFN-γ), all of which have been detected at increased plasma levels during and even 1 to 2 days prior to acute rejection episodes.[33, 34] Investigations of liver allograft biopsies by polymerase chain reaction (PCR) have confirmed the increased expression of these cytokines, as well as increased amounts of IL-5, especially in acute rejecting allografts.[35] Increased expression of ICAM-1 increases the avidity of binding of macrophages and lymphocytes to the vascular endothelium, which potentiates the inflammatory response.[36]

Immunocytochemical studies of normal liver and nonrejecting allografts have shown that few macrophages or Kupffer cells are making the cytokines TNF or IL-1. Vascular endothelium and bile ducts show no significant MHC or ICAM-1 expression. ICAM-1 is strongly expressed by the sinus endothelial cells and Kupffer cells but not by hepatic parenchymal cells. This pattern is significantly altered in the presence of cellular rejection. Inflammatory cells in portal areas and central venous spaces consist of macrophages with an immature phenotype, as well as lymphocytes expressing CD4 and CD8 in variable proportions. All these inflammatory cells strongly express MHC II, as do the bile ducts they are infiltrating. TNFα is strongly expressed by the macrophages in this infiltrate, indicating activation and secretion of this cytokine. Kupffer cells do not show increased expression, and neither cell type shows secretion of IL-1.

ICAM-1 continues to be strongly expressed by sinus endothelial cells but also shows upregulation on bile ducts, hepatocytes, and vascular endothelium.

The only significant change in these findings in severe acute rejection is the massive induction of IL-1 expression by various cell types, including macrophages, Kupffer cells, and vascular endothelial cells. These cells also show increased expression of ICAM-1. Hepatic parenchymal cells show strong staining with ICAM-1 and also with MHC II. Vascular endothelium shows increased expression of von Willebrand factor, also in the subendothelial space, suggesting vascular injury. In severe rejection, the phenotype of the macrophages also includes mature type. In chronic rejection, the same findings persist, although the majority of macrophages express mature phenotype, and the intensity of IL-1 and TNFα staining is diminished. ICAM-1 continues to be strongly expressed.[37]

These immunocytochemical observations indicate that the postulated role of cytokines made by macrophages in vascular endothelial activation is probably valid. TNF and later IL-1 probably cause the upregulation of ICAM and von Willebrand factor on vascular endothelium, which promotes inflammatory cell adhesion and migration. Within the graft, these and other cytokines activate cytotoxic effector cells (macrophages, T cells, and natural killer [NK] cells), resulting in tissue destruction. The specific inactivation of these cytokines in the initial stages of rejection by blocking monoclonal antibodies or genetically engineered soluble receptor molecules could be a powerful tool for immune intervention. Initial applications of monoclonal antibodies against TNF, soluble IL-1 receptor, ICAM-1, and leukocyte function–associated antigen-1 (LFA-1) appear promising in animal models (Chapter 11, pp. 223–224).

EFFECTS OF DRUGS ON THE ALLOGRAFT

Drugs may have a direct toxic effect on the allograft, or an allergic drug reaction may occur. The patients are taking a number of medications, including cyclosporine A, azathioprine, OKT3, antibiotics, steroids, and in some cases hyperalimentation.[6] Toxic reactions to these drugs may be difficult or impossible to establish by biopsy because the findings are nonspecific.

Cyclosporine exerts a toxic effect on the liver, although this toxicity is considerably less common and less severe than that seen in the kidney. In experimental animals, especially in rats, cyclosporine levels greater than that needed for immunosuppression will have hepatotoxic manifestations, characterized by hyperbilirubinemia, elevated liver enzymes, increased alkaline phosphatase, and decreased serum albumin. Histologically, the changes in the liver are characterized by central degeneration with fatty change, single cell necrosis, and cholestasis.[38]

In humans, the effects of cyclosporine on the liver have been studied in patients treated with cyclosporine for uveitis. These were patients who had not had liver transplants and received doses of cyclosporine greater than that which would be used for immunosuppression.[39] In these cases, 58 per cent of the patients were noted to have at least one abnormal liver function test, including increased bilirubin, SGOT, or alkaline phosphatase. Of those having an abnormal liver function test, approximately one half resolved spontaneously within several weeks. The remaining cases showed persistence of the abnormal liver function tests. These abnormalities were mild and self-limited despite continuation of the therapy. No liver biopsies were examined.

In patients receiving cyclosporine for renal transplantation,[40] 50 per cent developed abnormal liver function tests; decreasing the cyclosporine levels corrected the abnormal liver function studies. It is of interest that 2.4 per cent of the cases developed biliary tract stones, usually in the gallbladder but also occasionally in the common duct. This is a greater frequency than would be expected in the general population.

In patients with liver transplants, it is difficult to identify cyclosporine toxicity since other factors, such as preservation injury and transplant rejection, will produce similar abnormalities of liver function tests. Also, reactions of drugs other than cyclosporine enter into the differential diagnosis. It has been suggested that some of the episodes in which there is a transient abnormality of liver function tests with essentially negative findings on liver biopsy may represent cases of cyclosporine hepatotoxicity.[41] Hepatotoxicity from cyclosporine usually occurs early following transplantation and is usually associated with high cyclosporine blood levels. Occasionally the hepatotoxicity occurs late and with cyclosporine levels at the usual therapeutic level. Some of these cases may require substituting another immunosuppressive agent for cyclosporine.[42] Azathioprine does not cause serious hepatotoxicity; its most common toxicity is bone marrow suppression. Cholestasis has been reported with azathioprine but is usually transient.[43]

RECURRENCE OF PRIMARY DISEASE IN THE ALLOGRAFT

The most common primary condition to recur in a transplanted liver is a malignant neoplasm. Most patients (as many as 89 per cent) with malignant neoplasms of the liver that have been treated with liver transplantation will have recurrence of the neoplasm.[44] The exception is fibrolamellar hepatoma, which may have a more favorable prognosis.[44] Hepatitis B will recur in the transplanted liver. This may or may not have associated inflammation and necrosis, and the liver may act as a carrier for the virus rather than develop a progressive infection. Withdrawal of immunosuppression has been associated with a fulminant course of hepatitis B in such cases. There may be recurrence of hepatitis C.

Primary biliary cirrhosis recurring in the transplanted liver has been reported.[45] Since the changes in bile ducts in transplant rejection are quite similar to those seen in primary biliary cirrhosis, it is difficult to make a distinction between the two processes. Recurrence of primary sclerosing cholangitis has been reported.[3] Some metabolic disorders, such as alpha$_1$-antitrypsin deficiency, do not recur and are curable by liver transplantation. One of our cases was a patient who had liver failure because of chronic active hepatitis that had been acquired through multiple transfusions for classic hemophilia. In this case, the hemophilia was completely corrected by the transplantation. Similar results have been reported by others.[46-48]

INFECTIONS AND NEOPLASMS IN THE ALLOGRAFT

Some types of infections can be evaluated in biopsies early in the post-transplant period. Bacterial infections pose a significant problem. The most common ones include ascending cholangitis and intra-abdominal and intrahepatic abscesses. Viral infections related to the immunosuppressed state include cytomegalovirus (CMV), Epstein-Barr virus (EBV), and herpes simplex virus (HSV) (see Figs. 10–34 and 10–35). Fungal infections may also occur. Later in the post-transplant period hepatitis C may occur. In some patients the EBV infection will result in a tumor-like proliferation of lymphocytes, termed *post-transplant lymphoproliferative disorder* (PTLD). These subjects are reviewed in Chapters 12 and 13, pages 239 and 262.

GRAFT VERSUS HOST DISEASE

Patients with liver allografts are considered to be at risk for graft versus host disease (GVHD), even though the acute form of GVHD is a rare occurrence.[49] The largest number of reticuloendothelial cells dwells in the liver, and it has been calculated that about 1 $\times$ 10^9 mononuclear cells persist within the parenchyma of liver allografts even after cold perfusion at procurement. It is conceivable that a large number of immunocompetent cells could lead to different interactions with the recipient's immune system, namely, graft versus host activities.[50] Consequently, a subclinical, self-limited form of GVHD after liver allografting could occur quite often. Patients with some form of bone marrow suppression before transplantation theoretically would be at higher risk. Since biopsy results are very often nonspecific, alternative technology is needed to prove the diagnosis. Also, skin biopsy findings are difficult to differentiate from erythema multiforme and drug toxicity. Recently, PCR has been suggested as a technique to prove GVHD.[51] This approach now surpasses serologic typing for speed, accuracy, and cost. Early HLA typing by PCR could contribute to early confirmation of this complication and provide timely treatment.[50]

SUMMARY OF HISTOLOGIC FINDINGS IN ALLOGRAFTS

Bile Duct Damage. Nuclear atypia and loss of epithelial cells with infiltration by lymphocytes are characteristic of rejection. Similar changes may be seen in hepatitis and large duct obstruction. The ductules in bile duct proliferation characteristically show atypical change and are usually infiltrated by PMNs. Proliferating bile ducts should not be used to evaluate cellular rejection.

Bile Duct Proliferation. This usually has an associated PMN infiltrate and is characteristic of large duct obstruction although it may be seen in other conditions, including rejection.

Central Balloon Cell Change. Marked cytoplasmic swelling with displacement of organelles to the pericanalicular end of cell is characteristic of preservation injury. This occurs in the first several weeks post-transplant and is reversible. Ballooning change occurring later, with associated cell dropout, collapse, and inflammatory infiltrate, is found in chronic rejection. This predicts ultimate allograft failure.

Cholestasis. Central cholestasis is a very common finding in the transplanted liver. It is entirely nonspecific. The differential diagnosis indicates acute and chronic rejection, bacterial and viral infections, biliary obstruction or infection, drug injury, and functional cholestasis, including preservation injury. Cholestasis in periportal ductules may indicate sepsis.

Endothelialitis. This is diagnostic of rejection if characteristic portal infiltrates and bile duct findings are present. This change is the first to disappear following treatment for rejection. The lymphocytes are attached to endothelial cells or are in groups beneath endothelial cells in portal and central veins.

Extensive Hepatic Necrosis. In a needle biopsy it will be difficult to distinguish between extensive infarction associated with hyperacute rejection versus localized subcapsular necrosis associated with localized ischemia. The clinical findings will aid in making this distinction.

Fatty Change. If this is severe in the day 0 biopsy, there is a strong likelihood of graft failure. Less severe changes may be associated with a prolonged recovery following transplantation.

Granulomas. These are often small, epithelioid cell clusters without necrosis (Fig. 10–32). The cause is usually not identified. There is a long list of conditions that may have hepatic granulomas. In the transplanted patient, the more common causes include drug reaction and CMV and EBV infections. Tuberculosis and fungal infections are possible but less likely.

Hematopoiesis. This is occasionally seen and must be differentiated from a lymphocytic infiltrate of hepatitis. Hematopoiesis has been observed in association with some cases of central loss of cells in chronic rejection[23] (Fig. 10–33).

Loss of Central Parenchymal Cells. This indicates ischemia, which may be vascular ischemia due to mechanical problems with the hepatic artery, or the ischemia may indicate vascular rejection and be evidence of chronic rejection. If there is associated lymphocytic infiltration, chronic rejection is more likely. This may predict eventual loss of the allograft.

Lymphocytic Infiltrates in Sinusoids or Around Individual Cells. This is characteristic of hepatitis and may be seen in hepatitis C non-A, non-B as well as hepatitis associated with EBV or CMV infection (Fig. 10–34). This must be differentiated from extramedullary hematopoiesis.

PMN Clusters in Lobules. These are tight

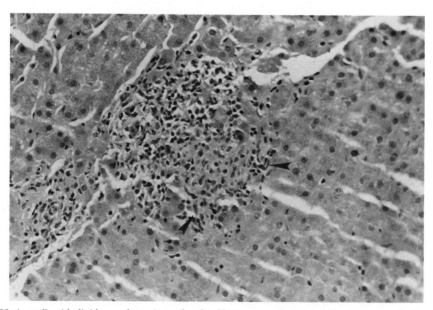

Figure 10–32. A small epithelioid granuloma (arrowheads). No cause was found for this. (Hematoxylin & eosin, × 400)

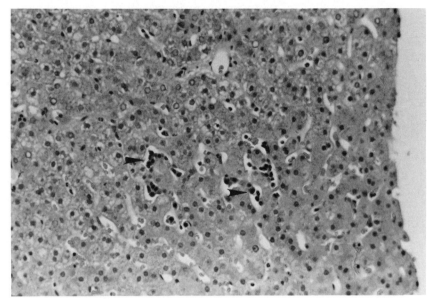

Figure 10–33. Extramedullary hematopoiesis occurring in a liver allograft. Note the groups of small, darkly stained cells in sinusoids (arrowheads). (Hematoxylin & eosin, × 250)

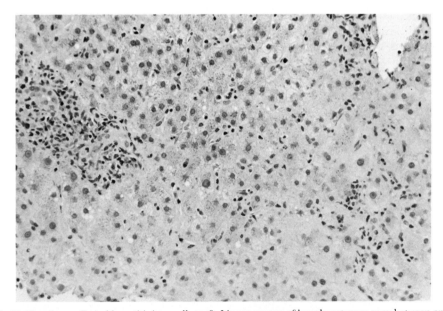

Figure 10–34. Non-A, non-B viral hepatitis in an allograft. Linear groups of lymphocytes are seen between and surrounding hepatic cells. (Hematoxylin & eosin, × 250)

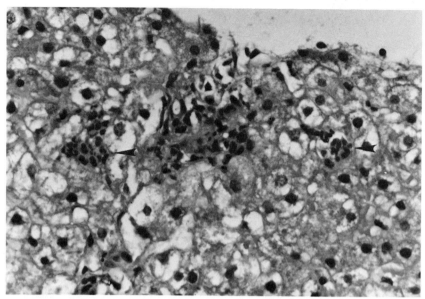

Figure 10–35. CMV hepatitis. There are clusters of neutrophils in the lobules (arrowheads). No viral inclusions are seen. (Hematoxylin & eosin, × 400)

clusters of PMNs, often no more than five or six cells (Fig. 10–35). This is strongly suggestive of CMV infection. Surgical hepatitis resembles this but will be found in the day 0 biopsy only.

Portal Inflammatory Infiltrates. A mixed cellular infiltrate consisting of lymphocytes, neutrophils, and eosinophils is characteristic of rejection. An infiltrate that is predominantly lymphoid suggests hepatitis or post-transplant lymphoproliferative disorder. A prominence

of neutrophils is associated with large duct obstruction and cholangitis, especially if the inflammatory cells are within the duct (Fig. 10–36). This may also be seen in rejection following OKT3 therapy in which the lymphocytes have been removed, leaving only the neutrophils. Eosinophils are characteristically found in acute rejection but may be seen in drug reactions. Plasma cells may be present in small numbers and are of no diagnostic value.

Rejection Vasculopathy. There is narrowing

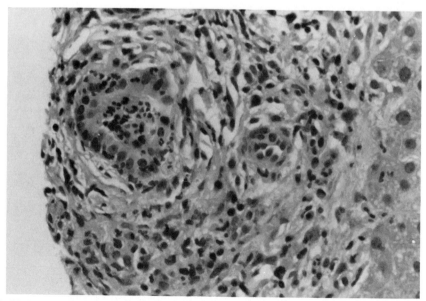

Figure 10–36. Acute cholangitis. Neutrophils are seen within the bile duct lumen. (Hematoxylin & eosin, × 400)

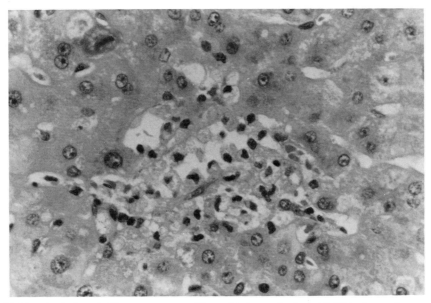

Figure 10–37. Chronic cholestasis. There are groups of foamy histiocytes in sinusoids. This change also occurs in chronic rejection. (Hematoxylin & eosin, × 400)

of the lumen by an accumulation of lipid-filled foamy macrophages within the intima. This occurs only in large arteries (those with external diameters greater than 300 μm) and is usually not seen in biopsies.[22] The small arteries seen in the portal triads may appear to have walls thicker than usual but with no foam cells. No conclusions can be drawn from the thicker-walled vessels, and they are usually considered to be within normal limits.

Single Cell Necrosis. This is a very common finding in transplanted livers and is of no diagnostic importance. It may be seen both early and late following transplantation. Usually no cellular infiltrate is associated with the necrotic cell. If inflammation is present, one should suspect some type of hepatitis.

Sinusoidal Foam Cells. These are clusters of foamy macrophages, usually in sinusoids (Fig. 10–37). They are commonly seen in chronic cholestatic liver disease. Because of chronic cholestasis being present in chronic rejection, foam cells are common in chronic rejection; but they are not diagnostic of chronic rejection.

Viral Inclusions. It is important to search for viral inclusions in every biopsy sample even though the biopsy may have other diagnostic findings.

REFERENCES

1. Wozney P, Zajko AB, Bron KM, et al. Vascular complications after liver transplantation: A five-year experience. Am J Radiol 147:657, 1968.
2. Snover DC, Freese DK, Sharp HL, et al. Liver allograft rejection: An analysis of the use of biopsy in determining outcome of rejection. Am J Surg Pathol 11:1, 1987.
3. Lerut J, Gordon RD, Iwatsuki S, et al. Biliary tract complications in human orthotopic liver transplantation. Transplantation 43:47, 1987.
4. Leopold JG, Parry TE, Storring FK. A change in the sinusoidal-trabecular structure of the liver with hepatic venous outflow block. J Pathol 100:87, 1970.
5. Shulman HM, McDonald GB, Matthews D, et al. An analysis of hepatic veno-occlusive disease and centrilobular hepatocyte degeneration following bone marrow transplantation. Gastroenterology 79:1178, 1980.
6. Snover DC. Liver transplantation. In Sale GE (ed). *Pathology of Organ Transplantation.* Boston, Butterworth's, 1990, pp 103–132.
7. Todo S, Demetris AJ, Makowka L, et al. Primary nonfunction of hepatic allografts with preexisting fatty infiltration. Transplantation 47:903, 1989.
8. D'Alessandro AM, Kalayoglu M, Sollinger HW, et al. The predictive value of donor liver biopsies for the development of primary nonfunction after orthotopic liver transplantation. Transplantation 51:157, 1991.
9. Adam R, Reynes M, Johann M, et al. The outcome of steatotic grafts in liver transplantation. Transplant Proc 23:1538, 1991.
10. Snover DC, et al. Orthotopic liver transplantation: A pathological study of 63 serial liver biopsies from 17 patients with special reference to the diagnostic features and natural history of rejection. Hepatology 4:1212, 1984.
11. Kakizoe S, Yanaga K, Starzl TE, Demetris AJ. Frozen section of liver biopsy for the evaluation of liver allografts. Transplant Proc 22:416, 1990.
12. Williams JW, Santiago V, Peters TG, et al. Cholestatic jaundice after hepatic transplantation. Am J Surg 151:65, 1986.
13. Howard TK, Klintmalm GBG, Cofer JB, Husberg BS, Goldstein RM, Gonwa TA. The influence of preservation injury on rejection in the hepatic transplant recipient. Transplantation 49:103, 1990.
14. Russo PA, Yunis EJ. Subcapsular hepatic necrosis in orthotopic liver allografts. Hepatology 6:708, 1986.

15. Medawar PB. Transplantation of tissues and organs. Br Med Bull 21:97, 1965.

16. Starzl TE, Demetris AJ, Murase N, et al. Cell migration, chimerism and graft acceptance. Lancet 339:1579, 1992.

17. Hanto DW, Snover DC, Noreen HJ, et al. Hyperacute rejection of a human orthotopic liver allograft in a presensitized recipient. Clin Transplant 1:304, 1987.

18. Knechtle SJ, Kolbeck PC, Tsuchimoto S, et al. Hepatic transplantation into sensitized recipients: Demonstration of hyperacute rejection. Transplantation 43:8, 1987.

19. Demetris AJ, Jaffe R, Tsakis, A, et al. Antibody-mediated rejection of human orthotopic liver allografts: A study of liver transplantation across ABO blood group barriers. Am J Pathol 132:489, 1988.

20. Takaya S, Iwaki Y, Starzl TE. Liver transplantation in positive cytotoxic crossmatch cases using FK506, high dose steroids and prostaglandin E1. Transplantation 54:927, 1992.

21. The First International Workshop and Colloquium on the Pathology of Liver Transplantation: Discussion. Transplant Proc 18(Suppl 4):144, 1986.

22. Grond J, Gouw ASH, Poppema S, Slooff MJH, Gips CH. Chronic rejection in liver transplants: A histopathologic analysis of failed grafts and antecedent serial biopsies. Transplant Proc 18:128, 1986.

23. Freese DK, Snover DC, Sharp HL, Gross CR, Savick SK, Payne WD. Chronic rejection after liver transplantation: A study of clinical histopathological and immunological features. Hepatology 13:882, 1991.

24. Ludwig J, Gross JB, Perkins JD, Moore SB. Persistent centrilobular necroses in hepatic allografts. Hum Pathol 21:656, 1990.

25. Ludwig J, Wiesner RH, Batts KP, Perkins JD, Krom RAF. The acute vanishing bile duct syndrome (acute irreversible rejection) after orthotopic liver transplantation. Hepatology 7:476, 1987.

26. Geoffrey L, Butany J, Wanless JR, et al. The vascular pathology of human hepatic allografts. Hum Pathol 24:182, 1993.

27. Vierling JM, Fennell RH Jr. Histopathology of early and late human hepatic allograft rejection: Evidence of progressive destruction of interlobular bile ducts. Hepatology 5:1076, 1985.

28. Hubscher SG, Buckels JAC, Elias E, McMaster P, Neuberger J. Vanishing bile-duct syndrome following liver transplantation—is it reversible? Transplantation 5:1004, 1991.

29. Noack KB, Wiesner RH, Batts K, et al. Severe ductopenic rejection with features of vanishing bile duct syndrome: Clinical, biochemical, and histologic evidence for spontaneous resolution. Transplant Proc 23:1448, 1991.

30. Wiesner RH, Ludwig J, Krom RAF, et al. Hepatic allograft rejection: New developments in terminology, diagnosis, prevention and treatment. Mayo Clin Proc 68:69, 1993.

31. Steinhoff G, Wonigeit K, Sorg C, et al. Analysis of sequential changes in major histocompatibility complex expression in human liver grafts after transplantation. Transplantation 45:394, 1988.

32. Adams DH, Shaw J, Hubscher SG, et al. Intercellular adhesion molecule 1 on liver allografts during rejection. Lancet 2:1122, 1989.

33. Imagawa DK, Millis JM, Olthoff K, et al. The role of tumor necrosis factor in allograft rejection. I. Elevated levels of tumor necrosis factor alpha predict rejection following orthotopic liver transplantation. Transplantation 50:219, 1990.

34. Tilg H, Vogel W, Aulitzky WE, et al. Evaluation of cytokines and cytokine induced secondary messages in sera of patients after liver transplantation. Transplantation 49:1074, 1990.

35. Martinez OM, Krams SM, Sterneck M, et al. Intragraft cytokine profile during human allograft rejection. Transplantation 53:449, 1992.

36. Pober JS, Cotran RS. The role of endothelial cells in inflammation. Transplantation 50:537, 1990.

37. Hoffman MW, Woniget K, Steinhoff G, et al. Production of cytokines (TNF-a and IL-1-beta) and endothelial cell activation in human liver allograft rejection. Transplantation 55:329, 1993.

38. Ryffel B, Donatsch P, Madorin M, Matter BE, Ruttimann G, Schon H, Stoll R, Wilson J. Toxicological evaluation of cyclosporin A. Arch Toxicol 53:107, 1983.

39. Kassianides C, Nussenblatt R, Palestine AG, Mellow SD, Hoofnagle JH. Liver injury from cyclosporine A. Dig Dis Sci 35:693, 1990.

40. Lorber MI, VanBuren CT, Flechner SM, Williams C, Kahan BD. Hepatobiliary and pancreatic complications of cyclosporine therapy in 466 renal transplant recipients. Transplantation 43:35, 1987.

41. Williams JW, Vera S, Peters TG, Van Voorst S, et al. Cholestatic jaundice after hepatic transplantation: A nonimmunologically mediated event. Am J Surg 151:65, 1986.

42. Klintmalm GBG, Iwatsuki S, Starzl TE. Cyclosporine A hepatotoxicity in 66 renal allograft recipients. Transplantation 32:488, 1981.

43. Georgii A, Wonigeit K, Worch KJ, Ringe B, et al. Infection after orthotopic grafting of liver. Transplant Proc 5:146, 1986.

44. Portmann B, O'Grady J, Williams R. Disease recurrence following orthotopic liver transplantation. Transplant Proc 18:136, 1986.

45. Polson RJ, Portmann B, Neuberger J, Calne RY, Williams R. Evidence for disease recurrence after liver transplantation for primary biliary cirrhosis: Clinical and histologic follow-up studies. Gastroenterology 97:715, 1989.

46. Bontempo FA, Lewis JH, Govene TS, et al. Liver transplantation in hemophilia. Blood 69:1721, 1987.

47. Delorme MA, Adams PC, Grant D, et al. Orthotopic liver transplantation in a patient with combined hemophilia A and B. Am J Hematol 33:136, 1990.

48. Gibas A, Dienstag JL, Schafet AI, et al. Cure of hemophilia A by orthotopic liver transplantation. Gastroenterology 95:192, 1988.

49. Jamieson JP, Joysey V, Friend PJ, et al. Graft versus host disease in solid organ transplantation. Transplant Int 4:67, 1991.

50. Mazzaferro V, Andreola S, Regalia E, et al. Confirmation of graft versus host disease after liver transplantation by PCR HLA typing. Transplantation 55:423, 1993.

51. Drobyski W, Thibodeau S, Truitt RL, et al. Third party mediated graft rejection and graft versus host disease after T-cell depleted bone marrow transplantation, as demonstrated by hypervariable DNA probes and HLA-DR polymorphism. Blood 74:2285, 1989.

Processes Common to All Solid Organ Allografts

III

In this section, immunosuppressive treatments and diseases common to all solid organ allografts are addressed. The mechanisms of action and the adverse effects of immunosuppressive drugs are considered in Chapter 11 by Drs. Norman and Costanzo. These physicians have extensive clinical experience dealing with immunosuppressive treatment involving a variety of allografts.

A chapter dealing with infections common to solid organ allografts has been written by Drs. Flinner and Classen. Dr. Flinner, a pathologist, and Dr. Classen, an infectious disease physician, have extensive practical experience treating these infections. The final chapter addresses malignancies found in transplant recipients, focusing on lymphoproliferative processes, since they are a unique aspect of malignancies involving allografts. Readers are encouraged to consult both the specific chapters on the site as well as the general discussion to obtain a complete picture of the features of these infectious and neoplastic processes.

11

ACTIONS, INTERACTIONS, AND TOXICITIES OF IMMUNOSUPPRESSIVE DRUGS AND TECHNIQUES: NEW AND OLD

Douglas J. Norman, MD, and Maria Rosa Costanzo, MD

OVERVIEW OF THE ALLOIMMUNE RESPONSE AND T CELL ACTIVATION

Allografts elicit an immune response that consists of cellular and sometimes humoral components. Cell-mediated rejection involves T cells predominantly,[1] but macrophages (delayed-type sensitivity)[2] and natural killer (NK) cells (antibody-dependent cell-mediated cytotoxicity, ADCC)[3] may also contribute. Antibodies capable of reacting with an allograft can be present before transplant, or they can develop afterward. For their normal function, cells that become cytolytic or antibody-producing depend upon a multitude of surface molecules (receptors for recognizing antigens or promoting cell adhesion), soluble proteins (cytokines), and intracellular mechanisms of activation (phosphorylation, transport, gene transcription, protein synthesis). The drugs and techniques used for immunosuppression following organ transplantation are aimed at blocking, inactivating, or neutralizing one or more of these components to render the immune response weak and inefficient.

T Cell Activation Pathways

T cells held captive in a test tube can be activated by lectins,[4] phorbol esters,[5, 6] mono-clonal antibodies,[7] calcium ionophores,[8] and alloantigens, or combinations of the above. Investigation of T cell activation in vitro has demonstrated calcium-dependent and independent pathways involving multiple accessory molecules and intracellular metabolic and synthetic processes.[9–11] Allograft-directed T cells are activated in vivo mainly through an interaction of alloantigen with its unique antigen receptor on T cells. The importance of this mode of activation is confirmed by the strong influence of major histocompatibility antigen disparity between a donor and recipient on T cell activation leading to rejection[12] and by the observation that T cell activation can be prevented simply by blocking the T cell antigen receptor.[13] Nevertheless, once activated, T cell proliferation and allograft-directed T cell killing depend upon secreted cytokines, cytokine receptors, and adhesion molecules, as well as upon normal gene transcription, translocation, and replication. At each step in the T cell activation-to-proliferation and differentiation cascade, blocking pharmacologic drugs or nonpharmacologic techniques can be employed to abrogate the immune response. These are now generally classified by where in the cascade they operate (Fig. 11–1). Some block cytokine synthesis, another inhibits the action of cytokines, and others inhibit DNA

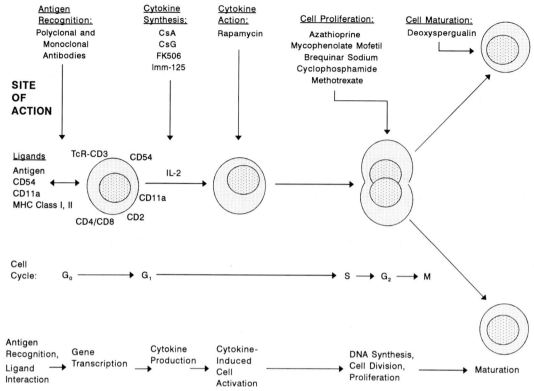

Figure 11–1. Sites of action of the immunosuppressive drugs. (Adapted from Morris, RE. Immunopharmacology of new xenobiotic immunosuppressive molecules. Semin Nephrol 12:306, 1992.)

synthesis. The anti-T cell monoclonal and polyclonal antibodies block antigen recognition or proliferation or deplete mononuclear cells by binding to cell surface molecules.

Role of Antibody (Humoral Immunity)

Stimulated by transfusions, pregnancies, or organ transplants,[14] antidonor antibodies can combine with donor endothelium and activate humoral (complement, fibrin)-mediated or cellular (polymorphonuclear cells [PMNs], platelets)-mediated mechanisms of cell damage. These mechanisms lead to vascular cell (endothelial, intimal smooth muscle) activation and proliferation, and/or necrosis and thrombosis.[15] Vascular rejection can be mediated by antibodies alone or by antibodies and mononuclear cells.[16, 17] In the latter scenario, the antibodies and cells can work independently or together in a type of immunity known as antibody-dependent cell-mediated cytotoxicity (ADCC).[3] The cells implicated in this type of immunity are known as NK (natural killer) or K (killer)[18]; when activated, they release perforins and other cell-damaging proteins. The specificity of this immune reaction is determined by the antibodies alone.

If present in a patient's serum prior to transplant, anti-HLA antibodies can be detected by testing for serum reactivity on a lymphocyte panel.[19] Donors against whom antibodies are present can be avoided through the use of a sensitive prospective cross-match.[20]

Role of Adhesion Molecules

For antigen-specific T cell interactions with an antigen-presenting cell (via the CD4+ T cell) or target cell (via the CD8+ T cell), the T cell receptor/CD3 complex–target antigen interaction is necessary[21, 22] but not sufficient. Other cell-surface molecules, currently called adhesion molecules, appear to be important also. These include intercellular adhesion molecule-1 (ICAM-1, CD54)[23, 24] and its ligand, leukocyte function–associated antigen (LFA)-1 (CD11a),[25] both on T cells and antigen-presenting cells (APC); CD2 (T cell–specific)[26] and its ligand LFA-3 (CD58),[27] present on APC and target cells; CD4 (helper T cell–specific)[28] and its ligand MHC class II; CD8 (cytolytic T cell–specific)[29] and its ligand MHC class I; and CD28 (T cell–specific)[30] and its ligand BB1/B7.[31] Interference with certain of these interactions involving CD4, ICAM, and CD28 can prevent T cell activation in vitro, which indicates their importance and suggests possible methods of immunosuppression for clinical organ transplantation.

Role of Cytokines

The cytokines interleukin (IL)-1[32] and IL-6[33] are important cofactors (with antigen) for activating T cells. Once activated by antigen and cofactors and driven from G_0 to G_1 of the cell cycle, a T cell is further activated and driven from G_1 to G_S by the cytokine IL-2.[34] IL-2 and IL-2 receptors (IL-2R) are produced by T cells during the initial activation (G_0 to G_1) of the T cell.[35] Resting T cells do not express IL-2R and will not respond to IL-2.[36] Differentiation of T cells to cytolytic cells requires IL-2.[37] Cytokines are also required for B cell growth and differentiation (IL-2, IL-4, IL-6).[38–41]

Role of Cell-Mediated Immunity

The dominant mechanism of rejection is T cell (CD8 +)–mediated cytolysis, as suggested by the finding of multiple T cells with the CD8 phenotype infiltrating rejecting allografts.[42] Delayed-type hypersensitivity (DTH) is T cell (CD4 +)– and macrophage-mediated and probably also plays a role in allograft rejection.[43]

PHARMACOLOGIC IMMUNOSUPPRESSION

For many years only a few drugs (corticosteroids, azathioprine and cyclophosphamide) were available for use as immunosuppressants. Today, many more are currently or soon to be available. These can be divided into several groups according to their site of action in the T cell activation cascade.

Inhibitors of Cytokine Synthesis

Cyclosporine (CSA) and FK506 both inhibit the production of cytokines. Cyclosporine is a fungal endecapeptide that works during an early stage of T cell activation by preventing the transcription of early genes necessary for the synthesis of cytokines, notably IL-2.[44] As a result, CSA blocks T cell activation by a variety of stimuli, including phytohemagglutinin (PHA), anti-CD3 monoclonal antibodies, ionomycin plus phorbol myristate acetate (PMA), and the allogeneic stimulus present in the mixed lymphocyte reaction (MLR).[45–48] Cyclosporine prevents T cells from progressing from G_0 to G_1 in the cell cycle; it blocks T cell proliferation, IL-2 production, and IL-2 receptor (IL-2R) expression.[44, 47, 49]

The precise mechanism of action of CSA is unknown. However, it is known to affect a subset of calcium-associated signaling events involved in the regulation of lymphokine gene expression, activation-driven cell death (apoptosis), and exocytosis.[50] Cyclosporine interacts with a 17-kD protein called cyclophilin that has peptidyl-prolyl *cis-trans* isomerase (PPIase) activity.[51, 52] The interaction of CSA with cyclophilin inhibits the activation of calcineurin, a calcium-dependent phosphoser/thr phosphatase. Calcineurin activity is necessary for the translocation to the nucleus of NFAT (nuclear factor of activated T cells)-B, which combines with NFAT-A in the nucleus and regulates the expression of the IL-2 gene.[53] The analogs of CSA, OG 37-325 and IMM-125, have activity similar to that of CSA and are immunosuppressive; however, other analogs that bind cyclophilin and block PPIase activity are not immunosuppressive, indicating that cyclophilin binding alone is insufficient to explain the immunosuppressive effects of CSA.[46]

FK506 is a bacterial macrolide that has a nearly identical pattern of T cell inhibition but is a hundredfold more potent than cyclosporine.[54] FK506 also inhibits IL-2 production, apoptosis, and IL2-R expression and proliferation in response to the same stimuli noted for CSA.[46, 48, 49] It also inhibits the transcriptional activation of NFAT[53] by binding to a unique immunophilin called FK binding protein (FKBP).[55] FK506 also prevents T cells from being activated to cycle from G_0 to G_1. The structures of both FK506 and FKBP are different from those of CSA and cyclophilin, yet their effects on T cell function are nearly identical.[44]

Inhibitors of Cytokine Action

Rapamycin (RAP) is an actinomycete macrolide lactone that inhibits cell cycle progression from G_1 to G_s, a later stage of T cell activation, in response to IL-2-driven activation.[45, 46, 48] Rapamycin blocks phosphorylation and activation of the 70-kD S6 protein kinases.[56] It has a structure very similar to that of FK506 and binds the same immunophilin, FKBP, but works at a different stage of T cell activation.[50] Rapamycin inhibits pathways of T cell activation that are insensitive to FK506, such as (1) IL-2-driven activation of IL-2-dependent cell lines, (2) IL-6-driven activation of IL-6-dependent cell lines, (3) activation by phorbol esters and anti-CD28, and (4) activation of murine B lymphocytes by bacterial polysaccharides.[57] Rapamycin only minimally blocks ionomycin + PMA-induced IL-2 production and IL2-R expression but prevents T cell proliferation from these stimuli.[52] Because they bind the same immunophilin, FKBP, RAP, and FK506 are antagonistic.[51, 58] In high doses, FK506 can reverse the inhibitory effects of RAP on IL-2-driven T cell proliferation. Cyclosporine and rapamycin appear to be synergistic and act at two separate sites.[47] Rapamycin potentiates CSA-induced inhibition of T cell activation by either anti-CD3 monoclonal antibodies, phytohemagglutinin, or alloantigen (MLR).

Inhibitors of Cell Proliferation

Azathioprine

Azathioprine (AZA) is a potent, nonspecific antimetabolite that, in the liver, is converted to 6-mercaptopurine and other metabolites that have variable immunosuppressive actions.[59] Azathioprine inhibits the synthesis of both DNA and RNA by blocking de novo purine synthesis and also produces breaks in the chromosomal DNA. Because of these antiproliferative effects, AZA decreases the expansion of allospecific clones of the T and B cells that mediate allograft rejection.[60, 61]

It is not known whether there is any correlation between the immunosuppressive effects of AZA and the degree of myelosuppression it induces. Leukopenia, anemia,[62] or thrombocytopenia[63] can occur together or alone. Because the enzyme xanthine oxidase is essential in controlling the level of 6-mercaptopurine, concomitant use of allopurinol requires that the dose of AZA be reduced by approximately 75 per cent to avoid severe myelotoxicity.[60]

Mycophenolate Mofetil

Mycophenolate mofetil (MM) is a semisynthetic morpholinoethyl ester of mycophenolic acid, a compound isolated from a corn mold. After gastrointestinal absorption, MM is quickly hydrolyzed to mycophenolic acid, the active compound. Mycophenolic acid undergoes metabolic elimination by hepatic conjugation with glucuronic acid to form an inactive metabolite, approximately 90 per cent of which is excreted in the urine or feces within 24 hours.[64] Mycophenolic acid selectively, noncompetitively, and reversibly inhibits inosine monophosphate dehydrogenase in the de novo pathway of guanosine nucleotide biosynthesis.[64] Inosine monophosphate (IMP) is converted to xanthine monophosphate (XMP) by the enzyme IMP dehydrogenase, and XMP is then converted to guanosine monophosphate (GMP) by the enzyme GMP synthetase. These target enzymes catalyze the de novo synthesis of purines, thereby inhibiting purine-dependent T and B cell functions (T and B cell proliferation, antibody formation, upregulation of cytotoxic T cells). Furthermore, inhibition of IMP dehydrogenase may decrease the intracellular guanosine triphosphate (GTP) pool, thereby reducing nucleotide availability for signal transduction and synthesis of cell surface proteins and receptors.[65–67]

In rodents, mycophenolate mofetil prolongs allo- and xenograft survival, reverses ongoing rejection, prevents cardiac allograft vasculopathy, and induces specific allounresponsiveness. The efficacy of MM in reversing ongoing rejection can be explained by the observation that activated T and B cells are richer than resting immune cells in β-glucuronidase, an enzyme that catalyzes the conversion of inactive mycophenolic acid glucuronide to the active compound.[68, 69]

Whereas some studies have shown that mycophenolate mofetil prolongs cardiac allograft survival synergistically with cyclosporine and 15-deoxyspergualin and cardiac xenograft survival with 15-deoxyspergualin and splenectomy, other studies have shown that CSA antagonizes the emergence of tolerance induced by MM alone. Clinical trials have shown that MM is an effective adjunct to CSA and steroids in preventing renal allograft rejection and reversing rejection refractory to conventional immunosuppression.[70] Use of MM for the treatment of refractory allograft rejection has also been reported.[71]

Mizoribine

Mizoribine (MZR), also called bredinin, is an imidazole nucleoside isolated from eupenicillum brefeldianum M-2166, which inhibits the enzymes inosine monophosphate dehydrogenase and guanosine monophosphate synthetase.[72] T and B cell proliferation and antibody production are inhibited owing to blockade of purine biosynthesis.[73–76] At high doses, MZR can decrease IL-2 production.[77] Mizoribine is highly water soluble, with a short elimination half-life. Elimination of MZR depends on renal function.[78] When compared with AZA, MZR appears to be less myelotoxic.[79–81]

In mice, MZR suppresses IgM production in vitro and prolongs allograft survival. Mizoribine is synergistic with CSA in rat heart/lung allograft models and canine heart, renal, and pancreas allograft models.

Mizoribine has been widely used as an alternative to AZA in Japanese patients for the prevention and treatment of renal allograft rejection.[82, 83] In this clinical setting, patients treated at the time of transplantation with MZR, CSA, and corticosteroids (CS), with or without antilymphocyte antibodies, have 2-year survival rate of more than 90 per cent. When used with cyclosporine, mizoribine has corticosteroid-sparing effects. As a selective inhibitor of purine biosynthesis, MZR offers several advantages, including better treatment and prophylaxis of humoral rejection, a decreased incidence of cardiac allograft vasculopathy, and perhaps a decreased incidence of post-transplant malignancy.

Brequinar Sodium

Brequinar sodium (BQR), a 4-substituted quinoline carboxylic acid derivative,[84, 85] inhibits the enzyme dihydro-orotate dehydrogenase, thus blocking the conversion of dihydro-orotate to orotate, resulting in inhibition of de novo pyrimidine biosynthesis. Thus, lymphocyte proliferation is impeded due to depletion of RNA and DNA precursors.[86] Brequinar sodium is hydrophobic[87] and undergoes triphasic elimination. The last phase of the decay lasts up to 24 hours.[87]

In murine transplantation models, the immunosuppressive potency of BQR is similar to that of FK506 and one hundredfold greater than that of MM. Brequinar is highly effective in reversing advanced murine heart allograft rejection and has synergistic immunosuppressive effects with CSA.[88] In rats, BQR prolongs heart allograft survival and induces tolerance to kidney and liver allografts.[89] Because MZR, MM, BQR, and AZA all inhibit nucleotide biosynthesis and are potentially myelotoxic, the

concomitant use of these drugs is unlikely. Because these new antiproliferative drugs have toxic effects distinct from those of CSA, FK506, and RAP, their most likely role will be that of AZA substitutes.[88–91]

Human dose-limiting toxicities of BQR have been myelosuppression, mucositis, skin rash, nausea, and vomiting. Angioneurotic edema has been reported. Most human trials have involved cancer patients, and the doses of BQR have been higher than those likely to be used for transplant immunosuppression.

Unlike azathioprine, mycophenolate mofetil and brequinar effectively reverse ongoing rejection, and thus they may be useful for both prevention and treatment of rejection. Because blockage of the enzymes in the purine and pyrimidine pathways by these drugs is rapidly reversible, it will be important to design a dose schedule to insure that sufficient blood levels of active drugs are maintained.[92]

Methotrexate

Methotrexate (MTX) is a folic acid analog that inhibits DNA synthesis and cell division by binding competitively with dihydrofolic reductase. Methotrexate is a weak organic acid and, as such, its primary route of elimination is through the kidney. After filtration and proximal tubular resorption, the drug undergoes tubular secretion.[93] Methotrexate is a potent cytostatic drug that has been used at high doses in malignancies characterized by rapid cellular proliferation and at lower doses in nonmalignant states characterized by rapid cell turnover, like psoriasis.[93–95] At a low dose, MTX has been extensively used for more than 15 years for the treatment of rheumatoid arthritis. The effectiveness of MTX in this setting and in graft versus host disease (GVHD) is not due to the cytostatic properties of MTX but to its potent inhibitory effects on cellular and humoral immunity.[96] Methotrexate and cyclosporine together are superior to CSA alone in the prevention of acute GVHD after bone marrow transplantation for leukemia.[97] Although the mechanism of action of MTX in autoimmune diseases is not completely understood, the disease-modifying potential of this drug appears associated with its effect on cellular and humoral immunity. The major short-term risk of MTX administration is significant myelosuppression.[98] The availability of a specific bone marrow stimulant, such as granulocyte colony-stimulating factor (G-CSF), may allow greater protection against dangerous leukopenia. The immunosuppressive activity of MTX may explain its success in several studies in which the drug was used to treat persistent cardiac allograft rejection.[98–101] It has not been tried for severe rejection and probably should not be used for this indication.

Inhibitor of Cell Maturation

Deoxyspergualin (DS) is a guanidine derivative isolated from *Bacillus laterosporus* that was first described as an antineoplastic agent and later found to be immunosuppressive.[102, 103]

15-Deoxyspergualin (15DS) acts primarily on accessory cells of the immune system. It reduces (1) class II HLA antigen expression of rat splenic and peritoneal macrophages,[104, 105] (2) macrophage IL-1 production upon stimulation with phorbol myristate acetate, (3) oxygen-derived free radical generation in monocytes, and (4) hydrolytic enzyme secretion by macrophages.[105, 106] 15-Deoxyspergualin blocks proliferative and cytotoxic responses of mouse and rat splenic lymphocytes in vitro.[107] These inhibitory effects are abolished completely by interferon-gamma (IF-γ) and partially by IL-2, suggesting that 15DS-induced immunosuppression is mediated by the inability of lymphocytes to produce IF-γ. Because 15DS inhibits immunization-induced production of IgG and IgM antibodies, it may suppress human antimouse antibody responses during monoclonal antibody therapy.[108, 109]

Prophylactic administration of 15-deoxyspergualin has prolonged the survival of rodent skin and vascularized organ grafts.[106, 110–114] It successfully reversed acute rejection of vascularized heart allografts[112, 115] but has not prolonged survival of repeat grafts in highly sensitized hosts unless given during sensitization.[116] The in vivo and in vitro immunosuppressive effects of 15DS are synergistic with those of cyclosporine[113] in allograft models and of FK506 in xenograft models.[117]

15-Deoxyspergualin has been used for prophylactic immunosuppression in clinical renal transplantation and for the treatment of acute rejection in renal and hepatic allografts. It reversed acute renal rejection in 70 per cent to 90 per cent of cases, especially when combined with corticosteroids. Since the mechanisms of immunosuppression of 15DS are distinct from those of other agents, its addition to any immunosuppressive regimen may offer significant advantages.[118–120] Because 15DS inhibits activated T and B cells, it may be useful to

prevent early rejection in patients undergoing repeat transplantation.

Corticosteroids

Corticosteroids (CS) are anti-inflammatory[121, 122] and lympholytic[123] and specifically block the production of cofactors (IL-1 and IL-6) by antigen-presenting cells that are necessary to activate T cells.[124] Corticosteroids exert an influence on cytokine gene transcription, perhaps by altering the expression of regulatory genes (early genes).[125] Corticosteroid-induced cell death (lymphocytolysis) perhaps is due to the induction of a lysis gene product (nuclease) that results in internucleosomal cleavage of the lymphocyte genome and eventual cell death.[126] The anti-inflammatory effects of CS relate to their ability to block release of tissue-damaging enzymes from PMNs and monocytes.[127, 128] These soluble mediators of inflammation are important effectors of irreversible cell damage and fibrosis. Corticosteroids remain a mainstay for maintenance immunosuppression and rejection therapy. They appear to be necessary for many patients.

BIOLOGIC IMMUNOSUPPRESSION WITH ANTIBODIES/FUSION MOLECULES

Antilymphocyte Antibodies

Antilymphocyte antibodies, the earliest form of biologic (versus chemical) immunosuppressive agents, have been used in transplantation since the 1960s. Polyclonal (PoAbs) and monoclonal antilymphocyte antibodies (MoAbs) are used commonly in solid organ transplantation, although probably less often in cardiac compared with other organ transplantation. Their dominant mechanisms of action are cell depletion and blocking of antigen recognition via interference with binding of the antibodies' target molecules with their respective ligands.[129]

There is a vast difference between PoAbs and MoAbs with regard to their manufacture, specificity, and potency. The polyclonal antilymphocyte antibodies are made in horses and rabbits by injecting thymocytes or lymphoblasts repeatedly until a high antibody titer develops.[130] These antibodies are nonspecific and must be adsorbed with stroma to remove activity against endothelium, red blood cells, and platelets. Monoclonal antibodies are made from hybridoma cells obtained by fusing antibody-producing cells of mice with myeloma cells.[131] These antibodies are highly purified and are directed to a single molecular target, as compared with many targets with the polyclonal preparations. Nonetheless, whereas most PoAbs are effective for immunosuppression,[130, 132–134] only a few of the MoAbs have proved useful.[129]

Polyclonal antibodies are panleukocytic; that is, they are directed against T cells, B cells, monocytes, and granulocytes. The targets of PoAbs can be characterized as multimolecular and panleukocytic, and these antibodies cross-react with tissue cells bearing similar molecules.[135] Many PoAb preparations are currently in use in the United States, Canada, Europe, and Asia. The most widely used of these are ATGam (Upjohn, Kalamazoo, MI), Fresenius (Fresenius AG, Bad Hamburg, Germany), Merieux Institute preparations (Pasteur Merieux, Sérums and Vaccines, Marcy L'Etoile, France), and Minnesota antilymphoblast globulin. In contrast, MoAbs can be selected so as to be directed to specific molecules on T cells, such as CD2, CD3, CD5, CD6, CD7, or subsets of T cells, such as CD4 and CD8, or even on activated subsets of T cells, such as CD25 (the IL-2 receptor). Monoclonal antibody targets are epitope-specific and cell-specific (T cell, T cell–subset, and so on), but MoAbs will cross-react with molecules bearing similar epitopes. As an example, it is known that an epitope

against which an anti-CD3 MoAb is directed is also found on cerebellar tissue. This MoAb is not used clinically, and the MoAb that is approved for use by the FDA has no anticerebellar or other antibrain tissue activity.

Many different MoAbs have been used in humans. These are best classified in groups according to their targets: panleukocytic, pan–T cell, lymphocyte subset–specific, activation antigen–specific or biased, costimulatory molecule-specific, and adhesion molecule–specific (Table 11–1). While MoAbs are much more specific than their PoAb counterparts, most of the MoAbs have proved not very effective, probably because the cell surface molecules to which they are directed are not critical for T and B cell function in vivo. Examples of the relatively unsuccessful MoAbs are anti-Tac,[136] Campath-6,[137] and 33B3.1,[138] which are all directed to the IL-2 receptor CD25; T12[139] directed to CD6, a molecule of unknown significance; and RFT2 directed to CD7, a molecule found in greater numbers on activated T cells and on natural killer cells.[140] In contrast, some monoclonal antibodies have proved very effective, and one in particular, OKT3, approved by the FDA for use in organ transplantation, is one of the most effective immunosuppressive drugs currently available.[141] This one and other MoAbs currently under investigation—T10B9,[142] WT32,[143] and BMA031[144]—are directed to the CD3/T cell receptor complex. Campath-1, a panleukocyte monoclonal antibody, appears to be effective and is more similar to the PoAbs in its reactivity patterns.[145]

Table 11–1. Classification of the Monoclonal Antibodies

Specificity	Name	Target Molecule/Function
Panleukocytic	Campath-1	Common leukocyte antigen
Pan–T Cell		
TcR-CD3	OKT3	Antigen recognition
	WT32	Antigen recognition
	BMA031	Antigen recognition
	T10 B9	Antigen recognition
CD6	T12	Unknown
CD5	Orthozyme H65	Unknown
Lymphocyte Subset		
CD25	Anti-Tac	Interleukin 2 receptor
	33B3.1	Interleukin 2 receptor
	Campath-6	Interleukin 2 receptor
CD7	RFT2	T cell leukemia antigen
		Ig gene super family member
CD4	OKT4A	Coactivation factor
		Ig gene super family member
Adhesion Molecule		
ICAM-1	Anti–ICAM-1	Cell adhesion
LFA-1	Anti–LFA-1	Cell adhesion

Monoclonal antibodies directed to intercellular adhesion molecules are just now entering clinical trials. The results of two such MoAbs, anti-ICAM[146] and anti LFA-1,[147, 148] appear promising in murine studies particularly when given together, but in humans they may not be any more effective than OKT4A, an anti-CD4 MoAb with great promise in animals[149, 150] that was disappointing in preliminary clinical studies.[151]

Possible mechanisms of action of the antilymphocyte antibodies include (1) opsonization and subsequent phagocytosis by mononuclear phagocytes residing in the spleen and liver, (2) antibody-dependent cell-mediated cytotoxicity, (3) complement-mediated cell lysis, (4) activation of cells, and (5) coating and subsequent blocking/inactivation of the function of cell surface molecules involved in antigen recognition, cell activation, or intercellular adhesion.[152] Polyclonal antibodies probably work predominantly by depleting T and B cells and coating their surface molecules. The most important mechanism of action of OKT3 is thought to be blocking, through modulation (removal), of cell surface CD3 and its closely associated molecule, the T cell receptor for antigen.[153] Cells without surface T cell receptors are probably not immunologically active. OKT3 also depletes T cells[154] initially and activates them.[7] The importance of these as reasons for the efficacy of OKT3 for immunosuppression is unknown.

A consequence of using heterologous antibodies for clinical transplantation is that they are immunogenic and stimulate the production of human antibodies against themselves.[155] Anti-OKT3 antibody production limits the prolonged or repeated use of OKT3.[156] Human antipolyclonal antibody production often results in serum sickness signs and symptoms;[157] however, serum sickness is rare following OKT3 use.

Fusion Molecules

Biotechnology has produced another approach to immunosuppression in the form of fusion molecules. Examples of fusion molecules proposed for use are monoclonal antibodies linked with ricin A chain (e.g., Orthozyme H65) and IL-2 linked with diphtheria toxin. Orthozyme H65 (anti-CD5, a pan–T cell molecule) has demonstrated efficacy following bone marrow transplantation for treating graft versus host disease. The ricin A chain enters the targeted T cell and blocks normal DNA synthesis.[158] The diphtheria toxin–linked IL-2 enters T cells via the IL-2 receptor (IL-2R) and has the theoretical advantage of entering only activated, not resting, T cells that express IL-2R. This fusion molecule has been used in T cell leukemia and rheumatoid arthritis studies and appears to have some efficacy.[159, 160]

Engineered Antibodies

Engineered antibodies and entirely human MoAb will be the MoAbs of the future. Complementarity-determining regions (CDR) of the parent mouse antibody that establish the specificity of an antibody can be fused with a human immunoglobulin backbone.[161] These antibodies have the potential for being less immunogenic, although the mouse CDR portion certainly elicits an antibody response. Human MoAb should not be at all immunogenic except minimally to allotypic differences. The problem with human MoAb is that human cells cannot be stimulated in vivo against human molecules, because the capacity for human B cells to respond to human proteins is limited. A promising new approach to MoAb production is the use of transgenic mice that have been given human immunoglobulin genes.[162] When inoculated with human proteins, the mice recognize them as non-self and respond by synthesizing human antibodies that are not immunogenic when injected into humans. It will be a few years before it is known how practical and effective this approach will actually be.

NONPHARMACOLOGIC METHODS OF IMMUNOSUPPRESSION

Total Lymphoid Irradiation

Total lymphoid irradiation (TLI) is the fractionated delivery of a widely variable amount of radiation (500 to 2000 cGy) to lymphatic tissues using a standard inverted Y-mantle field while shielding marrow-rich areas of long bones and iliac crests. Selective lymphoid irradiation (SLI) consists of the intravenous delivery of lymphoid tissues seeking isotopes in an effort to diminish bone marrow radiation further. Selected lymphoid irradiation is a definite advantage, but the current beta-emitting isotopes, after chelation to hematoporphyrin, do not localize efficiently in the thymus, and this may limit their ability to induce tolerance. Experimentally, TLI induces an initial period of nonspecific immunosuppression followed by gradual loss of broad spectrum immunosuppression and the evolution of a state of specific long-term allograft unresponsiveness, or tolerance.[163–166] A generalized depletion of lymphocytes occurs during and after TLI. In the intermediate post-TLI period there is a migration of lymphoid precursors, presumably from shielded bone marrow sites, and in situ re-emergence of radiation-resistant cells from spleen and lymphoid tissue. In the post-transplant post-TLI setting, additional repopulation of host lymphoid tissue and thymus by migrating donor antigen-presenting cells (APCs) may be a critical tolerogenic step. The attrition and repopulation period is associated with broad spectrum immunosuppression mediated by natural suppressor mechanisms[167] and manifested by an inability to reject either the allograft itself or unrelated third party alloantigenic challenges and by a lack of B cell response to appropriate antigens. Phenotypic analysis of circulating effector cells during repopulation reveals that the very slow re-emergence of CD3+ cells occurs, followed by emergence of weak CD3+ and CD8+ cells and then CD3+ and CD4+ cells.[168] The effects of TLI on intrathymic physiology remain largely unknown. A permissive window of "education" or deletion of potential allograft cytotoxic cells during recreation of the neonatal environment in thymic remnants during TLI may contribute to the tolerance induction mechanism.

Total lymphoid irradiation was used initially in humans as a pretransplant lymphoid depletion method. It is now known that the effects of TLI go beyond crude cell depletion. The most striking success with TLI strategy has been the induction of acquired immune tolerance to cadaveric renal allografts.[169] Three renal allograft recipients who had previously undergone a standard TLI regimen developed specific unresponsiveness to donor cells as assessed by either cell-mediated lympholysis (CML) or mixed lymphocyte culture (MLC). Moreover, these patients could be withdrawn from maintenance immunosuppression. Studies in primate renal transplantation have produced conflicting results on whether synergistic tolerance occurs with the combined use of cyclosporine and TLI.[170] Rat heart allograft survival was markedly prolonged when donor bone marrow cells were administered in conjunction with TLI, suggesting that TLI and sensitization of potential recipients to donor alloantigens are synergistic.[171] The combination of post-transplant TLI and antilymphocytic antibodies markedly prolonged allograft survival in dogs[172] and rats.[168]

Constraints in myocardial ischemia time and the unpredictability of organ availability preclude the use of preoperative TLI in cardiac transplantation and relegate this approach to renal and pancreatic transplantation. However, TLI has been successfully used to treat recurrent or recalcitrant cardiac transplant rejection in humans.[173] The introduction of a rapidly acting, potent lymphoid tissue–seeking radioisotope may make selective lymphoid irradiation (SLI) an effective peritransplant treatment modality.

Apheresis

Continuing improvement in fluid and cell separation technology has fostered creative uses of apheresis in clinical transplantation. On the horizon are two-step blood filtration methods that might allow for elective removal of cellular subsets, targeted antibodies, or regulatory cytokines.

The common clinical setting prompting the use of therapeutic plasma exchange (TPE) (removal of plasma and replacement with 4 per cent albumin salt solution) is the perceived need to remove pathogenic antibodies. The effects of therapeutic plasma exchange are complex, since plasma removal also depletes circulating cytokines and soluble antigens and enhances splenic clearance mechanisms, presumably by decreasing the level of circulating immune complexes. Therapeutic plasma exchange can be effective in reducing levels of pre-existing anti-HLA antibodies that are a barrier to transplantation in sensitized patients[174] and also is being used to attenuate acute humoral rejection, presumably antibody-mediated.[175, 176] Finally, depletion of circulating antimurine antibodies by TPE can possibly provide a treatment window for the reuse of antilymphocyte MoAbs.

Currently, there is no consensus on an absolute indication for therapeutic plasma exchange in cardiac transplantation, but certain clinical situations might prompt its consideration. In patients in urgent need of transplantation who have broadly reactive anti-HLA antibodies of either IgM or IgG isotypes of known, donor HLA-directed specificity, intensive TPE in the peritransplant period might allow successful transplantation. Intense perioperative conventional immunosuppression might abrogate the rapid reappearance of alloantibodies and subsequent rejection.[177] There is anecdotal evidence that vascular rejection can be reversed with TPE.

Immunoadsorption Techniques

An alternative method, the in-line interposition of a biocompatible matrix with irreversibly linked staphylococcal cell wall protein A over which TPE-separated plasma can be pumped, exploits the affinity of protein A for IgG. There is increasing interest in the use of this type of strategy to reduce pretransplant anti-HLA antibodies.[178] However, the future use of these global antibody adsorption techniques in transplantation appears limited in view of the rapid advances made in the production of specific column adsorbents that can be tailored to an individual patient's specific HLA sensitization pattern. For example, the coupling of specific HLA antigens such as HLA A2 to columns might allow the removal of antibodies directed specifically to this common HLA antigen.

Photopheresis

Photopheresis (PHO) is a new treatment modality that exploits ex vivo ultraviolet light (UV) activation of mononuclear cells (MNC) obtained by leukapheresis from a patient after ingestion of 8-methoxypsoralen (8-MOP). The mononuclear cells, presumably containing photomodulated allograft-directed cytotoxic cells, or APCs, are then reinfused. Photopheresis is effective in the treatment of cutaneous T cell lymphoma and is also being evaluated in scleroderma. Although the precise mechanism of PHO remains completely obscure, the originally proposed mechanism of irreversible DNA intercalation by 8-MOP seems too simplistic and is giving way to novel concepts of cell surface modulation. Ultraviolet-A–activated, MNC-bound 8-MOP may alter or compete with cell surface receptors, antigen-presenting structures, and adhesion molecules or other cytokine ligands so that immunoregulatory circuits are distorted and specific suppressor mechanisms are enhanced. However, while there is experimental evidence demonstrating

potent immunosuppressive and tolerogenic effects of UV-B light,[179] scant evidence, mostly clinical, supports the use of UV-A 8-MOP photomodulation of allograft rejection in human organ transplantation.

Photopheresis has been successfully used in the reversal of moderate, non-hemodynamically compromising cardiac transplant rejection[180] and recalcitrant rejection.[181] The use of UV-A or -B light for the induction of allograft tolerance is promising, but the unknown risk of mutagenicity after exposure in humans must be resolved. Probable future advances in photopheresis include (1) replacement of 8-MOP with its synthetic analog amino-methyltrimethylpsoralen (AMT), which has greater water solubility, affinity for DNA, and activity per molecule; (2) re-engineering UV lights since DNA cross-linking occurs most efficiently at 340 nm of UV-A; and (3) selective delivery of photoactivatable drugs to appropriate target cells in extracorporeally routed blood.

Although the fundamental concept of using UV light for tolerance induction holds promise in clinical transplantation, the current relatively cumbersome cell collection technique, ex vivo cell manipulation, and cost may relegate PHO to a passing note of interest as newer methods of delivering UV light to effector immune mechanisms are developed.

FUTURE APPROACHES TO TRANSPLANTATION ACCEPTANCE

Gene Transfer

An initial strategy of gene transfer in organ transplantation will presumably be to attempt to alter or suppress the expression of donor HLA and non-HLA antigens, the targets of the alloimmune response. Although many rodent species have constitutive HLA class I antigen expression on striated muscle cells, there is conflicting evidence whether similar HLA expression occurs or can be induced in human myocardial muscle cells. However, HLA class I antigens are constitutively expressed on vascular endothelium of the heart and other solid organs, and a large body of evidence supports both the constitutive and inducible presence of HLA class II determinants on vascular myocardial endothelium as well.

Perhaps the technology to use gene transfer techniques in this way will be available in the near future. Not only can successful plasmid transfer of gene expression to skeletal muscle be done,[182] but also transfer and stable expression of the reporter genes for beta-galactosidase and firefly luciferase occurred after the direct gene injection into the intravascular space of a rat cardiac isograft.[183] In the latter experiment, gene expression for the most part was limited in time and spatially restricted to the injection site; however, in two experimental animals, the expression of both genes was distributed to sites distant from apical gene injection.

The barriers that gene transplantation must overcome to become a clinically useful technique in cardiac transplantation are formidable. The technique of gene transfer would have to be highly efficient and rapid (occurring between donor explantation and recipient reimplantation), effective in cold ischemic conditions, or done prior to organ explantation. Genetic alteration of an intact donor is likely to raise ethical issues and might not be feasible. Moreover, genetic expression, even if established, would then have to be stable over a long period of time, and the expression of the genes transferred would have to be uniform throughout at least the endothelial surface of the coronary bed. The use of direct intracardiac gene transfer would also have to presume that passenger donor antigen-presenting cells with a rich density of class II HLA determinants have either been neutralized or removed from the graft during the transplant procedure.

To summarize, gene transfer, an exciting concept that may have relatively rapid application in cell transplantation, will require several more years of investigation before it becomes applicable to solid organ transplantation within the foreseeable future.

Tolerance

Tolerance is defined as indefinite host unresponsiveness to an allograft without the need for long-term immunosuppressive therapy. The potential mechanisms that may be able to induce allograft tolerance include (1) deletion from the T cell repertoire of clones reacting specifically against donor antigens, (2) functional inactivation of lymphocytes either by induction of anergy or paralysis of alloreactive T cell clones, and (3) activation of suppressive mechanisms that downregulate the activity of alloreactive T cell clones. Tolerance-inducing strategies currently being investigated in ex-

perimental and clinical transplantation include total lymphoid irradiation (TLI),[163] combined infusion of donor bone marrow cells and antilymphocyte globulin (ALG),[184, 185] establishment of mixed allogeneic chimerism,[156] blood transfusions,[186, 187] and combined administration of donor antigens with monoclonal antibodies against lymphocyte activation antigens or costimulatory molecules such as CD4.[188]

CURRENT USES OF IMMUNOSUPPRESSION

Immunosuppressive drugs are needed for three distinct phases of patient management following transplantation: (1) the immunosuppression induction phase, (2) the immunosuppression maintenance phase, and (3) treatment of acute rejection episodes.

Immunosuppression Induction

The induction phase of immunosuppression extends for approximately 2 weeks after transplantation. A number of issues are unique to this phase of therapy that require special consideration when choosing immunosuppressive drugs and their doses: (1) the immune response is normally strongest when an organ is just transplanted, because of a lack of adequate levels of immunosuppressive drugs and rapid activation of the immune response stimulated by passenger leukocytes emanating from the transplanted organ, (2) bacterial infections of the wound, lungs, and urinary tract are frequent, (3) surgical wounds must be able to heal, and this is especially a problem in diabetic, older, and obese patients, (4) native organs such as the liver and kidneys have marginal function because of cardiac failure, and commonly used immunosuppressive drugs can cause further dysfunction of these organs, and (5) transplanted organs are subjected to prolonged cold ischemia and retrieval trauma that can lead to their marginal function; their function can be further altered by drugs that have organ-specific toxicities.

Unquestionably, the induction phase of immunosuppression requires use of powerful drugs that can block the immune response specifically while allowing normal wound healing and mononuclear phagocyte function. Anti-T cell antibodies and cyclosporine (CSA) are more T cell–specific and phagocyte-sparing than are the antiproliferative drugs, although CSA's use is limited by its nephrotoxicity. Moreover, anti-T cell antibody use, while lymphocyte-specific, can promote viral infections[189] and lymphoproliferative disorders[190] in some settings and also must be used with caution. Most centers use a combination of an antisynthetic drug (CSA, FK506), an antiproliferative drug (AZA, MM), and corticosteroids for induction in doses that minimize their individual toxicities but still, together, can block the immune response. Still others add anti T-cell antibodies to allow for an even further reduction in cyclosporine and corticosteroid doses.

Maintenance

The maintenance phase of immunosuppression requires lower doses of fewer drugs, and patients can often be maintained on duotherapy with CSA + AZA or CSA + prednisone or even monotherapy with CSA alone. Long-term toxicities often dictate the need to reduce or eliminate one or more of the drugs; adaptation by the recipient to the allograft allows for this reduction to occur.

Rejection

Rejection episodes occur early after transplantation and when the adaptive state is lost due to infection or other stress or when the immunosuppressive drugs are reduced or stopped. Only in the latter cases do maintenance immunosuppressive drugs need to be increased. Rejection episodes occurring early generally respond to pulses of therapy alone without adjusting the schedule of maintenance immunosuppression. Pulse therapy with corticosteroids (CS) is usually sufficient. Later-occurring episodes are often reversible with very low doses of CS. Rejections that are resistant to CS are generally treated with anti-T cell antibodies, which usually succeed in reversing the episode. Rarely, mild rejections can be treated with a pulse of cyclosporine or of one of the inhibitors of cell proliferation (AZA, MTX, MM), but usually only when levels of these drugs have not been optimal. High doses of these drugs have unacceptable toxicities.

CONSEQUENCES OF OVERIMMUNOSUPPRESSION/ TOXICITIES OF IMMUNOSUPPRESSIVE DRUGS

Infection

The Registry of the International Society of Heart Transplantation reports that infection is the most common cause of postoperative death following transplantation.[191] A multicenter study of 24 very active transplant centers recently found that infection was the major cause of perioperative and postoperative mortality after cardiac transplantation. In this study of 814 patients, during a mean follow-up of 8.1 months, 409 serious infections occurred, of which 46 per cent were bacterial, 40 percent were viral, 7 per cent were fungal, and 5 per cent were protozoal.[192] Perioperative bacterial infections such as mediastinitis, pneumonia, urinary tract infections, and intravenous catheter-induced sepsis are treated conventionally.[193, 194] Opportunistic infections transmitted by the donor organ and blood products may result from reactivation of latent viruses or may be caused by air-, water-, or feces-borne organisms.[195]

Cytomegalovirus (CMV), a member of the herpesvirus group, is the infection most commonly transmitted by the donor organ. Fifty per cent to 80 per cent of adults have detectable IgG antibodies to CMV. Transmission of CMV from a CMV-seropositive donor to a CMV-seronegative recipient is common. The illness caused by a primary CMV infection is usually more severe than that caused by endogenous reactivation.[196] The infection usually occurs 4 to 12 weeks after transplantation. Localization to the lungs (pneumonia with fever and hypoxia), gastrointestinal tract (ulcerative disease), liver (hepatitis), heart (myocarditis), or eye (chorioretinitis, papillitis) may cause a life-threatening or sight-threatening illness.[197–199] Invasive CMV infection can be successfully treated with ganciclovir, a guanine analog that prevents viral replication by inhibiting virus-induced DNA polymerase.[200, 201]

Reactivation of herpes simplex or zoster, a bothersome but usually not life-threatening problem, may be prevented with oral low-dose acyclovir and treated with oral or intravenous acyclovir.[202]

The incubation period, latency, and pathogenesis of *Toxoplasma gondii* infections are similar to those of CMV.[203] Common manifestations of the primary infection, usually more severe than illness due to reactivation, include encephalitis, myocarditis, and pneumonitis. Infection with *Toxoplasma gondii* is treated and prevented by pyrimethamine and sulfadiazine, or clindamycin in patients allergic to sulfonamides.[204, 205] Prophylaxis is recommended when a seropositive donor organ is transplanted into a seronegative recipient.

Pneumocystis carinii, a protozoal infection, should be suspected in heart transplant recipients who have fever, dyspnea, profound hypoxemia, and radiographic evidence of diffuse pulmonary infiltrates.[206, 207] Early diagnosis of *Pneumocystis carinii* pneumonia (PCP) with methenamine silver stain of bronchial secretions or lavage specimens and aggressive treatment are lifesaving. Because CMV pneumonia often occurs concomitantly with PCP, CMV infection should be suspected in patients with PCP when hypoxemia persists despite institution of the appropriate antimicrobial therapy.[196]

Occasionally pneumonia in transplant recipients is due to *Legionella pneumophila.*[208] The diagnosis is easily overlooked unless a direct fluorescent antibody stain of appropriate sampling is performed. Fever and meningitis in heart transplant recipients may be caused by *Listeria monocytogenes.* Mucocutaneous candidiasis is not uncommon in heart transplant recipients. Solitary or multiple pulmonary nodules in immunosuppressed patients can be due to *Nocardia asteroides,* which can also cause retinitis, meningitis, and epididymitis. Debilitated heart transplant recipients receiving intensified immunosuppression for refractory or recurrent rejection or who have other opportunistic infections while taking multiple antibiotics are at higher risk of contracting aspergillosis. Infection may also occur in immunosuppressed patients exposed to high-density air-borne fungus and particularly to dust generated by construction. A solitary pulmonary lesion is treatable with antifungal drugs or surgical excision. Disseminated aspergillosis is usually fatal. See Chapter 12, p. 253.

After cardiac transplantation, the immunosuppressed recipient is never given live viral vaccines, which include MMR (mumps, measles, rubella) and Sabin oral polio vaccines. Diphtheria, pertussis, tetanus, pneumococcus, *Haemophilus influenzae,* and Salk vaccines do not contain live viruses and can be administered safely. Immunologically normal siblings and other household contacts of immunosuppressed recipients should not receive oral poliovirus immunization because the virus is transmissible. However, these siblings and household contacts can receive measles, mumps, and rubella immunization, because transmission of these viruses does not occur.[209] Also, these siblings and other household contacts should receive Salk polio immunization.[209] Immunization of the recipient with influenza vaccine is controversial.

Hypertension

Most heart transplant recipients develop CSA-induced hypertension. Their highest daily blood pressures will be in the morning because of increased salt retention at night.[210–214] Morning blood pressure values, therefore, should be used to guide antihypertensive therapy. Cyclosporine-induced hypertension is rarely controlled by diuretics alone. Nifedipine and other dihydropyridine calcium channel blockers are effective and appear to be better tolerated in the sustained-release preparation, which is less likely to cause wide fluctuations of blood pressure. Diltiazem and verapamil significantly decrease CSA requirements by increasing plasma levels.[215, 216]

Direct vasodilators (hydralazine) and β-blockers have been used to treat post-transplant hypertension with variable success. β-Blockers should be used with caution because the denervated transplanted heart relies on catecholamines to augment systolic performance, and the negative inotropic effect of these agents may be enhanced in the allografts. Angiotensin-converting enzyme inhibitors may also reduce blood pressure in CSA-treated patients.[217] The use of multiple antihypertensive agents frequently becomes necessary in most transplant recipients for adequate blood pressure control.

Renal Dysfunction

When cyclosporine is administered perioperatively, renal dysfunction may occur as a result of CSA-induced renal vasoconstriction superimposed on the effects of CSA renal hypoperfusion (due to congestive heart failure), third space loss of albumin and fluids (due to the use of extracorporeal circulation), and maldistribution of blood flow (due to anesthetic and inotropic drugs).[216] The incidence of acute CSA nephrotoxicity may be decreased by delaying initiation of CSA until 5 to 7 days after operation while antilymphocyte preparations are routinely administered or by reducing CSA loading doses.[218]

Chronic CSA nephrotoxicity is characterized by irreversible renal interstitial fibrosis.[219] Creatinine clearance will be reduced and serum creatinine elevated by 1 year after transplantation in virtually all CSA-treated patients.[220] Cyclosporine levels, endomyocardial biopsy findings, and the intensity of adverse effects are considerations in selecting a CSA dose that minimizes renal dysfunction but prevents rejection. Cyclosporine nephrotoxicity may not progress after 1 year, if CSA serum levels required to prevent rejection can be reduced. To minimize chronic nephrotoxicity, CSA doses should be adjusted when drugs that raise CSA levels are administered. In addition, fluid loss due to fever, vomiting, or excessive diuresis should be corrected promptly. Decreases in intravascular volume are poorly tolerated by the kidneys of CSA-treated patients and may result in a sharp increase in serum creatinine.

Gastrointestinal Complications

Hepatocellular enzyme abnormalities after transplantation may result from viral hepatitis due to cytomegalovirus (CMV) or hepatitis B or from the effects of drugs such as cyclosporine (CSA) and azathioprine (AZA). Cyclosporine hepatotoxicity is dose-dependent. The activation of AZA, which is converted to 6-mercaptopurine in the liver, is delayed in patients with hepatitis. Corticosteroid therapy may cause or aggravate cholelithiasis. Pancreatitis, which occurs in approximately 10 per cent of heart transplant recipients, may be related to hypoperfusion, inotropic agents, CMV infection, drugs (e.g., corticosteroid, AZA, CSA), or cholelithiasis.[221]

Endocrine and Metabolic Abnormalities

Metabolic abnormalities after transplantation are related primarily to corticosteroids and cyclosporine. Corticosteroid therapy may worsen glucose intolerance or induce diabetes mellitus. In insulin-dependent diabetics, higher insulin doses may be needed, and in diabetics treated with oral agents, insulin may be needed after transplantation.

Corticosteroids accelerate osteoporosis by increasing bone resorption and decreasing its formation. Older patients and postmenopausal women are at highest risk. Dietary calcium and vitamin D supplementation and low-dose estrogen therapy are widely used for prevention, but their efficacy has not been established. Corticosteroid therapy may cause aseptic necrosis of hips, knees, or shoulders. Accurate diagnosis can be made by magnetic resonance imaging. Symptoms of osteonecrosis may improve with dose reduction or discontinuation of CS, but joint replacement is frequently necessary.[222] The growth of most pediatric transplant recipients is retarded by CS.[223]

Sexual or menstrual dysfunction is common early after heart transplantation and often recurs when corticosteroid doses are increased. However, with resolution of the changes of congestive heart failure and with clinical stability, the loss of libido and sexual dysfunction so common in patients with end-stage heart failure usually resolves and fertility returns in most patients. There is no reported evidence of teratogenicity in children of male patients taking immunosuppressants.

An important minority of transplant recipients are young women, and it is important to address the advisability or safety of childbearing by such women. There are few data on childbearing by heart transplant recipients (five reported cases as of 1991); but, based on data from renal allograft recipients on similar immunosuppressive regimens, pregnancy in an allograft recipient is associated with a high incidence of premature births and of babies small for gestational age. However, there are no data suggesting teratogenicity or any long-term adverse sequelae in children of allograft-recipient mothers and no evidence of adverse effects of pregnancy on the health of the mother.[224] Methotrexate and cyclophosphamide may cause congenital anomalies, while CS and AZA are said to be safe in this regard. An increased incidence of spontaneous abortions, fetal anencephaly, and absence of the corpus callosum have been reported with CSA.

Both corticosteroids and cyclosporine cause hypercholesterolemia, the latter by impairing hepatic clearance of low density lipoproteins.[225, 226] Serum cholesterol levels are significantly lower in patients no longer taking CS.[227, 228] Treatment includes dietary restriction of fat and cholesterol, weight loss, and lipid-lowering agents. Lovastatin and other HMG CoA (3-hydroxy-3-methylglutaryl coenzyme A) reductase inhibitors are associated with an increased risk of rhabdomyolysis and renal injury when used by CSA-treated heart transplant recipients.[229] Concomitant gemfibrozil administration increases the likelihood of this adverse reaction.

Neurologic Complications

Seizures may occur after solid organ transplantation.[230] The multifactorial etiology of these seizures includes embolic, metabolic, and electrolyte disturbances, wide fluctuations in blood pressure, and arrhythmias. Cyclosporine and OKT3 may increase the likelihood of seizures. Additionally, encephalopathy has been reported in renal allograft recipients given OKT3 for induction, especially if there is delayed graft function.[231]

Malignancy

Transplant recipients have up to a 6 per cent risk of developing cancer, an age-controlled frequency 100 times greater than that of the general population.[232] Because skin cancer is the most common post-transplant malignancy,[233] dermatologic evaluation and protection from solar injury should be practiced routinely. In lymphoproliferative disorders there is a spectrum of abnormal B lymphocyte proliferation. The incidence of such disorders has been as high as 5 per cent in recipients of thoracic organs;[232] risk is correlated with the degree of total immunosuppression[234] and is believed to result from inadequate T cell control over Epstein-Barr virus–driven B cell proliferation.[235] Reactive lymphoid tissue or highly malignant tumors such as large cell non-Hodgkin's lymphomas may be detected histologically.[236] Both polyclonal and monoclonal proliferation have been identified by cell-surface immunoglobulin phenotype and immunoglobulin rearrangement.[237–243] Some of the lymphoproliferative disorders may have a fulminant clinical course with widespread tumor dissemination, organ failure, and sepsis.[232] For initial treatment of lymphoproliferative disorders, immunosuppression has been reduced with good results.[244] See Chapter 13, p. 269.

In summary, complications following heart transplantation affect several organ systems and vary in type and frequency over time. Because most are due to the effects of immuno-suppression, the successful outcome of heart transplantation requires a delicate balance between adequate immunosuppression and control of drug-related adverse effects.

CONCLUSIONS

There are many approaches to immunosuppression for organ transplantation. These include the use of pharmacologic agents, use of antibodies to lymphocytes, use of other biologic agents such as fusion molecules, and use of nonpharmacologic agents such as total lymphoid irradiation, apheresis, and photopheresis. It is important to consider the possibility that new drugs not only might prevent rejection but also might alter the appearance of rejection when it occurs. The future of immunosuppression might change significantly if genetic engineering or other techniques will allow for the induction of tolerance.

REFERENCES

1. Hall B, Dorsch S. The cellular basis of allograft rejection in vivo. I. The cellular requirements for first set rejection of heart grafts. J Exp Med 148:878, 1978.
2. MacPherson G, Christmas SE. The role of the macrophage in cardiac allograft rejection in the rat. Immunol Rev 77:143, 1984.
3. Thomas J, Thomas F, Kaplan AM, Lee HM. Antibody-dependent cellular cytotoxicity and chronic renal allograft rejection. Transplantation 22:94, 1976.
4. Hara T, Jung LK, Bjorndahl JM, Fu SM. Human T cell activation. III. Rapid induction of a phosphorylated 28 kD/32 kD disulfide-linked early activation antigen (EA 1) by 12-0-tetradecanoyl phorbol-13-acetate, mitogens, and antigens. J Exp Med 164(6): 1988, 1986.
5. Croll AD, Siggins KW, Morris AG, Pither JM. The induction of IFN-gamma production and m-RNAs of interleukin 2 and IFN-gamma by phorbol esters and a calcium ionophore. Biochem Biophys Res Commun 146(3):927, 1987.
6. Schlitt HJ, Kurrle R, Wonigeit K. T cell activation by monoclonal antibodies directed to different epitopes on the human T cell receptor/CD3 complex: Evidence for two different modes of activation. Eur J Immunol 19(9):1649, 1989.
7. Landegren U, Andersson J, Wigzell H. Mechanism of T lymphocyte activation by OKT3 antibodies: A general model for T cell induction. Eur J Immunol 14:325, 1984.
8. Chatila T, Silverman L, Miller R, Geha R. Mechanisms of T cell activation by the calcium ionophore ionomycin. J Immunol 143(4):1283, 1989.
9. Goronzy J, Weyand C, Imboden J, Manger B, Fathman CG. Heterogeneity of signal requirements in T cell activation within a panel of human proliferative T cell clones. J Immunol 138(1):3087, 1987.
10. Weiss A, Imboden JB. Cell surface molecules and

early events involved in human T lymphocyte activation. Adv Immunol 41:1, 1987.

11. Dobbs JF, Katz DR. Human T-cell activation: Comparative studies on the role of different phorbol esters. Immunology 63:133, 1988.

12. Opelz G. Influence of HLA matching on survival of second kidney transplants in cyclosporine-treated recipients. Transplantation 47:823, 1989.

13. Norman DJ, Kahana L, Stuart FP, et al. A randomized clinical trial of induction therapy with OKT3 in kidney transplantation. Transplantation 55(1):44, 1993.

14. Norman DJ, Barry JM, Boehne C, Wetzsteon P. Natural history of patients who make cytotoxic antibodies following prospective fresh blood transfusions. Transplant Proc 17:1041, 1985.

15. Jeannet M, Pinn VM, Flax MH, Winn HJ, Russell PS. Humoral antibodies in renal allotransplantation in man. N Engl J Med 282:111, 1980.

16. Colvin RB. The pathogenesis of vascular rejection. Transplant Proc 23(4):2052, 1991.

17. Salmela K, von Willebrand E, Kyllonen L, et al. Acute vascular rejection in renal transplantation. Transplant Proc 23(1):360, 1992.

18. Miltenburg AM, Jeijer-Paape ME, Weening JJ, Daha MR, van Es LA, van der Woude FJ. Induction of antibody-dependent cellular cytotoxicity against endothelial cells by renal transplantation. Transplantation 48(4):681, 1989.

19. Noreen HJ. Crossmatch Tests. *In* ASHI (ed). *ASHI Laboratory Manual,* 2nd ed. Lenexa, KS, 1990, p 307.

20. Fuller TC, Phelan D, Gebel HM, Rodey GE. Antigenic specificity of antibody reactivity in the antiglobulin-augmented lymphocytotoxicity test. Transplantation 34:24, 1982.

21. Sancho J, Silverman LB, Castigli E, et al. Developmental regulation of transmembrane signaling via the T cell antigen receptor/CD3 complex in human T lymphocytes. J Immunol 148(5):1315, 1992.

22. Brattsand G, Cantrell DA, Ward S, Ivars F, Gullberg M. Signal transduction through the T cell receptor-CD3 complex. Evidence for heterogeneity in receptor coupling. J Immunol 144(10):3651, 1990.

23. Diamond MS, Staunton DE, de Fougerolles AR, et al. ICAM-1 (CD54): A counter-receptor for Mac-1 (CD11b/CD18). J Cell Biol 111:3129, 1990.

24. Wang P, Vanky F, Li SL, Patarroyo M, Klein E. Functional characteristics of the intercellular adhesion molecule-1 (CD54) expressed on cytotoxic human blood lymphocytes. Cell Immunol 131(2):366, 1990.

25. Van Seventer GA, Shimizu Y, Horgan KJ, Shaw S. The LFA-1 ligand ICAM-1 provides an important costimulatory signal for T cell receptor-mediated activation of resting T cells. J Immunol 144(12):4579, 1990.

26. Suthanthiran M. T-cell differentiation antigen cluster 2 (CD2) is a receptor for accessory cells and can generate and/or transduce accessory signals. Cell Immunol 112(1):112, 1988.

27. Hahn WC, Rosenstein Y, Burakoff SJ, Bierer BE. Interaction of CD2 with its ligand lymphocyte function-associated antigen-3 induces adenosine 3′,5′-cyclic monophosphate production in T lymphocytes. J Immunol 147(1):14, 1991.

28. de Vries JE, Yssel H, Spits H. Interplay between the TCR/CD3 complex and CD4 or CD8 in the activation of cytotoxic T lymphocytes. Immunol Rev 109:119, 1989.

29. Wacholtz MC, Patel SS, Lipsky PE. Patterns of costimulation of T cell clones by cross-linking CD3, CD4/ CD8, and class I MHC molecules. J Immunol 142(12):4201, 1989.

30. Vandenberghe P, Freeman GJ, Nadler LM, et al. Antibody and B7/BB1-mediated ligation of the CD28 receptor induces tyrosine phosphorylation in human T cells. J Exp Med 175(4):951, 1992.

31. Koulova L, Clark EA, Shu G, Dupont B. The CD28 ligand B7/BB1 provides costimulatory signal for alloactivation of CD4+ T cells. J Exp Med 173:759, 1991.

32. Dinarello CA. Interleukin 1. Rev Infect Dis 6:51, 1984.

33. Vink A, Uyttenhove C, Wauters P, Van Snick J. Accessory factors involved in murine T cell activation. Distinct roles of interleukin 6, interleukin 1 and tumor necrosis factor. Eur J Immunol 20(1):1, 1990.

34. Gillis S, Mochizuki DY, Conlon DJ, et al. Molecular characterization of interleukin 2. Immunol Rev 63:167, 1982.

35. Lai KN, Leung JC, Lai FM. Soluble interleukin 2 receptor release, interleukin 2 production, and interleukin 2 receptor expression in activated T-lymphocytes in vitro. Pathology 23(3):224, 1991.

36. Miyawaki T, Yackie A, Uwadana N, Ohzeki S, Nagaoki T, Taniguchi N. Functional significance of Tac antigen expressed on activated human T lymphocytes: Tac antigen interacts with T-cell growth factor in cellular proliferation. J Immunol 129:2474, 1982.

37. Gonzalez-Gernandez A, Diaz-Espada F, Kreisler M, Gambon Deza F. Proliferative responses induced by the activation of protein kinase C during the development of human T lymphocytes. Eur J Immunol 21(1):115, 1991.

38. Xia X, Lee HK, Clark SC, Choi YS. Recombinant interleukin (IL) 2-induced human B cell differentiation is mediated by autocrine IL6. Eur J Immunol 19(12):2275, 1989.

39. Lipsky PE, Hirohata S, Jelinek DF, McAnally L, Splawski JB. Regulation of human B lymphocyte responsiveness. Scand J Rheumatol 76:229, 1993.

40. McHeyzer-Williams MG. Combinations of interleukins 2, 4 and 5 regulate the secretion of murine immunoglobulin isotypes. Eur J Immunol 19(11):2025, 1989.

41. Cardell S, Sander B. Interleukin 2, 4, and 5 are sequentially produced in mitogen-stimulated murine spleen cell cultures. Eur J Immunol 20(2):389, 1990.

42. Hall B, Dorsch S. Cells mediating allograft rejection. Immunol Rev 77:31, 1984.

43. Hall B, Bishop G, Farnsworth A, et al. Identification of the cellular subpopulations infiltrating rejecting cadaver renal allografts: Preponderance of the T4 subset of T cells. Transplantation 37:564, 1984.

44. Andersson J, Nagy S, Groth CG, Andersson U. Effects of FK506 and cyclosporine A on cytokine production studied in vitro at a single-cell level. Immunology 75(1):136, 1992.

45. Kahan BD, Gibbons S, Tejpal N, Stepkowski SM, Chou TC. Synergistic interactions of cyclosporine and rapamycin to inhibit immune performances of normal human peripheral blood lymphocytes in vitro. Transplantation 51(1):232, 1991.

46. Metcalfe SM, Richards FM. Cyclosporine, FK506, and rapamycin. Some effects on early activation events in serum-free, mitogen-stimulated mouse spleen cells. Transplantation 49(4):798, 1990.

47. Kimball PM, Kerman RH, Kahan BD. Production of synergistic but nonidentical mechanisms of immunosuppression by rapamycin and cyclosporine. Transplantation 51(2):486, 1991.

48. Sigal NH, Dumont FJ. Cyclosporin A, FK-506, and rapamycin: Pharmacologic probes of lymphocyte signal transduction. Annu Rev Immunol 10:519, 1992.

49. Henderson DJ, Naya I, Bundick RV. Comparison of the effects of FK-506, cyclosporine-A and rapamycin on IL-2 production. Immunology 73:316, 1991.

50. Bierer BE, Mattilla PS, Standaert RF, et al. Two distinct signal transmission pathways in T lymphocytes are inhibited by complexes formed between an immunophilin and either FK506 or rapamycin. Proc Natl Acad Sci USA 87(23):9231, 1990.

51. Metcalfe S, Milner J. Evidence that FK506 and rapamycin block T cell activation at different sites relative to early reversible phosphorylation involving the protein phosphatases PP1 and PP2A. Transplantation 51(6):1318, 1991.

52. Dumont FJ, Staruch MJ, Koprak SL, Melino MR, Sigal NH. Distinct mechanisms of suppression of murine T cell activation by the related macrolides FK-506 and rapamycin. J Immunol 144(1):251, 1990.

53. Flanagan WM, Corthesy B, Braun RJ. Nuclear association of a T cell transcription factor blocked by FK-506 and cyclosporine A. Nature 352:803, 1991.

54. Harding MW, Galat A, Uehling DE, Schreiber SL. A receptor for the immunosuppressant FK506 is a cis-trans peptidyl-prolylisomerase. Nature 341(6244): 758, 1989.

55. Schreiber SL. Chemistry and biology of the immunophilins and their immunosuppressive ligands. Science 251:283, 1991.

56. Kuo CJ, Chung J, Fiorentino DF, Flanagan WM, Blenis J, Crabtree GR. Rapamycin selectively inhibits interleukin-2 activation of p70 S6 kinase. Nature 358(6381):70, 1992.

57. Kay JE, Kromwel L, Doe SE, Denyer M. Inhibition of T and B lymphocyte proliferation by rapamycin. Immunology 72(4):544, 1991.

58. Dumont FJ, Melino MR, Staruch MJ, Koprak SL, Fischer PA, Sigal NH. The immunosuppressive macrolides FK-506 and rapamycin act as reciprocal antagonists in murine T cells. J Immunol 144(4):1418, 1990.

59. Calne RY, Alexandre GP, Murray JE. A study of the effects of drugs in prolonging survival of homologous renal transplants in dogs. Ann NY Acad Sci 99:743, 1962.

60. McCormack JJ, Johns DG. Purine antimetabolites. In Chabner B (ed). Pharmacologic Principles of Cancer Treatment. Philadelphia, WB Saunders, 1982, p 213.

61. Jensen MK. Chromosome studies in patients treated with azathioprine and amethopterin. Acta Med Scand 182:445, 1967.

62. Old CW, Flannery EP, Grogan TM, Stone WH, San Antonio RP. Azathioprine-induced pure red cell aplasia. JAMA 240:552, 1978.

63. Bennett WM, Norman DJ. Maintenance immunosuppression: Azathioprine and glucocorticoids. In Milford J (ed). Renal Transplantation. New York, Churchill Livingstone, 1989, p 97.

64. Sweene MJ, Hoffman DH, Esterman MA. Metabolism and biochemistry of mycophenolic acid. Cancer Res 32:1803, 1972.

65. Mustelin T. GTP dependence on the transduction of mitogenic signals through the T3 complex in T lymphocyte indicates the involvement of a G-protein. FEBS Lett 213:199, 1987.

66. Wilson BS, Deanin GG, Standefer JC, Vanderjagt D, Oliver JM. Depletion of guanine nucleotides with mycophenolic acid suppresses IgE-receptor-mediated degranulation in rat basophilic leukemia cells. J Immunol 143:259, 1989.

67. Kiguchi K, Collart FR, Henning-Chubb C, Huberman E. Cell differentiation and altered IMP dehydrogenase expression induced in human T-lymphoblastoid leukemia cells by mycophenolic acid and tiazofurin. Exp Cell Res 187(1):47, 1990.

68. Bou-Gharios G, Moss J, Abraham D, Partridge T, Olsen I. Ultrastructural studies of a lysosomal enzyme during lymphocyte activation. Br J Exp Pathol 69:661, 1988.

69. Aggarwal R, Batten S, Cockerell R, Tanner AR. Monocyte lysosomal enzyme release in response to naturally occurring circulating immune complexes. Scand J Immunol 19:159, 1984.

70. Sollinger HW, Deierhoi MH, Belzer FO, Diethelm AG, Kauffman RS. RS-61443—A phase I clinical trial and pilot rescue study. Transplantation 53:428, 1992.

71. Platz KP, Eckhoff DE, Hullett DA, Sollinger HW. Prolongation of dog renal allograft survival by RS-61443, a new potent immunosuppressive agent. Transplant Proc 23:497, 1991.

72. Hayashi R, Suzuki S, Shimatani K, et al. Synergistic effect of cyclosporine and mizoribine on graft survival in canine organ transplantation. Transplant Proc 22:1676, 1990.

73. Turka LA, Dayton J, Sinclair G, Thompson CB, Mitchell BS. Guanine ribonucleotide depletion inhibits T cell activation. Mechanism of action of the immunosuppressive drug mizoribine. J Clin Invest 87:940, 1991.

74. Hasunuma T, Yamanaka H, Terai C, et al. Selective inhibition of cytotoxic T lymphocyte proliferation by mizoribine (bredinin), an adenosine analog. Adv Exp Med Biol 253A:455, 1989.

75. Okubo M, Chen XM, Kamata K, Masaki Y, Uchiyama T. Suppressive effect of mizoribine on humoral antibody production in DBA/2 mice. Transplantation 41:495, 1986.

76. Gruber SA, Erdmann GR, Burke BA, et al. Mizoribine pharmacokinetics and pharmacodynamics in a canine renal allograft model of local immunosuppression. Transplantation 53:12, 1992.

77. Okubo M, Masaki Y, Kamata K, Sato N, Inoue K, Umetani N. Immunosuppressive mode of action of deoxyspergualin in mice, as compared with cyclosporine A and mizoribine. Transplant Proc 21(1):1085, 1989.

78. Okubo M, Kaneko Y, Mizukoshi M, et al. Decreased interleukin 2 production and increased LEU 2a-positive suppressor cells in renal transplant patients on triple therapy with mizoribine, cyclosporine A, and prednisone. Transplant Proc 19(1):1940, 1987.

79. Amemiya H, Suzuki S, Watanabe H, Hayashi R, Niiya S. Synergistically enhanced immunosuppressive effect by combined use of cyclosporine and mizoribine. Transplant Proc 21(1):956, 1989.

80. Gregory CR, Gourley IM, Cain GR, Patz JD, Imondi KA, Martin JA. Mizoribine serum levels associated with enterotoxicity in the dog. Transplantation 51:877, 1991.

81. Hayashi R, Kenmochi T, Fukuoka T, Suzuki S, Amemiya H. Synergistic effect of cyclosporine and mizoribine on canine pancreas allograft survival. Transplant Proc 23:1585, 1991.

82. Uchida H, Yokota K, Akiyama N, et al. Effectiveness of a new drug, Bredinin, on canine kidney allotransplant survival. Transplant Proc 11:865, 1979.

83. Mita K, Akiyama N, Nagao T, et al. Advantages of

mizoribine over azathioprine in combination therapy with cyclosporine for renal transplantation. Transplant Proc 22:1679, 1990.

84. Chen SF, Papp LM, Ardecky RJ, et al. Structure-activity relationship of quinoline carboxylic acids. A new class of inhibitors of dihydroorotate dehydrogenase. Biochem Pharmacol 40:709, 1990.

85. Peters GJ, Laurensse E, DeKant E, Nadal JC, Pinedo HM. The relationship between dihydroorotic acid dehydrogenase and in vitro and in vivo cytostatic effects of brequinar sodium (DUP-785; NSC 368390). Adv Exp Med Biol 253B:375, 1989.

86. DeKant E, Pinedo HM, Laurensse E, Peters GJ. The relation between inhibition of cell growth and of dihydroorotic acid dehydrogenase by brequinar sodium. Cancer Lett 46:123, 1989.

87. Schwartsmann G, van der Vijgh WJ, Van Hennik MB, et al. Pharmacokinetics of brequinar sodium (NSC 368390) in patients with solid tumors during a phase I study. Eur J Cancer Clin Oncol 25(12):1675, 1989.

88. Murphy MP, Morris RE. Brequinar sodium (DUP 785) selectively, effectively and potently suppresses allograft rejection in a heterotopic mouse heart transplant model. Transplant Proc (in press).

89. Cramer DV, Chapman FA, Jaffee BD, et al. The effect of a new immunosuppressive drug, brequinar sodium, on heart, liver, and kidney allograft rejection in the rat. Transplantation 53:303, 1992.

90. Morris RE. In vivo immunopharmacology of the macrolides FK506 and rapamycin: Toward the era of rational immunosuppressive drug discovery development, and use. Transplant Proc 23:2722, 1991.

91. Morris RE, Hoyt EG, Murphy MP, Eugui EM, Allison AC. Mycophenolic acid morpholinoethyl ester (RS-61443) is a new immunosuppressant that prevents and halts heart allograft rejection by selective inhibition of T- and B-cell purine synthesis. Transplant Proc 22:1659, 1990.

92. Morris RE, Wang J, Blum JR, et al. Immunosuppressive effects of the morpholinoethyl ester of mycophenolic acid (RS-61443) in rat and nonhuman primate recipients of heart allografts. Transplant Proc 23:19, 1991.

93. Healey LA. The current status of methotrexate use in rheumatic disease. Bull Rheum Dis 36(4):1, 1986.

94. Black RL, O'Brien WM, Wan Scott EJ, Auerbach R, Eisen AZ, Bunim JJ. Methotrexate therapy in psoriatic arthritis: Double blind study on 21 patients. JAMA 89:743, 1964.

95. Weinstein GD. Methotrexate. Ann Intern Med 86:199, 1977.

96. Gubner R, August S, Ginsber V. Therapeutic suppression of tissue reactivity: II. Effects of aminopterin in rheumatoid arthritis and psoriasis. Am J Med 22:176, 1951.

97. Storb R, Deeg J, Whitehead J, et al. Methotrexate and cyclosporine compared with cyclosporine alone for prophylaxis of acute graft versus host disease after marrow transplantation for leukemia. N Engl J Med 314:729, 1986.

98. Costanzo-Nordin MR, Grusk BB, Silver MA, et al. Reversal of recalcitrant cardiac allograft rejection with methotrexate. Circulation 78:III47, 1988.

99. Olsen SL, O'Connell JB, Bristow MR, Renlund DG. Methotrexate as an adjunct in the treatment of persistent mild cardiac allograft rejection. Transplantation 50:773, 1990.

100. Hosenpud JD, Hershberger RE, Ratkovec RM, et al. Methotrexate for the treatment of patients with multiple episodes of acute cardiac allograft rejection. J Heart Lung Transplant 11(4):739, 1992.

101. Bourge RC, Kirklin JK, White-Williams C, et al. Methotrexate pulse therapy in the treatment of recurrent acute heart rejection. J Heart Lung Transplant 11:1116, 1992.

102. Iwasawa H, Icondo S, Ikeda S. Synthesis of (−) deoxyspergualin and (−) spergualin-15phosphate. J Antibiot (Tokyo) 12:1665, 1982.

103. Dickneite G, Schorlemmer HU, Walter P. The influence of C(−) 15-deoxyspergualine on experimental transplantation and its immunopharmacological mode of action. Behring Inst Mitt 8:93, 1986.

104. Falk W, Ulrichs K, Muller-Ruchholtz W. 15-Deoxyspergualin (a new guanidine-like drug) blocks T lymphocyte proliferation. Transplant Proc 19:4239, 1987.

105. Dickneite G, Schorlemmer HU, Sedlacek HH, Falk W, Ulrichs K, Muller-Ruchholtz W. Suppression of macrophage function and prolongation of graft survival by the new guanidinic-like structure, 15-deoxyspergualin. Transplant Proc 19:1301, 1987.

106. Dickneite G, Walter P, Schorlemmer HU, Sedlacek HH. The influence of 15-DS on experimental skin and islet cell transplantation. In Ishigama J (ed). Recent Advances in Chemotherapy. Tokyo, University of Tokyo Press, 1985.

107. Nakata S, Ito T, Shirakura R, et al. Immunosuppressive mechanisms of 15-deoxyspergualin on heterotopic heart transplantation in rats. Transplant Proc 23:864, 1991.

108. Tepper MA, Petty B, Bursuker I, et al. Inhibition of antibody production by the immunosuppressive agent, 15-deoxyspergualin. Transplant Proc 23:328, 1991.

109. Schacter B, Petty B, Tepper MA, Spitalny G. 15-Deoxyspergualin inhibition of the humoral immune response. Presented at 13th International Transplant Congress, San Francisco, 1990.

110. Engemann R, Gassel HJ, Lafrenz E, Stoffregen C, Thiede A. Transplantation tolerance after short-term administration of 15-deoxyspergualin in orthotopic rat liver transplantation. Transplant Proc 19:4241, 1987.

111. Walter P, Dickneite G, Feifel G, Thies J. Deoxyspergualin induces tolerance in allogeneic kidney transplantation. Transplant Proc 19:3980, 1987.

112. Katayama Y, Takao M, Onodo K, et al. Immunosuppressive effects of FK506 and 15-deoxyspergualin in rat lung transplantation. Transplant Proc 23:349, 1991.

113. Schubert G, Stoffregen C, Loske G, Timmermann W, Schang T, Thiede A. Synergistic effect of 15-deoxyspergualin and cyclosporin A in pancreatic transplantation. Transplant Proc 21:1096, 1989.

114. Koyama I, Kadokura M, Hoshino T, Omoto R. Effective use of 15-deoxyspergualin in kidney transplantation. Transplant Proc 21:1088, 1989.

115. Suzuki S, Kanashiro M, Amemiya H. Immunosuppressive effect of a new drug, 15-deoxyspergualin, in heterotopic rat heart transplantation: In vivo energy metabolic studies by 31P-NMR spectroscopy. Transplant Proc 19:3982, 1987.

116. Li D, Kiang H, Takano Y. The effect of FK506 on heart allograft survival in highly sensitized rats in comparison with CYA and DSG. Presented at 13th International Transplant Congress, San Francisco, 1990.

117. Pruitt SK, Halperin EC, Bollinger RR. The effect of

15-deoxyspergualin on hamster-to-rat cardiac xenograft survival. Transplant Proc 23:585, 1991.

118. Amemiya H, Dohi K, Otsubo O. Markedly enhanced therapeutic effect of deoxyspergualin on acute rejection when combined with methylprednisolone in kidney recipients. Transplant Proc 23:1087, 1991.

119. Takahashi K, Tanabe K, Ooba S, et al. Prophylactic use of a new immunosuppressive agent, deoxyspergualin, in patients with kidney transplantation from ABO-incompatible or preformed antibody-positive donors. Transplant Proc 23:1078, 1991.

120. Koyama I, Amemiya H, Taguchi Y, et al. Prophylactic use of deoxyspergualin in a quadruple immunosuppressive protocol in renal transplantation. Transplant Proc 23:1096, 1991.

121. Kull FCJR. Reduction in tumor necrosis factor receptor affinity and cytotoxicity by glucocorticoids. Biochem Biophys Res Commun 153(1):402, 1988.

122. Rugstad HE. Antiinflammatory and immunoregulatory effects of glucocorticoids: Mode of action. Scand J Rheumatol 76:257, 1988.

123. Wielckens K, Delfs T, Muth A, Freese V, Kleeberg HJ. Glucocorticoid-induced lymphoma cell death: The good and the evil. J Steroid Biochem 27(1–3):413, 1987.

124. Waage A, Slupphaug G, Shalaby R. Glucocorticoids inhibit the production of IL6 from monocytes, endothelial cells and fibroblasts. Eur J Immunol 20(11):2439, 1990.

125. Kawahara RS, Deng ZW, Deuel TF. Glucocorticoids inhibit the transcriptional induction of JE, a platelet-derived growth factor-inducible gene. J Biol Chem 266(20):13261, 1991.

126. Compton MM, Caron LA, Cidlowski JA. Glucocorticoid action on the immune system. J Steroid Biochem 27(1–3):201, 1987.

127. Fitzke E, Dieter P. Glucocorticoids inhibit formation of inositol phosphates in macrophages. Biochem Biophys Res Commun 178(3):974, 1991.

128. Lemercier C, Julen N, Coulpier M, et al. Differential modulation by glucocorticoids of alternative complement protein secretion in cells of the monocyte/macrophage lineage. Eur J Immunol 22(4):909, 1992.

129. Norman DJ. Anti-lymphocyte antibodies in the treatment of allograft rejection: Targets, mechanisms of action, monitoring, and efficacy. Semin Nephrol 12(4):315, 1992.

130. Condie RM, Waskosky KE, Hall BL, et al. Efficacy of Minnesota antilymphoblast globulin in renal transplantation: A multicenter, placebo-controlled, prospective, randomized double-blind study. Transplant Proc 17(1):1304, 1985.

131. Kohler G, Milstein C. Continuous cultures of fused cells secreting antibody of predefined specificity. Nature 256:495, 1975.

132. Kreis H, Mansouri R, Descamps JM, et al. Antithymocyte globulin in cadaver kidney transplantation: A randomized trial based on T cell monitoring. Kidney Int 19:438, 1981.

133. Shield CF III, Cosimi AB, Tolkoff-Rubin N, Herrin J, Russell PS. Use of antithymocyte globulin for reversal of acute allograft rejection. Transplantation 28:461, 1979.

134. Fassbinder W, Bechstein PB, Stutte HJ, et al. Treatment of steroid-resistant rejections with ATG and/or plasma filtration improves graft survival rates after cadaveric kidney transplantation. Neth J Med 28:265, 1985.

135. Cerilli G, Brasile L, Clarke J, Haisch C, Cerilli J. Correlation of cell reaction patterns and in vitro immunosuppressive capabilities of six ATG products used clinically. Transplant Proc 17(6):2767, 1985.

136. Kirkman RL, Shapiro ME, Carpenter CB, et al. Early experience with anti-Tac in clinical renal transplantation. Transplant Proc 21(1):1766, 1989.

137. Friend PJ, Calne RY, Hale G, et al. Prophylactic use of an antilymphocyte monoclonal antibody following renal transplantation: A randomized controlled trial. Transplant Proc 19(1):1898, 1987.

138. Soulillou JP, Cantarovich D, Le Mauff B, et al. Randomized controlled trial of a monoclonal antibody against the interleukin-2 receptor (33B3.1) as compared with rabbit antithymocyte globulin for prophylaxis against rejection of renal allografts. N Engl J Med 322(17):1175, 1990.

139. Kirkman RL, Araujo JL, Burch CJ, et al. Treatment of acute renal allograft rejection with monoclonal anti-T12 antibody. Transplantation 36:620, 1983.

140. Raftery MJ, Lang CJ, Ivory K, et al. Use of RFT2 (CD7) monoclonal antibody as prophylaxis against renal allograft rejection. Transplant Proc 17:2737, 1985.

141. Ortho Multicenter Transplant Study Group. A randomized clinical trial of OKT3 monoclonal antibody for acute rejection of cadaveric renal transplants. N Engl J Med 313(6):337, 1985.

142. Waid TH, Lucas BA, Thompson JS, et al. Treatment of acute rejection with anti-T-cell antigen receptor complex αβ (T10 B9.1A-31) or anti-CD3 (OKT3) monoclonal antibody: Results of a prospective randomized double-blind trial. Transplant Proc 23:1062, 1991.

143. Frenken LAM, Hoitsma AJ, Tax WJM, Koene RAP. Prophylactic use of anti-CD3 monoclonal antibody WT32 in kidney transplantation. Transplant Proc 23:1072, 1991.

144. Land W, Hillebrand G, Illner WD, et al. First clinical experience with a new TCR/CD3-monoclonal antibody (BMA031) in kidney transplant patients. Transpl Int 1(2):116, 1988.

145. Waldmann H. Monoclonal antibodies for organ transplantation: Prospects for the future. Am J Kidney Dis 11:154, 1988.

146. Cosimi AB, Conti D, Delmonico FL, et al. In vivo effects of monoclonal antibody to ICAM-1 (CD54) in nonhuman primates with renal allografts. J Immunol 144(12):4604, 1990.

147. Talento A, Nguyen M, Blake T, et al. A single administration of LFA-1 antibody confers prolonged allograft survival. Transplantation 55:418, 1993.

148. Nakakura EK, McCabe SM, Zheng B, et al. Potent and effective prolongation by anti-LFA-1 monoclonal antibody monotherapy of non-primarily vascularized heart allograft survival in mice without T cell depletion. Transplantation 55:412, 1993.

149. Cosimi AB, Delmonico FL, Wright JK, et al. Prolonged survival of non human primate renal allograft recipients treated only with anti-CD4 monoclonal antibody. Surgery 108(2):406, 1990.

150. Wee SL, Stroka DM, Preffer FI, Jolliffe LK, Colvin RB, Cosimi AB. Primate renal allograft recipients. Transplantation 53(3):501, 1992.

151. Norman DJ, Bennett WM, Cobanoglu A, et al. The use of OKT4A (murine monoclonal anti-CD4 antibody) in human organ transplantation: The initial clinical experience. Transplant Proc 25:802, 1993.

152. Norman DJ. The clinical role of OKT3. Cardiol Clin 8(1):97, 1990.

153. Chang TW, Kung PC, Gingras SP, Goldstein G. Does OKT3 monoclonal antibody react with an antigen-recognition structure on human T cells? Proc Natl Acad Sci USA 78:1805, 1981.

154. Norman DJ, Shield CF III, Barry JM, Henell KR, Funnell MB, Lemon J. Therapeutic use of OKT3 monoclonal antibody for acute renal allograft rejection. Nephron 46(Suppl 1):41, 1987.

155. Chatenoud L, Jonker M, Goldstein G, Bach J-F, Villemain F. The human immune response against the OKT3 monoclonal antibody is oligoclonal. Science 232:1406, 1986.

156. Norman DJ, Shield CF III, Henell KR, Kimball JA, Barry JM, Bennett WM. Effectiveness of a second course of OKT3 monoclonal anti-T cell antibody for treatment of renal allograft rejection. Transplantation 46(4):525, 1988.

157. Shield CF III, Norman DJ, Marlett P, Fuccello AJ. Comparison of anti-mouse and anti-horse antibody production during the treatment of allograft rejection with OKT3 or ATG. Nephron 46(Suppl):48, 1987.

158. LeMaistre CF, Rosen S, Frankel A, et al. Phase I trial of H65-RTA immunoconjugate in patients with cutaneous T-cell lymphoma. Blood 78(5):1173, 1991.

159. Murphy JR, Kelley VE, Strom TB. Interleukin 2 toxin: A step toward selective immunomodulation. Am J Kidney Dis 11(2):159, 1988.

160. Bacha P, Williams DP, Waters C, Williams JM, Murphy JR, Strom TB. Interleukin 2 receptor-targeted cytotoxicity. Interleukin 2 receptor-mediated action of a diphtheria toxin-related interleukin 2 fusion protein. J Exp Med 167(2):612, 1988.

161. Woodle ES, Thistlethwaite JR Jr, Jolliffe LK, et al. Humanized OKT3 antibodies: Successful transfer of immune modulating properties and idiotype expression. J Immunol 148(9):2756, 1992.

162. MacQuitty JJ, Kay RM. GenPharm's knockout mice. Science 257(5074):1188, 1992.

163. Strober S. Natural suppressor (NS) cells, neonatal tolerance and total lymphoid irradiation: exploring obscure relationships. Annu Rev Immunol 2:219, 1984.

164. Modry DL, Strober S, Hoppe RT. Total lymphoid irradiation: Experimental models and clinical application in organ transplantation. Heart Transplant 2:122, 1983.

165. Hoppe RT, Strober S, Kaplan HS. Total lymphoid irradiation in the management of autoimmune diseases and organ transplantation. Radiat Oncol Annu 205, 1983.

166. Strober S. Total lymphoid irradiation: Basic and clinical studies in transplantation immunity. Prog Clin Biol Res 224:251, 1986.

167. Schwadron RB, Palathumpat V, Strober S. Natural suppressor cells derived from adult spleen and thymus. Transplantation 48:107, 1989.

168. Thomas J, Alquaisi M, Cunningham P, et al. The development of a posttransplant TLI treatment strategy that promotes organ allograft acceptance without chronic immunosuppression. Transplantation 53:247, 1992.

169. Strober S, Dhillon M, Schubert M, et al. Acquired immune tolerance to cadaveric renal allografts: A study of three patients treated with total lymphoid irradiation. N Engl J Med 321:28, 1989.

170. Myburgh JA. Total lymphoid irradiation in transplantation. Transplant Proc XX:118, 1988.

171. Florence LS, Ito T, Ang KK, et al. The synergistic effect of total-lymphoid irradiation with extracted donor alloantigen in inducing transplantation unresponsiveness. Transplantation 47:156, 1989.

172. Strober S, Modry DL, Hoppe RT, et al. Induction of specific unresponsiveness to heart allografts in mongrel dogs treated with total lymphoid irradiation and antithymocyte globulin. J Immunol 132:1013, 1984.

173. Frist WH, Winterland AW, Gerhardt EB, et al. Total lymphoid irradiation in heart transplantation: Adjunctive treatment for recurrent rejection. Ann Thorac Surg 48(6):863, 1989.

174. Robinson JA, Hubbell E, Costanzo-Nordin M, Pifarre R. Successful cardiac transplantation after allo-antibody removal by plasma exchange (abstract). Third World Apheresis Association Annual Meeting, April, 1990.

175. Partanen J, Nieminen MS, Krogerus L, Harjula ALJ, Mattila S. Heart transplant rejection treated with plasmapheresis. J Heart Lung Transplant 11:301, 1992.

176. Malafa M, Mancini MC, Myles JL, Gohara A, Dickinson JM, Walsh TE. Successful treatment of acute humoral rejection in heart transplant patients. J Heart Lung Transplant 11:486, 1992.

177. Caruana RJ, Zumbro GL, Hoff RG, Rao RN, Daspit SA. Successful cardiac transplantation across an ABO blood group barrier. Transplantation 46:472, 1988.

178. Kupin WL, Venkat KK, Hayashi H, Mozes MF, Oh HK, Watt R. Removal of lymphocytotoxic antibodies by pretransplant immunoadsorption therapy in highly sensitized renal transplant recipients. Transplantation 51:324, 1991.

179. Deeg HJ. Ultraviolet irradiation in transplantation biology. Manipulation of immunity and immunogenicity. Transplantation 45:845, 1988.

180. Costanzo-Nordin MR, Hubbell EA, O'Sullivan EJ, et al. Successful treatment of heart transplant rejection with photopheresis. Transplantation 53:808, 1992.

181. Wieland M, Randels MJ, Strauss RG, et al. Photopheresis: A promising therapy for intractable cardiac allograft rejection. J Clin Apheresis 7:42, 1992.

182. Wolff JA, Malone RW, Williams P, et al. Direct gene transfer into mouse muscle in vivo. Science 23:1465, 1990.

183. Ascadi G, Jiao A. Direct gene transfer and expression into rat heart in vivo. New Biologist 3:71, 1991.

184. Wood ML, Monaco AP. Suppressor cells in specific unresponsiveness to skin allografts in ALS-treated marrow-injected mice. Transplantation 29:196, 1980.

185. Wood ML, Monaco AP. Induction of unresponsiveness to skin allografts in adult mice disparate at defined regions of the H-2 complex. I. Effect of donor-specific bone marrow in ALS-treated mice. Transplantation 37:35, 1984.

186. Fabre JW, Morris PJ. The effect of donor strain blood pretreatment on renal allograft rejection in rats. Transplantation 14:608, 1972.

187. Norman DJ, Opelz G. Blood transfusions. _In Renal Transplantation_. New York, Churchill Livingstone, 1986, p 355.

188. Waldmann H. Manipulation of T-cell responses with monoclonal antibodies. Annu Rev Immunol 7:407, 1989.

189. Chou S, Norman DJ. Effect of OKT3 antibody therapy on cytomegalovirus reactivation in renal transplant recipients. Transplant Proc 17:2755, 1985.

190. Swinnen LJ, Costanzo-Nordin MR, Fisher SG, et al. Increased incidence of lymphoproliferative disorder after immunosuppression with the monoclonal anti-

body OKT3 in cardiac transplant recipients. N Engl J Med 323:1723, 1990.

191. Miller LW, Naftel DC, Bourge RC, et al. Infection following cardiac transplantation: A multi-institutional analysis. Personal communication, 1992.

192. Trento A, Domiher GS, Hardesty RL. Mediastinitis following heart transplantation: Incidence, treatment, and results. J Heart Transplant 3:336, 1984.

193. Miller R, Ruder J, Karwande SV, Burton NA. Treatment of mediastinitis after heart transplantation. J Heart Transplant 5:477, 1986.

194. Gottesdiener KM. Transplanted infections: Donor-to-host transmission with the allograft. Ann Intern Med 110:1001, 1989.

195. Dummer JS, White LT, Ho M, Griffith BP, Hardesty RL, Bahnson HT. Morbidity of cytomegalovirus infection in recipients of heart or heart-lung transplants who received cyclosporine. J Infect Dis 152:1182, 1985.

196. Smith CB. Cytomegalovirus pneumonia—State of the art. Chest 95:182S, 1989.

197. Bloom JN, Palestine AG. The diagnosis of cytomegalovirus retinitis. Ann Intern Med 109:963, 1988.

198. Gonwa TA, Capehart JE, Pilcher JW, Alivizatos PA. Cytomegalovirus myocarditis as a cause of cardiac dysfunction in a heart transplant recipient. Transplantation 47:197, 1989.

199. Watson FS, O'Connell JB, Amber IJ, et al. Treatment of cytomegalovirus pneumonia in heart transplant recipients with 9 (1,3-dihydroxy-2-proproxymethyl)-guanine (DHPG). J Heart Transplant 7:102, 1988.

200. Keay S, Petersen E, Icenogle T, et al. Ganciclovir treatment of serious cytomegalovirus infection in heart and heart-lung transplant recipients. Rev Infect Dis 10:S563, 1988.

201. Reed EC, Bowden RA, Dandliker PS, Litteby KE, Meyers JD. Treatment of cytomegalovirus pneumonia with ganciclovir and intravenous cytomegalovirus immunoglobulin in patients with bone marrow transplants. Ann Intern Med 109:783, 1988.

202. Seale L, Jones CJ, Kathpalia S, et al. Prevention of herpesvirus infections in renal allograft recipients by low-dose oral acyclovir. JAMA 254:3435, 1985.

203. Luft BJ, Naot Y, Araujo FG, Stinson EB, Remington JS. Primary and reactivated toxoplasma infection in patients with cardiac transplants. Clinical spectrum and problems in diagnosis in a defined population. Ann Intern Med 99:27, 1983.

204. Leport C, Raffi F, Matheron S, et al. Treatment of central nervous system toxoplasmosis with pyrimethamine/sulfadiazine combination in 35 patients with the acquired immunodeficiency syndrome. Efficacy of long-term continuous therapy. Am J Med 84:94, 1988.

205. Dannemann BR, Israelski DM, Remington JS. Treatment of toxoplasmic encephalitis with intravenous clindamycin. Arch Intern Med 148:2477, 1988.

206. Peters SG, Prakash UB. *Pneumocystis carinii* pneumonia. Review of 53 cases. Am J Med 82:73, 1987.

207. Franson TR, Kauffman HMJR, Adams MB. Cyclosporine therapy and refractory *Pneumocystis carinii* pneumonia. A potential association. Arch Surg 122:1034, 1987.

208. Favor A, Frazier OH, Cooley DA, et al. Legionella infections in cyclosporine-immunosuppressed cardiac transplants. Tex Heart Inst J 12:153, 1985.

209. American Academy of Pediatrics Report of the Committee on Infectious Diseases. Elk Grove Village, Illinois, Red Book, 1991.

210. Wenting GJ, Van den Minacker AH, Ritsemavan Eck JH, et al. Lack of circadian variation of blood pressure after heart transplantation. J Hypertens 4:S78, 1986.

211. Reeves RA, Shapiro AP, Thompson ME, Johnsen AM. Loss of nocturnal decline in blood pressure after cardiac transplantation. Circulation 73:401, 1986.

212. Thompson ME, Shapiro AP, Johnsen AM, et al. The contrasting effects of cyclosporine-A and azathioprine on arterial blood pressure and renal function following cardiac transplantation. Int J Cardiol 11:219, 1986.

213. Curtis JJ, Luke RG, Jones P, Diethelm AG. Hypertension in cyclosporine-treated renal transplant recipients is sodium dependent. Am J Med 85:134, 1988.

214. Ratkovec RM, Renlund DG, Bristow MR. Diltiazem treatment of cyclosporine-induced hypertension after cardiac transplantation (abstract). Cardiovasc Drugs Ther 3(2):622, 1989.

215. Bourge RC, Kirklin JK, Naftel DC, Figg WD, White-Williams C, Ketchum C. Diltiazem-cyclosporine interaction in cardiac transplant recipients: Impact on cyclosporine dose and medication costs. Am J Med 90:402, 1991.

216. McGiffin DC, Kirklin JK, Naftel B. Acute renal failure after heart transplantation and cyclosporine therapy. J Heart Transplant 4:396, 1985.

217. Jessup M, Cavarocchi N, Narins B, McClurken J, Kolff J. Antihypertensive therapy in patients after cardiac transplantation: A step care approach. Transplant Proc 20:I-801, 1988.

218. Greenberg A, Egel JW, Thompson ME, et al. Early and late forms of cyclosporine nephrotoxicity: Studies in cardiac transplant recipients. Am J Kidney Dis 9:12, 1987.

219. Myers BD, Ross J, Newton L, Luetscher J, Perlroth M. Cyclosporine associated chronic nephropathy. N Engl J Med 311:699, 1984.

220. Moran M, Tomlanovich S, Myers BD. Cyclosporine-induced chronic nephropathy in human recipients of cardiac allografts. Transplant Proc 17(4-S1):185, 1985.

221. Aziz S, Bergdahl L, Baldwin JC, et al. Pancreatitis after cardiac and cardiopulmonary transplantation. Surgery 97:653, 1985.

222. Ibels LS, Alfrey AC, Huffer WE, Weil R. Aseptic necrosis of bone following renal transplantation: Experience in 194 transplant recipients and review of the literature. Medicine 57:25, 1978.

223. Hyams JS, Carcy DL. Corticosteroids and growth. J Pediatr 113(2):249, 1988.

224. Hunt SA. Pregnancy in heart transplant recipients: A good idea? J Heart Lung Transplant 10:499, 1991.

225. Zimmerman J, Fainaru M, Eisenberg S. The effects of prednisone therapy on plasma lipoproteins and apolipoproteins: A prospective study. Metabolism 33:521, 1984.

226. Stamler JS, Vaughan DE, Rudd MA, et al. Frequency of hypercholesterolemia after cardiac transplantation. Am J Cardiol 62(17):1268, 1988.

227. Becker DM, Chamberlain B, Swank R, et al. Relationship between corticosteroid exposure and plasma lipid levels in heart transplant recipients. Am J Med 85:632, 1988.

228. Renlund DG, Bristow MR, Crandall BG, et al. Hypercholesterolemia after heart transplantation: Amelioration by corticosteroid-free maintenance immunosuppression. J Heart Transplant 8:214, 1989.

229. Norman DJ, Illingworth DR, Munson JL, Hosenpud

JD. Myolysis and acute renal failure in a heart transplant recipient on Lovastatin. N Engl J Med 318:46, 1988.

230. Grigg MM, Costanzo-Nordin MR, Celesia GG. The etiology of seizures after cardiac transplantation. Transplant Proc 20:937, 1988.

231. Shihab F, Barry JM, Norman DJ. Encephalopathy following the use of OKT3 in renal allograft transplantation. Transplant Proc 25(1):31, 1993.

232. Penn I. Cancers following cyclosporine therapy. Transplantation 43:32, 1987.

233. Batiuk T, Barry JM, Bennett WM, et al. The incidence and type of cancer occurring following the use of OKT3: A single center experience with 557 organ transplants. Transplant Proc 25:27, 1993.

234. Nalesnik MA, Makowka L, Starzl TE. The diagnosis and treatment of posttransplant lymphoproliferative disorders. Curr Probl Surg 25(6):365, 1988.

235. Penn I. Lymphomas complicating organ transplantation. Transplant Proc 15:2790, 1983.

236. Frizzera G, Hanto DW, Gajl-Peczalska KJ, et al. Polymorphic diffuse B-cell hyperplasias and lymphomas in renal transplant recipients. Cancer Res 41:4262, 1981.

237. Weintraub J, Warnke RA. Lymphoma in cardiac allotransplant recipients: Clinical and histological features and immunological phenotype. Transplantation 33:347, 1982.

238. Hanto DW, Frizzera G, Gaji-Peczalska KJ, et al. Epstein-Barr virus-induced B-cell lymphoma after renal transplantation: Acyclovir therapy and transition from polyclonal to monoclonal B-cell proliferation. N Engl J Med 306:913, 1982.

239. Cleary ML, Chao J, Warnke R, Sklar J. Immunoglobulin gene rearrangement as a diagnostic criterion of B-cell lymphoma. Proc Natl Acad Sci USA 81:593, 1984.

240. Arnold A, Cossman J, Bakhshi A, Jaffe ES, Waldmann TA, Korsmeyer SJ. Immunoglobulin-gene rearrangements as unique clonal markers in human lymphoid neoplasms. N Engl J Med 309:1593, 1983.

241. Nalesnik MA, Jaffe R, Starzl TE, et al. The pathology of posttransplant lymphoproliferative disorders occurring in the setting of cyclosporine A-prednisone immunosuppression. Am J Pathol 133:173, 1988.

242. Hanto DW, Birkenbach M, Frizzera G, Gajl-Peczalska KJ, Simmons RL, Schubach WH. Confirmation of the heterogeneity of posttransplant Epstein-Barr virus-associated B cell proliferations by immunoglobulin gene rearrangement analyses. Transplantation 47:458, 1989.

243. Cleary ML, Warnke R, Sklar J. Monoclonality of lymphoproliferative lesions in cardiac transplant recipients: Clonal analysis based on immunoglobulin-gene rearrangements. N Engl J Med 310:477, 1984.

244. Starzl TE, Nalesnik MA, Porter KA, et al. Reversibility of lymphomas and lymphoproliferative lesions developing under cyclosporine-steroid therapy. Lancet 1:583, 1984.

12

INFECTIONS IN TRANSPLANT PATIENTS

David C. Classen, MD, MS, and Robert L. Flinner, MD

Historically, infection has been the most morbid and lethal complication of organ transplantation.[1-11] Significant refinements have been made in the immunosuppression regimens used in transplant patients; however, the effects of this immunosuppression still lead to significant impairment of microbial defense mechanisms.[1-3] Dramatic narrowing of this immune modulation still appears distant. Thus, infections will remain one of the most common complications of organ transplantation for the foreseeable future.

There is considerable variability among infectious complications in organ transplant patients. The risk appears to be highest for bone marrow transplantation (which will not be covered in this chapter or in this book) and least for kidney transplantation, with the other transplanted solid organs falling in between.[2]

Table 12–1 outlines the relative risk of infection from the considerable experience at the University of Pittsburgh transplantation program. However, significant variability remains of infectious complications among solid organ transplants, which will be elucidated in this review.

OVERVIEW

Numerous factors contribute to the immunocompromised state that exists in transplant patients and that predisposes them to infectious complications. These factors are present to varying degrees throughout the life of the transplant patient. Many studies have shown that the risk of infection is highest within the first 4 months after transplant, declines stead-

Table 12–1. Frequency, Severity, and Type of Infections Occurring Among Solid Organ Transplant Patients

Type of Transplant	N	Infection per Patient	Infection-Associated Mortality (%)	Patients with Bacteremia (%)	Patients with Symptomatic CMV (%)	Patients with Invasive Fungal Infections (%)	Most Common Site	
							Site	All Infections (%)
Renal	64	0.98	0	5	8 (5)*	0	Urinary tract	41
Heart	119	1.36	15	13	16 (5)	8	Lung	27
Heart–lung	31	3.19	45	19	39 (32)	23	Lung	57
Liver	101	1.86	23	23	22 (5)	16	Abdomen, GI	23

*Percentage of all patients with CMV pneumonia.
From Ho M, Dummer JS, Peterson PK, Simmons RL. Infections in solid organ transplants. *In* Mandell GL, Douglas RG, Bennett JE (eds). *Principles and Practices of Infectious Diseases*, 3rd ed. New York, Churchill Livingstone, 1990, p 2292.

ily after that period, and then reaches a steady state for as long as the patients receive immunosuppressive agents. Four important factors in determining the risk of these infections are the net state of immunosuppression, host factors, transplantation factors, and epidemiologic exposures.[3]

The net state of immunosuppression is determined by several factors, the most important of which are the type, dose, and duration of immunosuppression therapy. Various immunosuppressive agents are used, such as corticosteroids, azathioprine, cyclosporine, and polyclonal and monoclonal antilymphocyte globulins. All these agents broadly suppress the immune system, especially when combined to treat episodes of rejection, which appears to increase dramatically the risk of infectious complications. In addition, the presence of granulocytopenia, the presence of foreign bodies (urinary, biliary, central line catheters), and metabolic factors such as uremia and hyperglycemia all contribute to further suppression of the immune system.[1] Certain viral infections such as cytomegalovirus (CMV) and Epstein-Barr virus (EBV) can modulate the immune system. Also important in determining the risk of infection are host factors, specifically underlying diseases such as diabetes, chronic renal failure, and chronic hepatic insufficiency. Certain transplant surgery–related factors can play a key role in causing infection; the stress and duration of surgery alone can have a dramatic impact on the immune system.[3] Finally, the transplanted organ can suffer from ischemic injury with resultant poor function, which can predispose the organ to early infectious complications.[2]

Epidemiologic exposure for transplant patients can be envisioned in three distinct ways.[3] First, remote exposure can include infections acquired months to years earlier that have been dormant up until the time of transplant and can be reactivated after transplant. These infections can include *Mycobacterium tuberculosis*, *Histoplasma capsulatum*, *Blastomyces dermatitides*, *Strongyloides stercoralis*, hepatitis B and C (HBV and HCV), *Toxoplasma gondii*, *Pneumocystis carinii*, and human immunodeficiency virus (HIV). Second, community-acquired exposure after the transplant can lead to a variety of infections, including influenza, primary varicella-zoster infection, salmonellosis, legionellosis, *Nocardia* infections, and cryptococcal infections. Third, hospital exposure can lead to nosocomial infections with typical and atypical mycobacterial infections, *Candida* species, As-

pergillus species, *Pseudomonas* species, *Enterobacter* species, and other gram-negative organisms. Hospital-related transmission of infection can also occur via transfused blood and blood products and transplanted tissues. Blood and blood products can transmit CMV, EBV, HIV, hepatitis A (HAV), HBV, HCV, and human T cell lymphotrophic virus-1 (HTLV-1). CMV and HIV have been transmitted by all solid organ transplant tissues; toxoplasmosis has been transmitted by kidney and heart tissue. Kidney tissue has been shown to transmit HBV and herpes simplex virus (HSV) infection.

INFECTION RISK

In all solid organ transplant patients the risk of infectious complications is highest in the few months after surgery and decreases steadily after this period. However, there is always some risk of infectious complications as long as the patient is receiving immunosuppressive agents to prevent rejection.[1–3, 10, 11] Figure 12–1 gives a rough guide to the chronology of potential infections in solid organ transplant patients. As a rule, conventional bacterial infections occur in the first month after transplant at the site of transplant and are often bacterial or fungal infections related to the patient's endogenous flora. Infections related to invasive devices occur commonly during the initial hospitalization; these include central line infections, urinary catheter infections, and pneumonia related to endotracheal tubes.

The greatest risk of opportunistic infections occurs from 1 to 6 months after transplantation. This is also a period with a significant risk of allograft rejection, with the requisite increased immunosuppression that entails treatment of rejection. In this setting, reactivation or primary infection with CMV can occur. Often these infections are manifested after a course of increased immunosuppression for rejection. Unfortunately, CMV infections can also lead to further immunosuppression, increasing the risk of other opportunistic infections such as disseminated fungal infections (*Candida* species, *Aspergillus* species, *Cryptococcus*, and endemic fungi), parasitic infections as with *Toxoplasma* or *Pneumocystis*, and viral infections such as EBV, varicella-zoster virus (VZV), papovavirus, and adenovirus infections.

Beyond 6 months after transplant the risk of infection decreases, in part because the risk of rejection has decreased and because the overall immunosuppression regimen has often

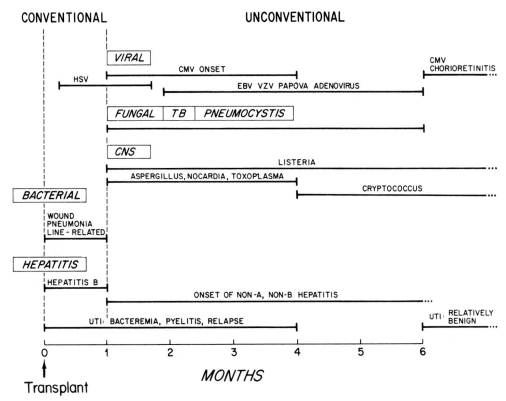

Figure 12–1. Chronologic occurrence of potential infections in solid organ transplant patients. (From Rubin RH, Wolfson JS, Cosimi AB, et al. Infection in the renal transplant recipient. Am J Med 70:405, 1981.)

been decreased by this point. Patients who are free of chronic rejection and thus on less immunosuppression are still susceptible to community-acquired infections such as pneumococcal pneumonia, influenza, and urinary tract infections. Those patients with chronic rejection usually are receiving greater immunosuppression and have a risk of infection similar to patients within the first 6 months after transplant. Finally, there are patients with chronic CMV infections, chronic HBV and HCV, and chronic EBV infection whose immune systems are modulated by these infections and hence are at the greatest long-term risk for opportunistic infections.

INFECTION DETECTION AND PREVENTION

A variety of strategies have been developed to diagnose, treat, and prevent potential infections before they become a problem in transplant patients.[1, 5, 7–9] This involves pretransplant screening of patients for a variety of active or latent infections, such as tuberculosis, HBV,

HCV, endemic fungal infections, toxoplasmosis, and EBV. It also involves vaccination strategies to prevent influenza, pneumococcal infections, measles, and potentially CMV and herpes virus (HSV) infections. Finally, pretransplant preparation involves the use of prophylactic agents after transplant to prevent development of infections with certain endogenous organisms such as *Pneumocystis*, HSV, CMV, and *Toxoplasma*. The net result of this approach has been a marked decrease in the occurrence of these infections in transplant patients over the last 10 years.

VIRAL INFECTIONS

Overall, viral infections are the most important infectious complications for transplant patients. They have a plethora of possible expressions: fever, pneumonia, diarrhea, hepatitis, meningitis, and encephalitis. They also can cause direct and significant damage to the allograft, and they potentially can play a role in rejection of the allograft. Some viruses can cause significant immunosuppression, and others can lead to the development of malignancies in transplant patients, such as the relationship between EBV and B cell lymphoma. The most common viruses causing disease in transplant patients are herpes viruses, hepatitis viruses, HIV, adenoviruses, and human papovaviruses.[1-3, 10, 11]

Herpes Viruses

Cytomegalovirus

The herpesvirus group includes cytomegalovirus, Epstein-Barr virus, varicella-zoster virus, and herpes simplex virus, which are all potential pathogens in transplant patients. Cytomegalovirus (CMV) is the most common cause of viral infections among transplant patients. Cytomegaloviral infections can occur as a primary infection or as a reactivated infection. Although CMV is usually a disseminated infection, there is great variability in its presentation, from clinically asymptomatic events to a mononucleosis-like syndrome to fulminant pneumonia leading to death. Primary infections tend to be more clinically apparent and more severe than reactivated latent infections in the immunocompromised host. Greater degrees of immunosuppression often lead to more serious manifestations of CMV infections. Cytomegalovirus does have a propensity to cause greater damage in the transplanted organ than in endogenous organs.

Although CMV can involve any organ, the most severe clinical manifestations occur with involvement of lung, liver, and gastrointestinal tract. Cytomegaloviral involvement of lung, especially in heart and lung transplants, leads to an interstitial pneumonia that can be severe, prolonged, and lethal.[5, 8] Cytomegaloviral hepatitis is often mild, but more dramatic involvement, including hepatic necrosis, can occur in liver transplant patients. Gastrointestinal involvement can include most of the alimentary tract; more commonly, it causes esophagitis and gastritis, although severe colonic involvement can cause bloody diarrhea and massive bleeding. Less common sequelae of CMV infections include myocarditis, renal involvement, transverse myelitis, and encephalitis.

Pathologic Findings in CMV Infections. Cytomegalovirus-infected cells that are diagnostic of a CMV infection must have both cytomegaly and characteristic large basophilic intranuclear inclusions[12] (Fig. 12–2). Often small granular eosinophilic cytoplasmic inclusions are also present. These cytoplasmic inclusions occurring in cells showing cytomegaly are virtually diagnostic of CMV infection even if no intranuclear inclusion is present. This is especially the case in infected endothelial cells in gastrointestinal biopsies (Figs. 12–3 and 12–4). Even in a severe infection only small numbers of diagnostic cells are seen, and a careful search must be conducted. Clusters of polymorphonuclear leukocytes in hepatic sinu-

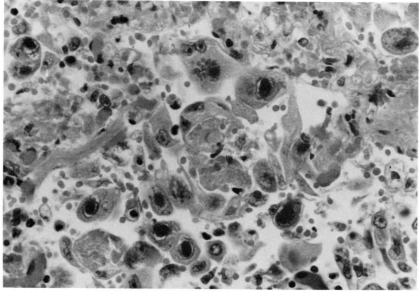

Figure 12–2. CMV pneumonitis. Enlarged cells with large intranuclear inclusions and granular cytoplasmic inclusions are seen. (Hematoxylin & eosin, × 450)

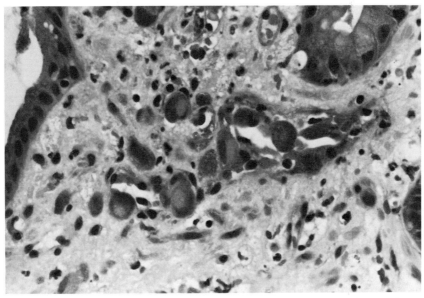

Figure 12–3. CMV gastritis, showing enlarged endothelial and stromal cells with ill-defined intranuclear and cytoplasmic inclusions. In the gastrointestinal tract, these cells, rather than epithelial cells, show the diagnostic findings; the inclusions are usually not of the classic type shown in Figure 12–1. (Hematoxylin & eosin, × 450)

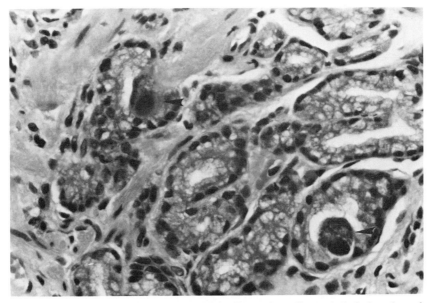

Figure 12–4. In the duodenum, Brunner's gland epithelial cells may have diagnostic inclusions (arrowheads). (Hematoxylin & eosin, × 450)

soids are good evidence of CMV infection, although there are exceptions to this.[13] Rarely, there may be epithelioid granulomas, although CMV inclusions are not present in the granuloma.[14] There is a report of fibrin ring granulomas in the bone marrow with CMV infection. In this unusual form of granuloma, there is a clear space within a peripheral fibrin ring within the granuloma.[15] The presence of the virus can also be detected by immunofluorescence and immunoperoxidase methods and electron microscopy.[16] A viral genome may be identified by gene probes, such as polymerase chain reaction, but this does not discriminate between a latent and an active infection.[16] In situ hybridization studies may detect infection in the absence of diagnostic inclusions.[17, 18]

Herpes Simplex

Herpes simplex virus (HSV) infections are a common but usually self-limited problem in transplant patients. Most infections are due to reactivation in seropositive patients, and they tend to occur in oral or genital mucocutaneous regions. However, the appearance of the lesions can be atypical, and they can look more like ulcers than vesicles. They can be more problematic in transplant patients than in normal patients. HSV infections can disseminate in transplant patients; however, these infections usually respond well to appropriate therapy. Herpes simplex virus can cause a se-

vere and rapidly progressive hepatitis. A liver biopsy is usually needed to make the diagnosis. Other uncommon presentations include tracheal or esophageal involvement and meningoencephalitis.[2] Serologic studies are not the common diagnostic method because infection with HSV is easily demonstrated by culture, pathologic examination, or immunofluorescent techniques.

Pathologic Findings in HSV Infections. In practice, herpes simplex virus is most often seen in biopsies from the esophagus. These are ulcerated areas, and the diagnostic cells are usually at the margin of the ulcer. A biopsy sample that consists only of ulcer bed would not be expected to be diagnostic. The diagnostic change occurs in the squamous cells that are often detached from the underlying tissue and that show multinucleation with intranuclear inclusions[12, 19] (Fig. 12–5). These inclusions are homogeneous eosinophilic material that entirely fills the nucleus,[19] or they may have a nonstaining rim at the periphery. The infected cells do not show the enlargement seen with CMV infection.

Varicella-Zoster

Varicella-zoster virus (VZV) infections usually occur in transplant patients as reactivation in the form of dermatomal zoster. Dissemination is uncommon in solid organ transplants in this setting, although if it occurs it usually

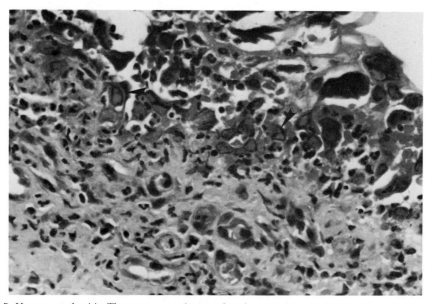

Figure 12–5. Herpes esophagitis. There are many intranuclear homogeneous inclusions in an esophageal ulceration (arrowheads). (Hematoxylin & eosin, × 450)

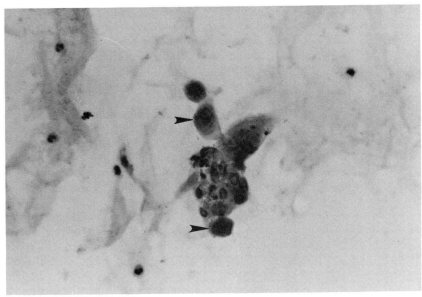

Figure 12–6. Tzanck smear from a herpes vesicle of the skin, showing multinucleated epithelial cells (arrowheads) with homogeneous intranuclear inclusions. (Hematoxylin & eosin, × 450)

responds to treatment. In contrast, in nonimmune transplant patients a primary VZV infection can be rapidly fatal, with pneumonia, hepatitis, pancreatitis, disseminated intravascular coagulation, and in some cases encephalitis. Hence the serologic status of all patients for VZV is usually determined before transplant. Diagnosis depends on the clinical presentation and examination of skin biopsy material.

Pathologic Findings in VZV Infection. Varicella-zoster pathologic changes are the same as those seen in herpes simplex virus infection.[12] Tzanck smears can be used in examining fluid from a vesicle infected with the herpes virus. In these smears, characteristic herpes-type inclusions can be found in the desquamated epithelial cells (Fig. 12–6). These can be stained with the usual stains, including Wright's, Papanicolaou's (Pap), or hematoxylin & eosin. The virus is difficult to grow in culture but can be suspected based on the pathologic appearance in skin biopsies, combined with appropriate serologic studies.[12]

Epstein-Barr Virus

Epstein-Barr virus (EBV) infections, like CMV, can occur as a primary infection or as reactivation of latent infection in solid organ transplant patients. Less than 5 per cent of adults are seronegative for EBV; thus, primary infection is more common in pediatric transplant patients. The usual clinical presentation is a mononucleosis-like syndrome, with pharyngitis, lymphadenopathy, fever, and biochemical hepatitis. The most important syndrome associated with EBV in these patients is a lymphoproliferative syndrome that occurs most frequently within the first 3 months after transplant. This syndrome usually presents with a B cell lymphoproliferative disorder that appears to have a spectrum from benign polyclonal B cell hyperplasia to a malignant monoclonal B cell lymphoma.[1-3] This entity is more common with primary than reactivated EBV infections and also is more commonly seen with increased degrees of immunosuppression. (See Chapter 13, page 265, which deals with this topic.) Diagnosis of EBV infections can be made serologically.

Hepatitis Viruses

Hepatitis B (HBV) and hepatitis C (formerly non-A, non-B hepatitis; HCV) are both significant problems in solid organ transplant patients.[20, 21] Although usually a problem that precedes transplantation, both these infections can be transmitted by transplanted organs and potentially by blood products; the risk of this latter mechanism of transmission appears low. Acquisition of either of these agents in the peritransplant period can lead to rapidly progressive liver disease and death. However, more commonly, these agents cause chronic liver disease that can progress to cirrhosis. Patients with both HBV and HCV can be expected to have recurrences of disease after liver transplantation, and in some centers these agents are considered contraindications to transplantation. Diagnosis of these diseases can be suspected after liver biopsy and confirmed with serologic tests for the presence of antibody or antigen or both.

Pathologic Findings in Viral Hepatitis. Acute viral hepatitis caused by HAV, HBV, or HCV is characterized histologically by various forms of liver cell damage accompanied by a lymphocytic infiltrate.[22] The hepatic cells show swelling of their cytoplasm (ballooning degeneration), which is a reversible change. Irreversible changes consist of necrosis with shrinkage and eosinophilia of cytoplasm and pyknosis of nuclei. Another form of cell death is a rounded cell with intensely eosinophilic cytoplasm and absence of a nucleus. This necrotic cell often appears to be dissociated from the liver cell plates. This is commonly referred to as an acidophilic body. These findings of cell damage and loss are accompanied by regenerative activity of liver cells with mitoses and double-layered hepatic cords. Cholestasis is common. The inflammatory infiltrate is predominantly lymphocytic and located in the lobules with smaller numbers of cells in portal triads. Later there may be accumulation of groups of lipochrome-pigmented macrophages in sinusoids that have phagocytized material from necrotic cells. More severe cases may develop more extensive cell necrosis, with bridging necrosis between portal and central areas. Fulminant and subfulminant forms have broad zones of cell loss with collapse of the reticulum framework.

Chronic hepatitis, caused by the hepatitis B and C viruses, is characterized by inflammation found in portal rather than lobular areas.[22] If the hepatitis is progressive (chronic active hepatitis), there is piecemeal necrosis. This type of cell loss is identified by the portal lymphocytic infiltrate that extends into the adjacent liver cords surrounding and isolating individual cells. There are findings in chronic hepatitis C infection that, though not diagnostic, are seen more frequently than in hepatitis A and B. It is generally felt that fatty change is not a feature of viral hepatitis. However, hepatitis C often may have mild fatty change. The inflammatory infiltrate often is in the sinusoids with single cells or with rows or beads of cells.[22] Necrotic cells are infrequent and may take the form of triangular shrunken cells. HCV usually develops 3 to 4 months post-transplant and

becomes chronic or results in subfulminant liver failure.[23] Liver disease caused by HCV accounts for 8 per cent to 28 per cent of deaths in transplant recipients, long-term.[24]

Reinfection with HBV may appear, similar to hepatitis in nontransplant patients.[21] In the acute phase, the inflammation is panlobular whereas in the chronic phase there is portal and periportal inflammation with piecemeal necrosis.[22] The most important process to differentiate from hepatitis is acute cellular rejection of the liver (see Chapter 10, page 194). Cellular rejection can usually be readily distinguished from the changes of hepatitis; in cellular rejection, the inflammation is portal (not lobular), and characteristic change occurs in the bile ducts. Furthermore, venules show endothelialitis in rejection, which is not seen in hepatitis.[25] Most episodes of acute rejection occur during the first month post-transplant, whereas hepatitis occurs from the second month onward. Occasionally, cellular rejection and hepatitis may occur in the same liver, which will produce histologic findings difficult to interpret.[26] Furthermore, the use of immunosuppression may modify the histologic picture: the inflammatory infiltrate may not be as prominent as expected. It has been observed that hepatitis B carriers are at risk of developing fulminant hepatitis with liver failure when immunosuppressive therapy or chemotherapy is withdrawn.[27–29] This occurs in transplant patients as well as in patients receiving chemotherapy for malignancy.[30] There is evidence that in some of these cases of fulminant hepatitis B infection, the delta agent is responsible for the fulminant course of the hepatitis.[28, 31]

Adenoviruses and Papovaviruses (Human Papilloma Virus)

Adenovirus can cause mild-to-moderate infections in transplant patients, usually involving respiratory tract, conjunctiva, hepatitis, and hemorrhagic cystitis. Over 25 per cent of transplant patients develop human papilloma virus (HPV) infections with either BK or JC, the two major human pathogens.[32]

Although the spectrum of disease with these two agents is incompletely defined and subclinical infections are probably common, they have been associated with ureteral stenosis, renal allograft dysfunction, endocrine and exocrine pancreatic dysfunction, and accelerated atherosclerosis.[2, 3] There also has been an association with papovavirus (HPV) and a variety of malignancies. Diagnosis of these infections depends on culture and pathologic examination of affected tissues.

Pathologic Findings in Adenovirus and HPV Infections. Cells infected with adenovirus show no enlargement or multinucleation. The nuclei contain basophilic smudged viral inclusions.[32]

Examples of HPV-induced proliferations include verruca vulgaris and condyloma. Verruca vulgaris is characterized by epidermal hyperplasia producing a verrucoid, hyperkeratotic surface.[33] There is a rounded, noninvasive interface between the epithelium and underlying dermis. There is no cell atypia.

Condyloma acuminatum involving the genital epithelium has a verrucoid, hyperkeratotic surface with epidermal hyperplasia.[33] The upper layers of squamous cells often have cytoplasmic vacuolization (koilocytosis) with wrinkled hyperchromatic nuclei (raisinoid nuclei) (Fig. 12–7). A similar change is seen with condyloma of the uterine cervix except that most often there is no verrucoid or keratotic change. No viral inclusions are seen.

Human Immunodeficiency Virus

Unfortunately, transplant patients have not been spared infections with human immunodeficiency virus (HIV). Although most transplant programs screen potential transplant patients for infection with HIV, the screening of donors has not been completely effective in preventing the use of organs from an HIV-infected donor. Several examples of this method of transmission have been documented, with the efficiency of transmission approaching 100 per cent. Transplant patients have much the same clinical symptoms as normal patients after primary infection. Unlike the case in normal patients, immunosuppression can significantly delay seroconversion in transplant patients.[1]

Pathologic features of infection are similar to those described in other infected individuals and will not be covered here.[1-5]

BACTERIAL INFECTIONS

Early Infections

Transplant patients develop a broad spectrum of bacterial infections. Initially in the peritransplant period, these patients develop nosocomial infections related to the surgical procedure and to the placement of invasive devices. The transplanted organ is subject to surgery-related trauma, subsequent wound infection, infected periorgan fluid collections, ischemia, and rejection.[1-5] Thus it is a common site of bacterial infection, especially in the early transplant period. Among liver transplants, bacterial infections are often intra-ab-

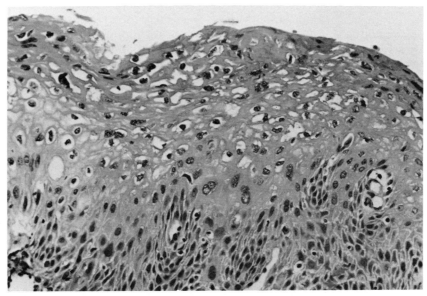

Figure 12–7. Condyloma of the uterine cervix. Note the enlarged, hyperchromatic, wrinkled nuclei. (Hematoxylin & eosin, × 450)

dominal (biliary tract or peritoneal cavity) and commonly involve gram-negative and anaerobic bacteria. Among heart and lung transplant patients, the chest is a frequent site of bacterial infections, usually manifested as a mediastinitis or pneumonia. In these patients bacteria are the most common cause of infections in the chest. The bacterial etiologies of these infections are similar to those of other patients undergoing open heart surgery. Staphylococcal and gram-negative species predominate. Hospital-acquired agents such as *Pseudomonas* species and *Legionella* species can also cause infections in the chest. In addition, *Mycoplasma hominis* has been shown to be a cause of mediastinitis in these patients.[5] Kidney transplant patients can develop bacterial wound infections. However, urinary tract infections are far more common, usually with gram-negative organisms.[9]

Invasive devices act as a portal and conduit for infection in transplant patients. In renal transplant patients, the urinary catheter is a common source of gram-negative urinary tract infections. Among liver transplant patients, a biliary catheter with an external drain is commonly used and is virtually always colonized by gram-negative organisms, enterococci, or both. This is the common source of organisms that are found in those patients who develop cholangitis or liver abscesses.

Late Infections

Beyond this peritransplant (usually the first month) period, transplant patients are at risk for routine community-acquired bacterial infections, such as *Streptococcus pneumoniae*, and they are also at risk for *Listeria monocytogenes* infections. Listeria can cause pneumonia, bacteremia, and meningitis in transplant patients. However, these patients are also susceptible to more subacute bacterial infections, such as *Nocardia* species and typical and atypical mycobacterial infections. This risk probably continues for the full period of immunosuppression, which is usually for the life of the transplanted organ. *Nocardia* infections usually begin in the lung as a subacute and often subclinical process from which they can disseminate to skin, bones, joints, liver, and brain. Diagnosis virtually always requires tissue culture and examination, usually by bronchoscopy of the lung or biopsy of involved tissue. Treatment is usually quite effective, especially early in the

course of the disease, before the infection has spread.

Pathologic Findings in Bacterial Infections. Bacteria may be seen with Gram stains and often with Gomori methenamine silver, Grocott modification (GMS) stains. Gram-negative organisms are often difficult to see in sections. There may be an associated PMN infiltrate with tissue necrosis.[12]

Nocardial Infections

A biopsy specimen of an affected area shows a necrotizing and suppurative response in the acute phase. Chronic infection may have a mixed suppurative and granulomatous response, although well-defined granulomas with caseation are not found.[12] The organisms are randomly distributed in the inflammatory infiltrate and do not form aggregates, as is seen in *Actinomyces* infections. The organisms are bacterial in size (1 millimicron wide), filamentous, gram-positive, and, most importantly, show branching[34] (Fig. 12–8). This characteristic branching must be distinguished from bacterial organisms lying on top of one another. The morphology is best demonstrated with Gram and GMS stains. *Nocardia* are also partially acid-fast positive.[35] With acidfast stains, using the standard acid alcohol decolorization the organism is usually negative, but with a weak acid for the decolorization *Nocardia* will be acid-fast positive. This is helpful in differentiating *Nocardia* from other acid-fast organisms. *Nocardia* can also be demonstrated in bronchoalveolar lavage (BAL) specimens with use of the proper stains. The *Nocardia* organisms are usually not seen in the routine hematoxylin & eosin sections.

Mycobacterial Infections

Mycobacterial infections are much more common in transplant patients than in the general population. Both *M. tuberculosis* and atypical mycobacteria cause infection in transplant patients. Mycobacterial infections in transplant patients can present in a wide spectrum of forms, including localized pulmonary disease, progressive pulmonary disease, granulomatous hepatitis, gastrointestinal disease, bone and joint involvement, meningitis, and brain abscesses. Disseminated disease characterized as a miliary pattern can often present

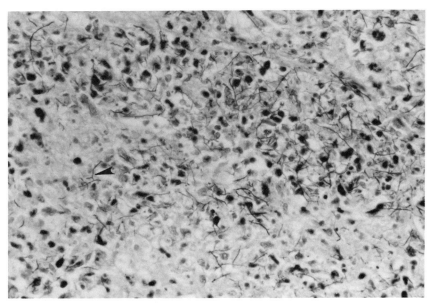

Figure 12–8. *Nocardia* abscess of the lung. Note the filamentous bacteria-sized organisms. Branching is evident at the arrowhead and elsewhere. (Gram stain, × 450)

in a very benign and insidious fashion. Among atypical mycobacteria, *M. avium-intracellulare, M. kansasii,* and *M. chelonei* are most common, but a wide variety of species can cause disease.[2, 3] Unfortunately, atypical mycobacteria can be a common contaminant in sputum cultures; thus a tissue diagnosis of infection is preferred. Diagnosis of mycobacterial infections is made through culture and staining of tissue from involved areas and in the setting of a history of prior skin test reactivity. Unfortunately, primary infections after transplant often do not lead to reactive skin tests because patients are often anergic at this time.

Pathologic Findings in Mycobacterial Infections. As a routine procedure, all specimens should be stained with acid-fast stains: GMS, periodic acid–Schiff (PAS), and Gram stains. Mycobacterial acid-fast organisms must be distinguished from *Nocardia* organisms. *Nocardia* characteristically show branching and are only partially acid-fast positive (see Fig. 12–8). Also, *Nocardia* are strongly gram-positive and are readily seen with GMS stain. Mycobacterial organisms may stain with GMS but are characteristically negative with Gram stain.

In *M. tuberculosis* infections, the affected area contains granulomas with central caseation or coagulation necrosis.[35] The granulomas are made up of many epithelioid histiocytes with multinucleated giant cells and with small numbers of lymphocytes. Acid-fast stains are necessary for diagnosis. The section must be searched carefully with high dry magnification (× 400). Only a few or at times no organisms will be found, although they may be recovered in cultures. The organisms are slender, non-branching, beaded rods 4 millimicrons in length. An incredible number of organisms may be present (as many as 10^6 bacilli per ml) and yet not be detected in the acid-fast stains.[12] In some biopsies, noncaseating granulomas of sarcoid type may be seen in tuberculosis. On the other hand, in immunosuppressed patients the reaction in the tissue may not be typically granulomatous. Instead there may be areas of necrosis or accumulation of foamy macrophages. All biopsies should be stained for organisms regardless of the histologic picture.

Atypical mycobacterial infections, such as those produced by *Mycobacterium kansasii,* may produce lesions similar to those seen in *M. tuberculosis* infections.[12] *Mycobacterium kansasii* may be recovered from bronchial washings in some patients with chronic pulmonary disease and not represent the etiologic agent.[12] The organisms, therefore, ideally should be found in the granulomatous lesion. *Mycobacterium kansasii* may be slightly larger than *M. tuberculosis,* but this distinction cannot be made reliably by morphology alone. The other atypical acid-fast organism of importance is *M. avium-intracellulare* (MAI).[12] In the immunosuppressed patients, many organisms will be found in aggregates of foamy macrophages. In addition to the MAI organisms being acid-fast-positive, they are also strongly PAS-positive. Granulomas are usually not formed.

PARASITIC INFECTIONS

As in the general population, transplant patients are at risk for numerous parasitic infections, depending on their particular epidemiologic exposure. For patients in the United States, three parasitic infections are common. In descending importance, the parasites are *Pneumocystis carinii*, *Toxoplasma*, and *Strongyloides*.[1, 3]

Pneumocystis carinii

Pneumocystis carinii pneumonia (PCP) is so common in transplant patients within the first 6 months after transplanation that almost all transplant patients are placed on prophylactic trimethoprim-sulfamethoxazole to prevent this infection. The presentation of this disease is often subacute, with nonproductive cough, progressive dyspnea, and fever. A chest radiograph usually reveals an interstitial infiltrate, although many other findings have been described. Many diagnostic techniques have been developed, the most reliable of which is bronchoscopy with transbronchial biopsy or alveolar lavage with pathologic examination. Frequently, this disease occurs in concert with cytomegalovirus and can also present at extrapulmonary sites.

Pathologic Findings in *Pneumocystis carinii* Infection. The *Pneumocystis* organism has been classified as a protozoan in the past. Electron microscopic studies and ribosomal RNA analysis have suggested that the organism is a yeastlike fungus.[36] However, the current terminology used for this organism is that used for protozoans.

Pneumocystis organisms are found most commonly free in the alveolar spaces of the lung. They may be attached to type II pneumocytes or within macrophages. Less commonly they may be found in other tissues, including spleen, lymph node, bone marrow, and liver.[37] The life cycle is characterized by trophozoites developing into cysts within which intracystic bodies develop.[36] When the intracystic bodies are released from the cyst, they become trophozoites. The trophozoites measure from 2 to 8 microns in diameter and contain a small

nucleus within the cytoplasm. In hematoxylin & eosin (H&E) sections of lung containing *Pneumocystis* organisms, the nuclei of the trophozoite are often seen as small dots in the frothy material found in alveoli (Fig. 12–9).

The cysts occur in various stages of development and vary from 6 to 8 microns in diameter. The stages include a precyst, a cyst containing up to 8 intracytoplasmic bodies (sporozoites), and an empty cyst that has lost its intracystic body. The cyst wall stains with GMS whereas intracystic bodies and trophozoites do not stain with GMS.[38] The intracystic bodies may show nuclear staining with Giemsa stain.[38] The cyst characteristically has a localized area of thickening that stains strongly with GMS and appears as a darkly stained dot[39] (Fig. 12–10). Depending on the orientation of the cyst, this thickened area may appear to be within the cyst but is in fact on the membrane overlying the contents of the cyst. This thickened area of the membrane is a useful diagnostic finding and aids in distinguishing *Pneumocystis* from yeastlike organisms such as *Histoplasma*. Often, especially in tissue sections, the cyst wall is collapsed or indented, giving the appearance of an indented Ping-Pong ball, crescent, or cup structure; these shapes can be very useful diagnostically. In H&E sections, the cysts and trophozoites are indistinguishable from one another and form part of the foamy alveolar exudate in lungs heavily infected with *Pneumocystis*. Approximately 30 per cent to 40 per cent of the intra-alveolar material consists of organisms;[40] the remainder consists of surfactant, cellular debris, and fibrin. The inflammatory reaction to *Pneumocystis* infection is scant and often consists mainly of alveolar macrophages[41] with no neutrophilic response. In addition, there may be findings of diffuse alveolar damage characterized by septal edema, active fibroplasia, and lymphocytes with hyaline membranes and type 2 pneumocyte proliferation. Rarely a necrotizing granulomatous response has been observed.[37]

The trophozoites are quite sensitive to treatment with trimethoprim-sulfamethoxazole, whereas the cysts may survive such treatment. Although the trophozoites are the most prevalent form in clinical material, they are difficult to identify with certainty since they are negative with the GMS stain. Therefore, one is dependent upon identifying the cysts for a definitive diagnosis.

In bronchoalveolar lavage (BAL) specimens, one may at times encounter a mass of organisms, which represents the intra-alveolar cast

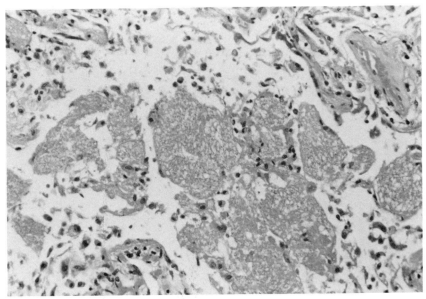

Figure 12–9. *Pneumocystis* pneumonia. Frothy aggregates of organisms in the alveoli are seen, as well as barely discernible nuclear dots. (Hematoxylin & eosin, × 250)

of foamy material that is characteristically found in lung biopsies (Fig. 12–11). The H&E and Pap stains do not stain either the trophozoite or cyst very well. However, if frothy intra-alveolar casts are present in a BAL specimen, H&E and Pap stains will outline the characteristic frothy pattern and stain the small dots representing the nuclei of trophozoites. Trophozoites are stained with Giemsa stain, with

the nucleus red and cytoplasm pale blue. In addition, the DIFF-QUIK stain also stains trophozoites as well as the intracystic bodies. The cyst will also stain positive with PAS stain. Gram and acid-fast stains are negative.

The most reliable and widely used stain for *Pneumocystis* is the GMS stain (Gomori methenamine silver, Grocott modification).[42] This silver stain stains the wall of the cyst form and,

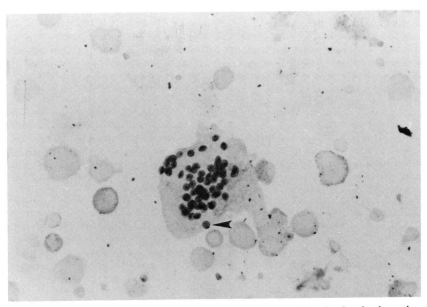

Figure 12–10. *Pneumocystis* pneumonia. There are cysts with prominent dots. Note the dot clearly on the cyst membrane (arrowhead). (Gomori methenamine silver, × 450)

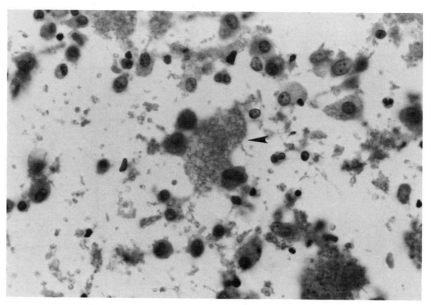

Figure 12–11. *Pneumocystis* pneumonia, showing intra-alveolar casts of foamy material (arrowhead). (Hematoxylin & eosin, × 450)

very importantly, stains the capsular dot, which is the thickened zone of the cyst wall. Trophozoites and intracystic bodies are not stained with GMS. The GMS can be done rapidly by microwave methods and can be accurately interpreted.[43] The morphologic features include round to indented structures (6 to 8 microns), with black staining of the cyst wall but with no internal staining. There are one or two darkly stained dots in the cell wall. When the thickened, dotlike area is in profile, it is easy to see that this is a structure occurring in the cell wall of the organism. However, if the cyst is oriented in other ways, the capsular dot appears to be within the cyst, suggesting a nucleus. It is, therefore, important to find cysts oriented in a manner where this thickening can be seen in the cyst wall, since this finding is diagnostic.

Yeast forms of fungi will show similar GMS staining of their capsules. *Histoplasma* and *Cryptococcus* yeastlike organisms may be in the same size range as *Pneumocystis*. Absence of the cyst wall dot and the presence of budding yeast forms will identify the organism as yeast forms of a fungus. Also, *Histoplasma* and *Cryptococcus* often have a granulomatous reaction that can appear with *Pneumocystis* but is much less common.[37] Staining of debris by GMS poses a problem in many specimens. Attention to details of the *Pneumocystis* morphology should prevent misdiagnosis.

Immunocytochemical stains can be used to identify organisms.[40] However, these are not significantly more sensitive than the GMS stain, and many of these stains will stain both viable and nonviable organisms.[38] The same organisms may also be detected by immunofluorescent techniques and by electron microscopy.

Toxoplasma

Toxoplasmosis is a less common disease than PCP. It can occur in all transplant patients but is most common in heart transplant patients. This is because it can be transmitted most effectively in transplanted heart where more cyst forms reside than in other transplanted organs. In immunocompetent individuals, this disease presents as a primary infection with a mononucleosis type of syndrome. However, in transplant patients it usually presents as reactivated infection with neurologic involvement; myocarditis or pneumonitis has been described. The usual manifestations are fever, visual disturbances, headache, photophobia, focal neurologic manifestations, and seizures. Cerebrospinal fluid examination reveals a slight mononuclear pleocytosis, with elevated protein and normal glucose levels. Diagnosis can be suspected on the basis of prior seropositivity and on brain imaging studies demonstrating intracerebral lesions. Ultimately the diagnosis relies on tissue biopsy.[44]

Pathologic Findings in *Toxoplasma* Infec-

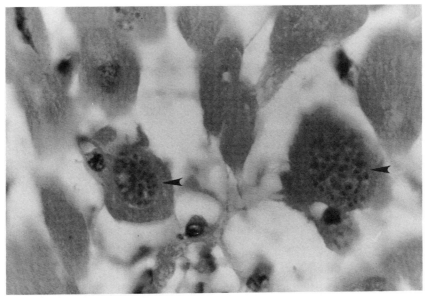

Figure 12–12. *Toxoplasma* cysts in myocardial fibers (arrowheads). Note the many trophozoites with the cysts. (Hematoxylin & eosin, × 450)

tions. In heart transplant patients, the organism can be found in endomyocardial biopsies[44] (Fig. 12–12). Infected cells contain a *Toxoplasma* cyst (up to 100 microns) that contains trophozoites. These trophozoites are usually ovoid or banana shaped and measure 4 to 6 microns in length.[45] No inflammation is present. When the infection is activated, there may be dissemination to various organs, including brain, with necrosis and inflammation. The organisms may be difficult to find in biopsies. Sensitivity and specificity of detection may be increased by immunohistochemical stains using antibodies against *Toxoplasma*.[46] A simpler approach is examining cytocentrifuged spinal fluid using Wright Giemsa stains.[47]

Strongyloides

Strongyloides stercoralis is another potential pathogen in transplant patients. This infection most commonly occurs in the southern parts of the United States, where the parasite is found and where immigrants from Central and South America often settle.[12, 45] This infection can have a very long latency, up to 40 years, from initial infection to presentation. The initial infection occurs when the round worm penetrates the skin from the soil. The organism migrates to the lungs and then is coughed up and swallowed. The adult lives in the duodenum, where mating occurs, and the eggs are released and excreted in the stools.

In some immunocompromised patients, the eggs can hatch in the gut and autoreinfection can occur. This is commonly referred to as hyperinfection syndrome; it often presents with bacterial sepsis or bacterial meningitis associated with a gram-negative organism. Diagnosis can be accomplished by examining stool specimens for typical eggs or by finding the worm in stained sputum samples. Gastric or duodenal biopsies may identify larvae in the mucosa (Fig. 12–13). Serologic assays are available.

FUNGAL INFECTIONS

Invasive fungal infections among transplant patients are often life-threatening complications. They are occurring with greater frequency. The reason for this increasing incidence reflects the effectiveness of complex multidrug immunosuppressive regimens on cell-mediated immunity. Unfortunately, fungal infections disseminate very quickly in transplant patients and can be very difficult to diagnose, often leading to very advanced disease by the time they are recognized.[1–3] Therefore, fungal infections can be very difficult to cure because of the late stage of progression at the time of detection. Patients can acquire primary infection with fungi or they can experience a reactivation. Primary infection usually occurs with opportunistic pathogens such as *Candida*

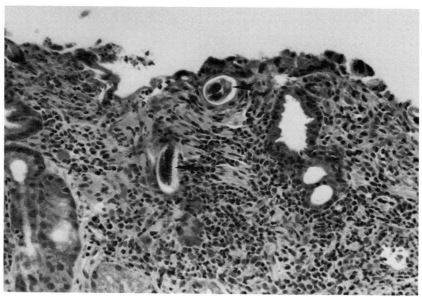

Figure 12–13. *Strongyloides* larva in gastric mucosa. The organism is seen in two cross-sections within the mucosa (arrowheads). (Hematoxylin & eosin, × 250)

species, *Aspergillus* species, *C. neoformans,* and the Mucoraceae. Reactivation of infection usually occurs with the geographically endemic fungi *Histoplasma, Coccidioides,* and *Blastomyces,* although primary infection with these agents is also possible given the proper epidemiologic exposure. A variety of superficial fungal infections can occur in transplant patients, but they are usually mild and self-limited.[1–5]

Candida

Candida species, including *Torulopsis* species, are the most common fungal pathogens in transplant patients. Indeed, it is such a common pathogen that many transplant patients are given prophylaxis with antifungal agents. A wide spectrum of disease is possible, including superficial skin involvement, urinary tract infections, and invasive disease with involvement of perineum, blood stream, liver, eye, and central nervous system. Various invasive devices can act as a portal of entry for this organism. Disseminated *Candida* infections can be notoriously difficult to detect. In *Candida* fungemia, blood cultures are only positive about 50 per cent of the time. Diagnosis requires a high index of suspicion and the isolation of the organism from culture or the identification of the organism on pathologic examination. *Candida* species can be a contaminant from various sources, including skin, sputum, surgical wounds, and catheter drainage. The organism can also be seen as a contaminant in speci-

mens obtained during bronchoscopy. Cultures from blood and sterile sites often reflect true disease. Therefore, a combined modality approach to diagnosis is important in the diagnosis of *Candida* infections in transplant patients.

Aspergillus

Aspergillus species are serious pathogens that often lead to disseminated infection and death among transplant patients. As in *Candida* infections, the disease can evade diagnosis until widespread progression has occurred. Unlike *Candida,* which is an endogenous organism, *Aspergillus* species are usually acquired from the environment. Several studies have related outbreaks to hospital construction projects, presumably by aerosolizing the *Aspergillus.* The portal of entry is the upper respiratory tract with involvement of the lungs or sinuses. Pre-existing lung cavities can be colonized with this organism, leading to the classic presentation of a fungus ball. However, this is not a common presentation in transplant patients, who more commonly develop a diffuse pneumonia with patchy infiltrates on chest radiographs, although consolidation of a particular lobe or segment is possible, which can mimic a bacterial process. Fever, nonproductive cough, dyspnea, and hemoptysis can all be presenting symptoms. Fungemia with dissemination to skin, joints, bone, and central nervous system is possible. Central nervous system involvement usually takes the form of single or multiple brain abscesses.

Diagnosis requires a high degree of suspicion: blood cultures are rarely positive, and no reliable serologic assay is available. *Aspergillus* can be cultured from sputum, but this does not always indicate pathogenicity since it occurs as a contaminant; its isolation should dramatically raise the index of suspicion. The diagnosis is made by pathologic examination of tissue from sites of involvement.[48, 49]

Cryptococcus

Cryptococcal infections are the next most common opportunistic fungal infection in transplant patients. The portal of entry is the lung, where primary infection can cause fever, nonproductive cough, and shortness of breath. Chest radiograph findings usually reveal a focal infiltrate, although a diffuse infiltrate is possible. Pulmonary involvement in transplant patients can be silent, with dissemination occurring and presenting with skin and central nervous system involvement. Cutaneous manifestations include rash and nodules; central nervous system involvement can present with fever, headache, and malaise, although the symptoms can be very mild. Focal neurologic findings are uncommon. Diagnosis requires cultures of pulmonary secretions and cerebrospinal fluid examination, which can reveal lymphocytic pleocytosis, elevated protein levels, and low glucose levels. Tests of cerebrospinal fluid and blood for cryptococcal antigen are most helpful in the diagnosis.[48, 49]

Phycomycoses

Phycomycoses due to *Mucor* and *Rhizopus* species can produce locally destructive rhinocerebral infections that are notoriously resistant to treatment. Infection can progress rapidly and involve the central nervous system. Extension to the brain leads to death without exception. These organisms can also cause infection in surgical wounds. A variety of other saprophytic fungi can cause disease in transplant patients. These organisms rarely cause death and respond to local therapy.[1-5]

Endemic Fungi

The endemic fungi *Histoplasma, Blastomyces,* and *Coccidioides* all occur in transplant patients, but only after the appropriate geographic ex-

posure. Primary infection is reported in transplant patients, but reactivation is far more common. Thus many transplant programs screen patients pretransplant for evidence of prior infection with these organisms. Such serologic studies will provide evidence of prior infection with these agents and allow a concerted surveillance for manifestations of reactivation. Reactivation presents with dissemination, which can lead to insidious syndromes including very mild symptoms of fever, malaise, and fatigue. However, patients can also present with pancytopenia or with more focal manifestations such as diffuse chest radiographic findings, mucocutaneous involvement, or central nervous system involvement. Diagnosis can be quite difficult, and knowledge of prior exposure or positive serologic results can be most helpful. Diagnosis is usually established by pathologic examination of involved tissues or by cultures of involved sites.[1-5]

Pathologic Findings in Fungal Infections. The most common fungi encountered are *Aspergillus* and *Candida* species.[48, 49] *Aspergillus* hyphae are slightly larger than those in *Candida* with a diameter of 3 to 6 microns.[35] The hyphae of *Aspergillus* are septate and show acute angle branching (Fig. 12–14). They may be seen in routine H&E stains but often are obscured by purulent exudate and necrosis. GMS and PAS stains should be done on all specimens from the lung and gastrointestinal tract. The abscesses that are formed in infected livers are usually not sampled for microscopic examination. It is uncommon for conidia (spores) to be present unless the organism is growing in a pulmonary cavity. Conidia are small, 2 to 3 microns, and often are lightly pigmented.[35] *Candida* pseudohyphae are smaller than those of *Aspergillus,* with a diameter of 3 to 4 microns.[35] They are septate branching and may have bulbous enlargements along the hyphal segments (Fig. 12–15). Conidia are commonly present and provide additional morphologic evidence that the organism is a *Candida* species.

Other organisms with morphology similar to that of *Aspergillus* may occur. One example we observed is *Chrysosporium* occurring in the lung of a renal transplant patient (Fig. 12–16). This is ordinarily a commensal organism.[35] Less commonly occurring organisms can be seen, such as *Coccidioides* and *Cryptococcus.*[50] As an example, a liver transplant patient was seen who had disseminated coccidioidomycosis. The organism was identified in a BAL specimen. Characteristically, round organisms that vary considerably in size may be seen with

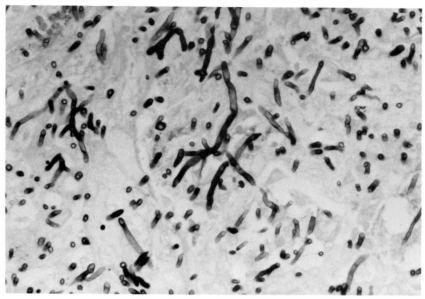

Figure 12–14. *Aspergillus* pneumonia. The hyphae show septa and acute angle branching. (Gomori methenamine silver, × 450)

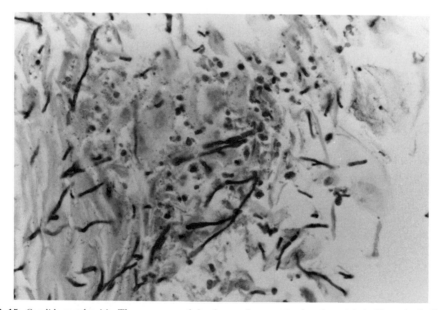

Figure 12–15. *Candida* esophagitis. There are pseudohyphae and spores in the ulcer debris. Note the bulbous enlargements of the hyphae. (Periodic acid–Schiff, × 450)

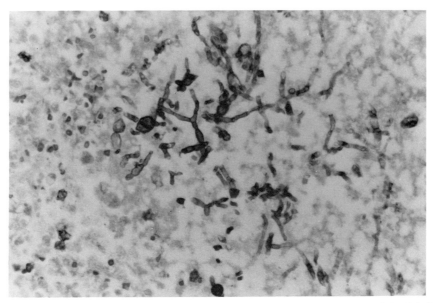

Figure 12–16. *Chrysosporium* species in a lung abscess. There are features of both *Aspergillus* and *Candida*. The organism was identified by culture. (Gomori methenamine silver, × 450)

H&E, GMS, and PAS strains. The largest forms seen are the spherules (30 to 100 microns), which are often filled with endospores[35] (Fig. 12–17). Free endospores (2 to 5 microns) and various-sized spores at various levels of development are present. *Cryptococcus* is 2 to 20 microns in size, with yeastlike budding forms and a PAS-positive, mucicarmine-positive capsule (Fig. 12–18).

Phycomycosis is an infection most often caused by *Rhizopus* species.[35] This organism has a propensity to invade blood vessels, resulting in thrombosis of the blood vessel and ischemic infarction of the surrounding tissue. The hyphae in tissue sections are approximately the size of those of *Aspergillus* (5 to 20 millimicrons in diameter) and can be confused with the latter. *Rhizopus* and *Mucor* differ from *Aspergil-*

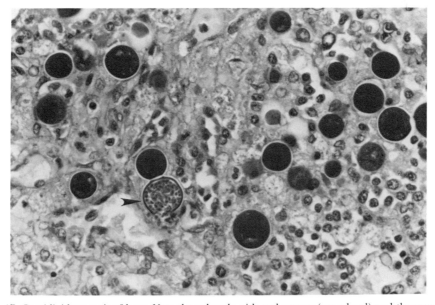

Figure 12–17. Coccidioidomycosis of lung. Note the spherule with endospores (arrowhead) and the many developing spherules of various sizes. (Periodic acid–Schiff, × 450)

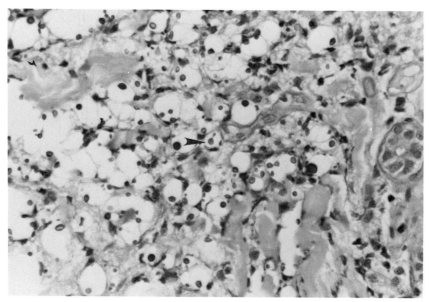

Figure 12–18. Cryptococcal subcutaneous abscess. Budding yeastlike organisms are visible (arrowhead). The space around the organism is the capsule. (Periodic acid–Schiff, × 450)

lus by the former being nonseptate, showing right angle branching, and having irregular, wrinkled hyphal walls. *Aspergillus* is septate, shows acute angle branching, and has parallel walls. *Rhizopus* is easily seen in routine H&E sections since it is stained basophilic with hematoxylin. Fungal stains such as PAS and GMS are very useful in finding the organisms. Spores produced by this organism are not seen in tissue sections unless the hyphae are growing in air-filled cavities.

DIAGNOSTIC CONSIDERATIONS IN INFECTIONS IN TRANSPLANT RECIPIENTS

In infections occurring in transplanted patients, it is common for more than one agent to be present in an infected area.[1, 2, 51] Therefore, one cannot stop searching after one agent is identified. Routine H&E stains as well as special stains for acid-fast organisms, fungi, *Pneumocystis*, and bacteria should be done on all specimens and each stain searched carefully for organisms. For example, it is not at all uncommon for a lung biopsy to contain both cytomegalovirus-infected cells and *Pneumocystis*.

When an infectious agent is present, only a few diagnostic cells may be present. These may not be evident on either the routine or special stains and may require gene probes, immuno-

peroxidase, or other methods. Depending on the site involved, different cell types will be found to contain diagnostic findings. For example, in CMV infections of the liver, characteristic inclusions are found in the epithelial cells, whereas infection in the gastrointestinal tract characteristically shows the inclusions in endothelial and mesenchymal cells.

Sites Most Commonly Examined for Infections

The sites most commonly examined for infections include the lung, liver, stomach, colon, and skin.[1, 2] The following considerations are specific for histologic examination of these sites for various infectious agents:

Lung

Open lung biopsies, transbronchial biopsies, and bronchoalveolar lavage specimens (BAL) may be done. The BAL specimen usually yields an excellent specimen that provides material for both culture and microscopic examination[52] and is usually the first invasive approach for evaluating pulmonary infiltrates. In CMV infections, alveolar lining cells, macrophages, and endothelial cells may be infected (see Figure 12–2). In *Pneumocystis* infections, there may be clusters of organisms or merely single organisms (see Figures 12–9, 12–10, and 12–

11). Lung specimens can also include fungi, especially *Aspergillus* and *Candida,* other viral infections such as herpes and adenovirus, as well as bacteria (see Figures 12–14, 12–16, and 12–17). Acid-fast organisms may also occur, including *Mycobacterium tuberculosis, M. avium-intracellulare,* and *Nocardia* (see Figure 12–8). Rarely, pulmonary alveolar proteinosis has been reported in transplant patients.[53] This intra-alveolar acellular substance has a granular eosinophilic appearance and may resemble *Pneumocystis* pneumonia (Fig. 12–19). No pneumocystic organisms are seen, although GMS stain may stain particles of the material. In immunosuppressed patients, an alveolar proteinosis change may occur in the presence of a variety of infections, including bacterial, fungal, and viral.[54]

Liver

In the liver, viral inclusions may be seen either in hepatic parenchymal cells or in bile duct cells. In CMV-infected parenchymal cells, there may be a cluster of neutrophils around the affected cell. The presence of a microcluster of neutrophils in the liver is strongly suggestive of a CMV infection.[13, 55] A specimen with this finding should be further sectioned to search for a diagnostic inclusion. Less commonly, an epithelioid cell granuloma may occur in the liver related to CMV infection.[14]

Non-necrotizing epithelioid cell granulomas in the liver may occur in association with many different things.[14] Most often the cause is not established. Other organisms such as bacteria and fungi produce abscesses in the liver, which are usually not sampled as biopsies.

Gastrointestinal Tract

In the esophagus, *Candida* and herpes infections may occur in immunocompetent patients. However, the most common setting is the immunocompromised host. Cytomegalovirus occurs in the esophagus exclusively in immunocompromised hosts.[56, 57] In the stomach and colon, the diagnostic CMV-infected cells are most often endothelial and mesenchymal cells.[19] Less commonly, epithelial cells will show the characteristic change. However, duodenal biopsy may show involvement of Brunner gland epithelium[58] (see Figure 12–4). In the lamina propria or submucosa of the gastrointestinal tract, capillaries and arterioles are often infected, manifested by strikingly enlarged endothelial cells. Inclusions in the cells often are not classic and may be ill defined or not evident at all. However, the presence of markedly enlarged endothelial cells should be considered strongly suggestive of CMV infection. The affected area shows stromal edema; inflammatory cells are present in scant number; these do not obscure the diagnostic cells

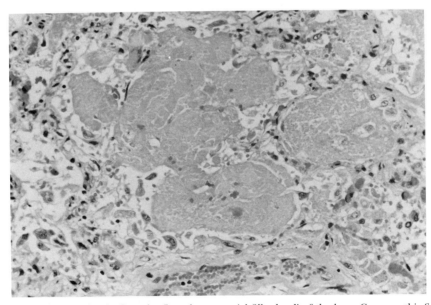

Figure 12–19. Alveolar proteinosis. Granular flocculent material fills alveoli of the lung. Compare this figure with the *Pneumocystis* pneumonia shown in Figure 12–9. Special stains showed *Aspergillus* organisms with the material; see Figure 12–14. (Hematoxylin & eosin, × 250)

(see Figure 12–3). *Candida* is the most frequently seen fungus in the gastrointestinal tract and is most commonly seen in esophageal ulceration, at times in conjunction with herpetic lesions.[19] Gastric biopsies may also show *Candida* organisms in the superficial part of an ulcer. Gastric involvement by *Candida* is most often considered to be colonization of a pre-existing ulceration, whereas in the esophagus the organism may be the cause of the ulceration[59, 60] (see Figure 12–5).

Skin

Punch biopsies of the skin may identify viral or fungal infections. Cytologic examination of vesicle fluid can identify viral inclusion bodies (Tzanck preparation)[12] (see Figure 12–6).

REFERENCES

1. Ho M, Dummer JS. Risk factors and approach to infections in transplant recipients. *In* Mandell GL, Douglas RG, Bennett JE (eds). *Principles and Practices of Infectious Diseases*, 3rd ed. New York, Churchill Livingstone, 1990, p 2284.
2. Ho M, Dummer JS, Peterson PK, Simmons RL. Infections in solid organ transplants. *In* Mandell GL, Douglas RG, Bennett JE (eds). *Principles and Practices of Infectious Diseases*, 3rd ed. New York, Churchill Livingstone, 1990, p 2292.
3. Tolkoff-Rubin NE, Rubin RH. Infection in organ transplant patients. *In* Gorbach SL, Bartlett JG, Blacklow NR (eds). *Infectious Diseases*. Philadelphia, WB Saunders, 1992, p 1040.
4. Dunn DL, Najarian JS. Infectious complications in transplant surgery. *In* Davis JM, Shires GT (eds). *Principles and Management of Surgical Infections*. Baltimore, Williams & Wilkins, 1985, p 425.
5. Petri WA. Infections in heart transplant recipients. *In* Mandell GL, Douglas RG, Bennett JE (eds). *Principles and Practices of Infectious Diseases, Update # 4*. New York, Churchill Livingstone, 1991.
6. Markin RS, Stratta RJ, Woods GL. Infection after liver transplantation. Am J Surg Pathol 14(suppl):64, 1990.
7. Paya CV, Hermans PE, Washington JA, et al. Incidence, distribution, and outcome of episodes of infection in 100 orthotopic liver transplantations. Mayo Clin Proc 64:555, 1989.
8. Dummer JS, Montero CG, Griffith BP, et al. Infections in heart-lung transplant recipients. Transplantation 41:725, 1986.
9. Dunn DL, Simmons RL. Opportunistic infections after renal transplant. Infection Surg 8:164, 1989.
10. Rubin RH, Tolkoff-Rubin NE. Infection: The new problems. Transplant Proc 21:1440, 1989.
11. Brayman KL, Stephanian E, Matas AJ, et al. Analysis of infectious complications occurring after solid-organ transplantation. Arch Surg 127:38, 1992.
12. von Lichtenberg F. *Pathology of Infectious Diseases*. New York, Raven Press, 1991, p 302.
13. DelBuono EA, Frank TS, Wilson M, Appelman HD. Post-transplant minimicroabscess disease. Lab Invest 66:96A, 1992.
14. Ishak KG. Granulomas of the liver. *In* Ioachim HL (ed). *Pathology of Granulomas*. New York, Raven Press, 1983, p 307.
15. Young JF, Goulian M. Bone marrow fibrin ring granulomas and cytomegalovirus infection. Am J Clin Pathol 99:65, 1993.
16. Arbustini E, Grasso M, Diegoli M, et al. Histopathologic and molecular profile of human cytomegalovirus infections in patients with heart transplants. Am J Clin Pathol 98:205, 1992.
17. Millett R, Tomita T, Marshall HE, et al. Cytomegalovirus endomyocarditis in a transplanted heart: A case report with in situ hybridization. Arch Pathol Lab Med 115:511, 1991.
18. Masih AS, Linder J, Shaw BW, et al. Rapid identification of cytomegalovirus in liver allograft biopsies by in situ hybridization. Am J Surg Pathol 12:362, 1988.
19. Lewin KJ, Riddell RH, Weinstein WM (eds). *Gastrointestinal Pathology and Its Clinical Implications*. New York, Igaku-Shoin, 1992, p 123.
20. Thung SN, Shim K, Shieh YSC, et al. Hepatitis C in liver allografts. Arch Pathol Lab Med 117:145, 1993.
21. Demetris AJ, Todo S, Van Thiel DH, et al. Evolution of hepatitis B virus liver disease after hepatic replacement. Am J Pathol 137:667, 1990.
22. Snover DC (ed). *Biopsy Diagnosis of Liver Disease*. Baltimore, Williams & Wilkins, 1992.
23. Pereira BJG, Milford EL, Kirkman RL, Levey AS. Transmission of hepatitis C virus by organ transplantation. N Engl J Med 325:454, 1991.
24. Pereira BJG, Milford EL, Kirkman RL: Prevalence of hepatitis C virus RNA in organ donors positive for hepatitis C antibody and in the recipients of their organs. N Engl J Med 327:910, 1992.
25. Demetris AJ, Jaffe R, Sheahan DG, et al. Recurrent hepatitis B in liver allograft recipients: Differentiation between viral hepatitis B and rejection. Am J Pathol 125:161, 1986.
26. Demetris AJ, Jaffe R, Sheahan DG, et al. Hepatitis B virus infection and liver transplantation. Hepatology 7:973, 1987.
27. Hanson CA, Sutherland DE, Snover DC. Fulminant hepatic failure in an HBsAg carrier renal transplant patient following cessation of immunosuppressive therapy. Transplantation 39:311, 1985.
28. Kharsa G, Degott C, Degos F, et al. Fulminant hepatitis in renal transplant recipients: The role of the delta agent. Transplantation 44:221, 1987.
29. Thomas HC. Acute liver decompensation on withdrawal of cytotoxic chemotherapy and immunosuppressive therapy in hepatitis B carriers: Implications for the treatment of chronic HBV carriers. Q J Med 270:873, 1989.
30. Pinto PC, Hu E, Bernstein-Singer M, Pinter-Brown L, Govindarajan S. Acute hepatic injury after the withdrawal of immunosuppressive chemotherapy in patients with hepatitis B. Cancer 65:878, 1990.
31. Marinucci G, Valeri L, Alfani D, et al. Delta infection and liver disease recurrence in hepatic allografts. Transplant Proc 18:1402, 1986.
32. Koneru B, Jaffe R, Esquivel CO, et al. Adenoviral infections in pediatric liver transplant recipients. JAMA 258:489, 1987.
33. Rosai J. *Ackerman's Surgical Pathology*. St. Louis, Mosby, 1989, pp 54–56, 1023.
34. Chapman SW, Wilson JP. Nocardiosis in transplant recipients. Semin Respir Infect 5:74, 1990.
35. Chandler FW, Watts JC (eds). *Pathologic Diagnosis of Fungal Infections*. Chicago, ASCP Press, 1987.

36. Gutierrez Y. The biology of *Pneumocystis carinii.* Semin Diagn Pathol 6:203, 1989.
37. Saldana MJ, Mones JM. Cavitation and other atypical manifestations of *Pneumocystis carinii* pneumonia. Semin Diagn Pathol 6:273, 1989.
38. Bedrossian CWM, Mason MR, Gupta PK. Rapid cytologic diagnosis of *Pneumocystis:* A comparison of effective techniques. Semin Diagn Pathol 6:245, 1989.
39. Watts JC, Chandler FW. *Pneumocystis carinii* pneumonitis: The nature and diagnostic significance of the methenamine silver–positive intracystic bodies. Am J Surg Pathol 9:744, 1985.
40. Bedrossian CWM. Ultrastructure of *Pneumocystis carinii:* A review of internal and surface characteristics. Semin Diagn Pathol 6:212, 1989.
41. Lanken PN, Minda M, Pietra GG, et al. Alveolar response to experimental *Pneumocystis carinii* pneumonia in the rat. Am J Pathol 99:561, 1980.
42. Amin MB, Mezger E, Zarbo RJ. Detection of *Pneumocystis carinii:* Comparative study of monoclonal antibody and silver staining. Am J Clin Pathol 98:13, 1992.
43. Brinn NT. Rapid metallic histological staining using the microwave oven. J Histotech 6:125, 1983.
44. Cuft BJ, Naut Y, Aranjo FG, et al. Primary and reactivated *Toxoplasma* infection in patients with cardiac transplants. Ann Intern Med 99:27, 1983.
45. Noble ER, Noble GA (eds). *Parasitology: The Biology of Animal Parasites.* Philadelphia, Lea & Febiger, 1982, p 80.
46. Conley FK, Jenkins HT, Remington JS. *Toxoplasma gondii* infection of the central nervous system. Hum Pathol 12:690, 1980.
47. McCabe RE, Remington JS. *Toxoplasma gondii. In* Mandell GL, Douglas RG, Bennett JE (eds). *Principles and Practices of Infectious Disease,* 3rd ed. New York, Churchill Livingstone, 1990, p 2090.
48. Wajszczuk CP, Dummer JS, Ho M, et al. Fungal infections in liver transplant recipients. Transplantation 40:347, 1985.
49. Ho M. Laboratory evaluations of infections in immunosuppressed transplant patients. Clin Lab Med 11:715, 1991.
50. Dodd LG, Nelson SD. Disseminated coccidioidomycosis detected by percutaneous liver biopsy in a liver transplant recipient. Am J Clin Pathol 93:141, 1990.
51. Paya CV, Hermans PE, Washington JA, et al. Incidence, distribution and outcome of episodes of infection in 100 orthotopic liver transplantations. Mayo Clin Proc 64:555, 1989.
52. Pisani RJ, Wright AJ. Clinical utility of bronchoalveolar lavage in immunocompromised hosts. Mayo Clin Proc 67:221, 1992.
53. Bedrossian CWM, Luna MA, Conklin RH, Miller WC. Alveolar proteinosis as a consequence of immunosuppression. A hypothesis based on clinical pathologic observations. Hum Pathol 11:527, 1980.
54. Colby TV, Lombard C, Yousem SA, Kitaichi M (eds). *Atlas of Pulmonary Surgical Pathology.* Philadelphia, WB Saunders, 1991, p 372.
55. Snover DC, Hutton S, Balfour HH, Bloomer JR. Cytomegalovirus infection of the liver in transplant recipients. J Clin Gastroenterol 9:659, 1987.
56. Alexander JA, Brouillette DE, Chien MC, et al. Infectious esophagitis following liver and renal transplantation. Dig Dis Sci 33:1121, 1988.
57. McDonald GB, Sharma P, Hackman RC, et al. Esophageal infections in immunosuppressed patients after marrow transplantation. Gastroenterology 88:1111, 1985.
58. Franzin G, Muolo A, Griminelli T. Cytomegalovirus inclusions in the gastroduodenal mucosa of patients after renal transplantation. Gut 22:698, 1981.
59. Gotlieb-Jensen K, Andersen J. Occurrence of *Candida* in gastric ulcers. Significance for the healing process. Gastroenterology 85:535, 1983.
60. DiFebo G, Miglioli M, Calo G, et al. *Candida albicans* infection of gastric ulcer. Gastroenterol Clin Biol 30:178, 1985.

13

NEOPLASMS OCCURRING IN SOLID ORGAN TRANSPLANT RECIPIENTS

ROBERT L. FLINNER, MD

Organ transplantation with immunosuppression is associated with an increased incidence of neoplasms occurring in the recipient.[1] Early reported incidences of malignancy varied from 2 per cent to 7 per cent.[2] In many early series, short survival of the patient precluded time for development of a neoplasm. More recent studies have reported malignancy incidences of from 3 per cent to 11 per cent within the first year and up to 21 per cent after 5 years.[2] Up to 5 per cent of transplanted patients will develop more than one neoplasm.[2] If the cause were simply due to suppression of immune surveillance, one would expect a general increase in all tumors rather than the very selective increase that occurs (lymphoproliferative disease, skin cancer, cervical and vulvar cancer). This selection suggests that there must be another factor (or factors) responsible.

One factor is the effect of oncogenic viruses; viral infections are very common in transplant patients, especially Epstein-Barr virus (EBV), herpes simplex virus (HSV), and cytomegalovirus (CMV). The frequency of EBV infections in a transplant population varies from 16 per cent to 38 per cent, with lower incidences in renal allograft recipients.[3] In contrast, CMV infection in transplanted populations is much higher: 77 per cent in renal transplants, 66 per cent in liver transplants, and 96 per cent in heart and heart-lung recipients.

What determines whether the virus produces an infectious disease or a neoplasm is not known. The most extensively studied virus-tumor relationship is Burkitt's lymphoma. The EBV virus plays a central role in the genesis of this tumor. However, it is apparent that a cofactor is necessary. In African Burkitt's lymphoma, the cofactor has been shown to be the chronic antigenic stimulation resulting from chronic infection with malaria.[1] A viral infection may be activated either by immunosuppression or immune stimulation. In the case of organ transplantation, the key cofactor may be chronic immune stimulation by the allograft.

In skin cancer, herpes simplex virus I (HSV) and herpes zoster virus (HZV) have been implicated.[1] Ultraviolet light may transform HSV-I from infectious to oncogenic activity. Cytomegalovirus has been suspected, though not established, in the pathogenesis of Kaposi's sarcoma.[4–6] Papilloma virus is related to cervical and vulvar intraepithelial neoplasm/carcinoma in a similar manner (Table 13–1).

There is abundant evidence that Epstein-Barr virus (EBV) plays a central role in the pathogenesis of post-transplant lymphoproliferative disorder (PTLD).[3, 7–9] This may be either a primary or reactivation infection, although primary infections result in a higher frequency of PTLD at shorter intervals after transplant.[6] In the great majority of cases of PTLD, evidence can be found of EBV infection. The EBV genome has been demonstrated in the proliferating B cells in PTLD by in situ hybridization techniques.[10, 11] Immunohisto-

Table 13–1. Types of Malignancies Related to Immunosuppressive Regimens

Type	Before CsA (%)	After CsA (%)
PTLD	12	41
Skin cancer	40	15
Kaposi's sarcoma	3	8
Cervix	6	2
Vulva/perineum	3	>1

chemical studies demonstrate evidence of a latent EBV infection.[12, 13]

POST-TRANSPLANT LYMPHOPROLIFERATIVE DISORDER

Although post-transplant lymphoproliferative disorder (PTLD) is a common neoplastic process in patients with solid tumor allografts, there has been no change in the absolute incidence of PTLD since the advent of cyclosporine use in the early 1980s.[14] There has been a change in incidence relative to other tumors (from 12 per cent to 41 per cent; see Table 13–1) because of the dramatic drop in the incidence of skin cancer. The overall incidence has remained approximately 1.7 per cent.[3] There is a difference in the incidence related to the type of organ (allograft) trans-planted; heart-lung recipients have an increased incidence over other solid organs.[7, 15] The striking incidence in heart-lung transplants may be related to several specific factors, including the propensity to develop multiple severe episodes of infections and/or rejection, frequent occurrence of primary EBV infections, and increased intensity of immunosuppression in heart-lung cases compared with other allografts.[7]

Relationship of PTLD to Type of Allograft

The incidence of PTLD is directly related to the type of allograft.[7] In renal transplants, up to 50 per cent of reported cases have been in the central nervous system, although the majority of these reports deal with patients in the precyclosporine era. By contrast, in liver transplants, there is nodal involvement in 48 per cent, gastrointestinal tract involvement in 26 per cent, and rare central nervous system or allograft involvement. In heart-lung transplants, 60 per cent of PTLD is primarily pulmonary. A much lower incidence of lung involvement is seen in other types of allografts. Involvement by PTLD of the allograft occurs in 17 per cent of kidneys and in 8.6 per cent of livers; there are rare cases in heart transplants[7] (Figs. 13–1, 13–2, and 13–3).

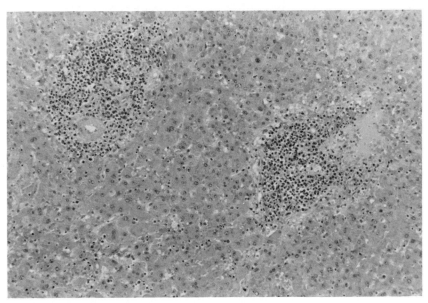

Figure 13–1. PTLD involving the liver. The portal triads are expanded by a dense lymphoid infiltrate. (Hematoxylin & eosin, × 100)

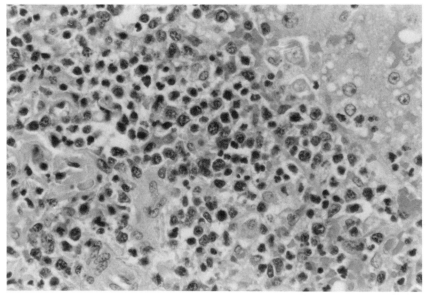

Figure 13–2. PTLD involving the liver. A polymorphous dense lymphoid infiltrate is seen. (Hematoxylin & eosin, × 450)

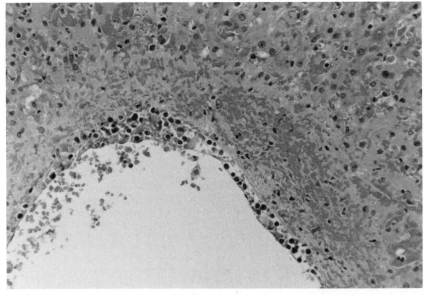

Figure 13–3. PTLD involving the liver. The large lymphoid cells infiltrate beneath the endothelium of a vein. This resembles endothelialitis seen in cellular rejection. (Hematoxylin & eosin, × 250)

Relationship of PTLD and Type of Immunosuppression

The incidence of PTLD varies considerably in relation to the drug regimens used for immunosuppression. With precyclosporine agents such as antilymphocyte globulin (ALG), prednisone, and azathioprine (AZ), an incidence of PTLD of from 1.0 per cent to 4.9 per cent has been reported.[16-18] With high doses of cyclosporine A (CSA), there is a much higher incidence of from 9 per cent to 13 per cent.[19, 20] However, with lower doses of CSA and close monitoring of CSA blood levels, the reported incidence varies from 0 per cent to 1.5 per cent.[21, 22] A combination of CSA, AZ, and prednisone has a reported incidence of 5.3 per cent.[22] With the addition of OKT3 there was a reported incidence of 11.4 per cent in cardiac transplants.[23] Thus it appears that the incidence of PTLD, in part, depends on the immunosuppressive regimen employed.

With CSA, the PTLD occurs at a shorter interval after transplantation (average, 20 months)[6, 15] compared with conventional immunosuppressive therapy (ALG, AZ) (average, 42 months). The distribution of involvement also differs with CSA-treated cases; in CSA-treated recipients, lymph node and small bowel tumors are more frequent. In AZ-treated cases central nervous system involvement is more frequent.[15, 17]

Relationship of EBV, Cyclosporine Therapy, and PTLD

Epstein Barr virus (EBV) infects B cells and causes them to proliferate.[24] In the immunologically competent patient, activated cytotoxic and suppressor T lymphocytes then function and remove the virally infected B cells, thus ending the clinical infection.[25] There may be a less important role for humoral antibodies,[26] natural killer cells,[27] T lymphocytes, and cytokines like interferon-gamma.[27] Cyclosporin A specifically inhibits the proliferation of T lymphocytes and thus allows unopposed proliferation of EBV-infected B lymphocytes.[28] Thus, post-transplant lymphoproliferative disorders are more likely to emerge with CSA immunosuppression, and they are potentially reversible with the removal of CSA therapy.[28] A similar mechanism is observed with azathioprine.[29] A number of other factors contribute to the development of PTLD. These include type of

EBV infection (primary or reactivation), route of infection,[30] interaction of other viruses with EBV,[31, 32] types of drugs used,[22] and degree of immunosuppression.[23]

Pathogenesis of PTLD (Fig. 13–4)

1. The Epstein-Barr virus infects the B lymphocytes, causing them to proliferate in a polyclonal manner.[24] In the normal, immunologically competent person, there is a concomitant proliferation of cytotoxic T cells that prevents uninhibited proliferation of the infected B cells.[25] In reactivation infections,[14] memory T cells are present that proliferate and react early to the infection.

2. Chronic immune stimulation by the allograft acts as a cofactor by activating the oncogenic virus.

3. Immunosuppression (especially the direct effect of CSA[14]) prevents proliferation of T cells and their inhibiting effect on EBV-infected B cells. This results in rapidly proliferating clones of infected B cells (polyclonal PTLD, polymorphous proliferation).

4. Clonal selection, genetic alterations, or both[33] result in the emergence of one or more clones of cells in the proliferating population (monoclonal/oligoclonal,[34] monomorphic proliferation).

5. Chromosomal translocations or activation of host cell oncogenes then may lead to malignant transformation of the cells (monomorphic proliferation). Therefore, the emergence of malignant monoclonal PTLD lesions depends not only on the viral transformation of EBV-infected B cell populations but also on occurrence of chromosomal translocations.[3]

6. Removal or decrease in immunosuppression will result in complete regression in some of the polyclonal as well as monoclonal proliferations.[35]

Clinical Presentations of PTLD

Post-transplant lymphoproliferative disorder has three different clinical presentations:[15]

1. Prominent head and neck involvement with infectious mononucleosis-like findings.[14] This includes cervical lymphadenopathy, pharyngitis, and fever. This occurs in about 47 per cent of cases. The lymph nodes of head and neck will show PTLD on biopsy. In one half of these patients, the PTLD is self-limited,

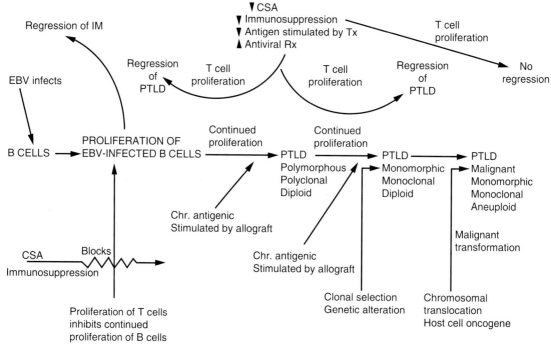

Figure 13–4. Diagram of the pathogenesis of post-transplant lymphoproliferative disorder (PTLD).

whereas in the other 50 per cent it is rapidly fatal. The patients are usually young (average, 21 years), and the condition develops soon after transplantation (4.5 to 9 months).[14, 15]

2. Extranodal tumor masses involving the gastrointestinal tract, liver, lung, oral cavity, and central nervous system. This type of presentation occurs in 53 per cent of cases. The gastrointestinal involvement (small intestinal masses) may perforate, producing acute abdominal symptoms. This form is seen in older age groups (average, 47 years) and occurs at a longer interval from transplantation (up to several years).[15]

3. Allograft failure may occur due to infiltration by PTLD. This especially will involve the allografted lung.[14]

Pathologic Findings in PTLD[15]

Grossly, PTLD may either diffusely infiltrate the organ or form tumor masses.[15, 35] Microscopically, the lymphoid proliferation consists of B lymphocytes that may be polymorphic or monomorphic. In the polymorphic type, there is a range of lymphocytes representing all levels of differentiation (activation), including small lymphocytes, small and large cleaved and noncleaved cells, immunoblasts, plasmacytoid

lymphocytes, and plasma cells[35] (Fig. 13–5). This type occurs in approximately 56 per cent of the cases.[15] Other cases are monomorphic, consisting of a uniform population of cells at one level of differentiation (Fig. 13–6). These vary from large, noncleaved cells (large cell lymphoma); small, noncleaved types (Burkitt-like); and immunoblastic type. The monomorphic type was found in 15 per cent of cases (Figs. 13–7 and 13–8). An intermediate group of cases showed slight polymorphism (29 per cent of cases).

In one study of the clonality of PTLD lesions, it was found that 28 per cent were monoclonal, 30 per cent polyclonal, and 12 per cent both monoclonal and polyclonal (in separate lesions) in the same patients. In an additional 30 per cent, the clonality was indeterminant. Some of the cases showing monoclonal PTLDs had several monoclonal proliferations but not always with identical immunoglobulin gene rearrangement patterns (oligoclonal). This suggests that either multiple independent lesions were occurring or there was a continuing process of gene rearrangement in the tumor. It has been suggested that PTLD lesions represent a spectrum of lesions from polymorphous to monomorphic and polyclonal to monoclonal and that the lesions may evolve and progress along this pathway.[4, 35] Thus, in some cases the

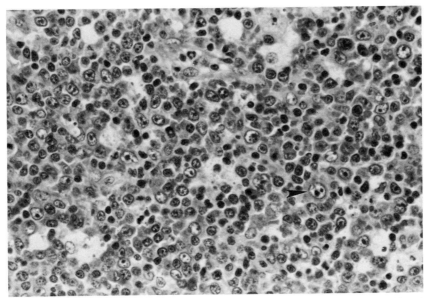

Figure 13–5. PTLD involving a lymph node. This is a polymorphous type, with a wide range of lymphoid cells from immunoblasts (arrowhead) to small lymphocytes and plasma cells. The infiltrate was polyclonal on immunoperoxidase studies. (Hematoxylin & eosin, × 400)

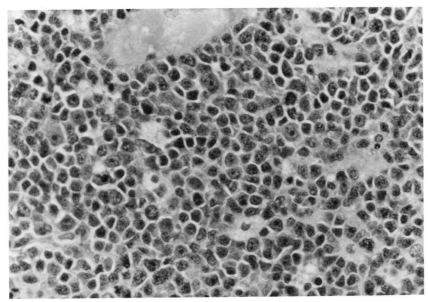

Figure 13–6. PTLD. A monomorphic population of large lymphoid cells is seen. Immunoperoxidase stain indicated that cells were monoclonal. (Hematoxylin & eosin, × 400)

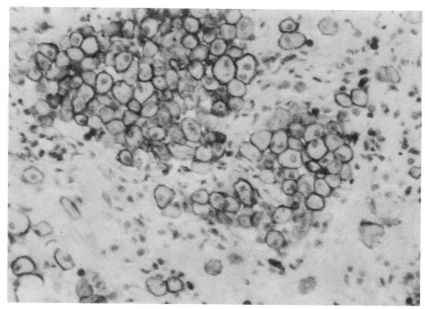

Figure 13–7. PTLD. Monomorphic staining of the large lymphoid cells of Figure 13–5. CD 20, a pan B marker, is diffusely positive on the membranes of all the cells. Cells all expressed kappa light chain. (Immunoperoxidase, × 400)

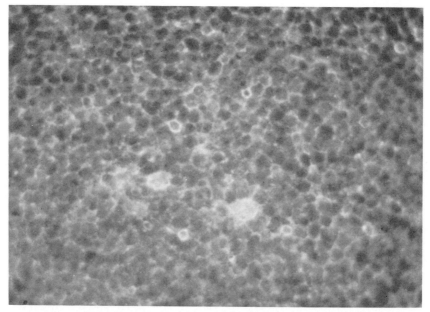

Figure 13–8. PTLD; monomorphic staining of the lymphoid cells comprising this monomorphic infiltrate in a lymph node. Some intracytoplasmic as well as membrane staining is seen. Cells were labeled with kappa light chain using an immunofluorescence procedure. (× 250)

Table 13–2. Histologic and Clonal Findings in PTLD

Histology	Clonality	Therapy (see text)
Polymorphous	55% polyclonal	Acyclovir
	45% monoclonal	Stop immunosuppression
Minimal polymorphism	18% polyclonal	Stop immunosuppression
	78% monoclonal	± Cytotoxic chemotherapy
Monomorphic	100% monoclonal	Cytotoxic chemotherapy
		Radiation therapy

process is reactive with polyclonality. At the other extreme are cases that are clearly malignant based on morphologic, immunologic, and genetic evidence.

Of the cases showing a polymorphic histology, 55 per cent are polyclonal and 45 per cent monoclonal.[15] Of those showing minimal polymorphism, 18 per cent are polyclonal and 78 per cent monoclonal. Of those showing a monomorphic proliferation, all are found to be monoclonal. Thus, the polymorphic lesions can be either monoclonal or polyclonal, while the monomorphic lesions appear to be uniformly monoclonal. Gene rearrangement studies confirm these findings of clonality (Table 13–2). A practical approach to diagnosis is to divide the cases into either polymorphic or monomorphic types. Studies of clonality will help support the histologic findings of type of lesion. It is recommended that all these lesions be called PTLD rather than malignant lymphoma, since many are potentially reversible by decreasing immunosuppression.

Response to Treatment in PTLD

The first line of treatment in patients with PTLD consists of withdrawing or decreasing the immunosuppression.[4] The majority of cases that either regress (23 per cent) or resolve (44 per cent) on withdrawal of immunosuppression are polymorphous, with histology and clonality identical to the remaining cases that had no response. These latter cases often involved multiple sites. Gene rearrangements showed that the monoclonal tumors among the nonresponsive group were likely to have clonal rearrangement, with strong intensity of rearranged bands. Although many cases of PTLD are potentially reversible, the histologic appearance of the PTLD and its clonality do not predict the clinical course or outcome upon reduction of immunosuppression.[3]

Another therapeutic approach is the use of acyclovir for the polymorphous, polyclonal

types of PTLD.[14] This agent acts by blocking viral replication; the effectiveness of the agent in PTLD has yet to be established. In cases with evidence of malignant transformation, chemotherapy and radiation are used in conjunction with decreasing or discontinuing the immunosuppression[34] (see Table 13–2).

OTHER LYMPHOPROLIFERATIVE PROCESSES OCCURRING IN TRANSPLANT RECIPIENTS

Although most lymphoproliferative processes in allograft recipients appear to be EBV-induced B cell proliferations that we designate as PTLD, in a small number of cases association with EBV is not found.[17, 36] A small number of peripheral T cell lymphomas occur in allograft recipients.[37, 38] These have been suppressor, helper, or null phenotypes, lymphoblastic lymphoma, or T cell lymphoma/leukemia.[38] The T cell lymphomas behave as fully malignant lesions, with no cases showing regression. Hodgkin's disease in post-transplant patients is notable by its rarity.[39]

Finally, there is a group of patients with findings suggesting hyersensitivity lymphadenopathy.[40–42, 44] A florid immunoblastic proliferation of polyclonal B cells resembles the forms of PTLD described earlier. This has associated prominent lymphadenopathy. Some patients have fever, arthralgia, and skin rash. In all such patients, the lymphadenopathy and associated findings subside quickly with or without withdrawal of immunosuppression.[41, 43] It is felt that these cases represent a hypersensitivity reaction to foreign proteins such as OKT3. Some patients treated with such foreign proteins make anti-idiotypic antibody responses to these agents, which creates a serum sickness–like illness. If this mechanism can be established to be the cause of the lymphadenopathy, additional therapy is not needed since the process is self-limited or will improve upon withdrawal from the sensitizing agent.

OTHER NEOPLASMS IN TRANSPLANTATION

In addition to PTLD, other neoplasms show an increased incidence in transplanted patients.[44] These include squamous cell carcinoma of the skin and lip; carcinoma of the cervix, especially carcinoma in situ; squamous cell carcinoma of the vulva and perineum; and Kaposi's sarcoma. These neoplasms are related to activation of oncogenic viruses by the immunosuppression or by chronic immunologic stimulation of the transplanted organ.

Neoplasms Transplanted with the Allograft

In the early experience with transplantation, especially renal transplants, cases occurred in which carcinomas developed related to transplantation of malignant cells from the donor.[2] These were either primary tumors of the kidney or, more often, metastases to the kidney from other primary tumors in the donor. Most of these were bronchogenic carcinomas, malignant melanomas, and breast cancer. Some of these tumors showed regression following removal of the transplanted kidney and the stopping of immunosuppression. Because of this experience, patients are not acceptable as donors if they have malignant neoplasms, with the exception of skin cancer and primary brain tumors. It was noted that there was up to a 40 per cent chance of a transplanted kidney containing malignant cells from a person who had a primary malignant tumor elsewhere in the body.[2]

Pre-existing Neoplasms in the Host

Patients transplanted for malignant hepatic or renal neoplasms do poorly, with a high incidence of recurrence of the tumor.[2] Exceptions are small, incidentally found hepatomas or renal cell carcinomas.[2] One cardiac patient was transplanted for a widely invasive hemangioendothelioma of the heart. He is doing well 5 years post-transplant (author's case).

Skin and Lip Carcinoma

Squamous cell carcinoma has a high incidence in transplant recipients[44] (Fig. 13–9). These tumors occur in sun-exposed areas, just as is seen in nontransplant patients, although there is also an increased incidence in nonsun-exposed areas. There is evidence that herpes simplex I virus is important in the pathogenesis of these tumors. Most of the squamous cell carcinomas of the skin are of low-grade malignancy and can be treated by local excision without reducing immunosuppression. Use of sun screens may greatly reduce the incidence of these lesions. Other cutaneous lesions that may occur include hyperkeratoses, keratoacanthomas, and porokeratosis of Mibelli.[45]

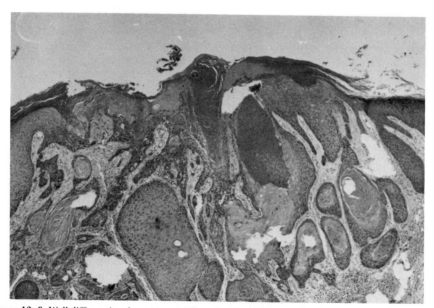

Figure 13–9. Well-differentiated squamous cell carcinoma of the lip. (Hematoxylin & eosin, × 250)

Basal cell carcinomas also occur, but squamous cell carcinoma is considerably more common in transplant recipients. This is the reverse of the case in the general population. The skin tumors are often multiple (43 per cent of cases).[44] Although the tumors are usually low grade, some do show aggressiveness; in some cases lymph node metastases and death from the skin cancer have occurred. Other non-neoplastic lesions that could be confused with carcinoma include viral warts and chronic ulcers of the lower lip.

Malignant melanoma of the skin also has an increased incidence in transplant recipients.[44]

Cervical and Perineal Carcinomas

There is an increased incidence of carcinoma of the cervix, especially carcinoma in situ or dysplasia, in transplant recipients. An increased incidence of carcinomas of the vulva, perineum, penis, and scrotum is also seen.[44]

Kaposi's Sarcoma

Kaposi's sarcoma shows an increased incidence in transplant recipients.[11, 12] The incidence is not nearly as high as has been observed in patients with AIDS (acquired immune deficiency syndrome).[46] Complete regression of the lesions has been observed in some cases following decrease of immunosuppression.[44, 47]

Evidence has been presented suggesting an etiologic role for cytomegalovirus (CMV) in the pathogenesis of Kaposi's sarcoma.[48, 49] Recent studies using more specific gene probes have failed to confirm this.[50] Another undetected virus may still play a role in this process. The observed predilection of the Kaposi lesions in the oropharynx and rectum in homosexual men with AIDS suggests transmission of a viral agent by oral or anal routes of inoculation.[51] An oncogene has been found in Kaposi's sarcoma that may produce fibroblast growth factor activity.[51, 52] The growth factor produced by the tumor cells may induce other sites of proliferation. Multifocal lesions may be produced by this mechanism rather than by metastatic spread of the proliferating cells: the lesion is not observed to spread in a contiguous or metastatic pattern but appears at multiple unrelated sites, often simultaneously.[50]

Pathologically, these lesions consist of proliferating spindle cells arranged in fascicles with frequent clefts containing red blood cells (Figs. 13–10 and 13–11). Hemosiderin is commonly present. The degree of nuclear anaplasia varies.[50] Early lesions may consist of prominent vascularity resembling inflammatory or granulation tissue that may be nondiagnostic. In transplanted patients, the most common sites of involvement are skin and gastrointestinal tract.

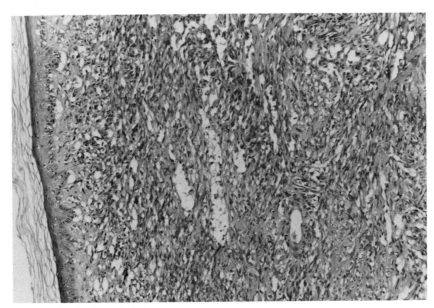

Figure 13–10. Kaposi's sarcoma of the skin. A spindle cell lesion is expanding the dermis. (Hematoxylin & eosin, × 100)

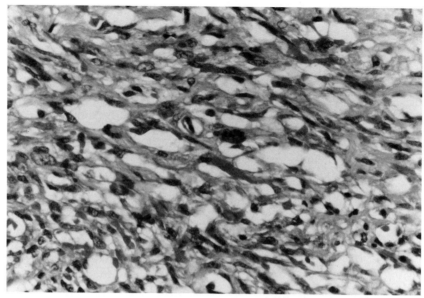

Figure 13–11. Kaposi's sarcoma of the skin. The lesion consists of atypical spindle cells with prominent spaces between the cells. (Hematoxylin & eosin, × 400)

Other Tumors

All the neoplasms occurring in the general population will occur in transplanted patients but with no increased incidence. Thus, tumors commonly found in nontransplanted patients, such as lung, breast, prostate, and colorectal carcinoma, will be found as frequently in the transplanted patient.[2] Since most transplanted patients are younger than patients developing those common neoplasms, the patient's age will determine the incidence of these lesions.

REFERENCES

1. Matas AJ, Simmons RL, Najarian JS. Chronic antigenic stimulation, herpesvirus infection, and cancer in transplant recipients. Lancet 1:1277, 1975.
2. Penn I. Tumor incidence in human allograft recipients. Transplant Proc 11:1047, 1979.
3. Ho M, Miller G, Atchinson RW, et al. Epstein-Barr virus infections and DNA hybridization studies in post-transplantation lymphoma and lymphoproliferative lesions: The role of primary infection. J Infect Dis 152:876, 1985.
4. Little PJ, Khader AA, Farthing CF, et al. Kaposi's sarcoma in a patient after renal transplantation. Postgrad Med J 49:325, 1983.
5. Harwood AR, Osoba D, Goldstein MB, et al. Kaposi's sarcoma in recipients of renal transplants. Am J Med 67:759, 1979.
6. Penn I. Cancers following cyclosporine therapy. Transplantation 43:21, 1987.
7. Randhawa PS, Yousem SA, Paradis IL, et al. The clinical spectrum, pathology, and clonal analysis of Epstein-Barr virus-associated lymphoproliferative disorders in heart-lung transplant recipients. Am J Clin Pathol 92:177, 1989.
8. Randhawa PS, Markin RS, Starzl TE, Demetris AJ, et al. Epstein-Barr virus-associated syndromes in immunosuppressed liver transplant recipients. Am J Surg Pathol 14:538, 1990.
9. Hanto DW, Frizzera G, Pertilo DT, et al. Clinical spectrum of lymphoproliferative disorders in renal transplant recipients and evidence for the role of Epstein-Barr virus. Cancer Res 41:4253, 1981.
10. Weiss LM, Movahed LA. In situ demonstration of Epstein-Barr viral genomes in viral-associated B cell lymphoproliferations. Am J Pathol 134:651, 1989.
11. Borisch-Chappuis B, Nezelof C, Muller H, Muller-Hermelink HK. Different Epstein-Barr virus expression in lymphomas from immunocompromised and immunocompetent patients. Am J Pathol 136:751, 1990.
12. Thomas JA, Hotchin NA, Allday JJ, et al. Immunohistology of Epstein-Barr virus associated antigens in B cell disorders from immunocompromised individuals. Transplantation 49:944, 1990.
13. Young L, Alfieri C, Hennessy K, et al. Expression of Epstein-Barr virus transformation-associated genes in tissues of patients with EBV lymphoproliferative disease. N Engl J Med 321:1080, 1989.
14. Hanto DW, Frizzera G, Gajl-Peczalska KJ, Simmon RL, et al. Epstein-Barr virus, immunodeficiency, and B cell lymphoproliferation. Transplantation 39:461, 1985.
15. Nalesnik MA, Jaffe R, Starzl TE, et al. The pathology of post-transplant lymphoproliferative disorders occurring in the setting of cyclosporine A-prednisone immunosuppression. Am J Pathol 133:173, 1988.
16. Hanto DW, Gajl-Peczalska KJ, Frizzera G, et al. Epstein-Barr virus (EBV) induced polyclonal and monoclonal B-cell lymphoproliferative diseases occurring after renal transplantation. Clinical, pathologic and virologic findings and implications for therapy. Ann Surg 198:356, 1983.
17. Perry JA, Jacobson JO, Conti D, Delmonico F, Harris NL. Lymphoproliferative disorders and hematologic malignancies following organ transplantation. Mod Pathol 2:583, 1989.

18. Weintraub J, Warnke RA. Lymphoma in cardiac allotransplant recipients: Clinical and histological features and immunological phenotype. Transplantation. 33:347, 1982.
19. Calne RY, Rolles K, White DJG, et al. Cyclosporin A initially as the only immunosuppressant in 34 recipients of cadaveric organs: 32 kidneys, 2 pancreases and 2 livers. Lancet 2:1033, 1979.
20. Bieber CP, Heberling RL, Jamieson SW, et al. Lymphoma in cardiac transplant recipients: Associated with the use of cyclosporine A, prednisone and antithymocyte globulin. *In* Purtilo DT (ed). *Immune Deficiency and Cancer: Epstein-Barr Virus and Lymphoproliferative Malignancies.* New York, Plenum Press, 1983, p 309.
21. Kahan BD, Flechner SM, Lorber MI, Jensen C, Golden D, Van Buren CT. Complications of cyclosporin therapy. World J Surg 10:348, 1986.
22. Wilkinson AH, Smith JL, Hunsicker LG, et al. Increased frequency of posttransplant lymphomas in patients treated with cyclosporine, azathioprine and prednisone. Transplantation 47:293, 1989.
23. Swinnen LJ, Costanzo-Nordin MR, Fisher SG, et al. Increased incidence of lymphoproliferative disorder after immunosuppression with the monoclonal antibody OKT3 in cardiac transplant recipients. N Engl J Med 323:1723, 1990.
24. Brown N, Smith D, Miller G, et al. Infectious mononucleosis: A polyclonal B cell transformation in vivo. J Infect Dis 150:517, 1984.
25. Klein E, Ernberg I, Masucci MG, et al. T-cell response to B-cells and Epstein-Barr virus antigens in infectious mononucleosis. Cancer Res 41:4210, 1981.
26. Henle G, Henle W, Horwitz CA. Antibodies to Epstein-Barr virus-associated nuclear antigen in infectious mononucleosis. J Infect Dis 130:231, 1974.
27. Blazar B, Patarroya M, Klein E, Klein G. Increased sensitivity of human lymphoid lines to natural killer cells after induction of the Epstein-Barr viral cycle by superinfection or sodium butyrate. J Exp Med 151:614, 1980.
28. Bird AG, McLachlan SM. Cyclosporine A and Epstein-Barr virus. Lancet 2:418, 1980.
29. Gaston JSH, Rickinson AB, Epstein MA. Epstein-Barr virus–specific T-cell memory in renal allograft recipients under long-term immunosuppression. Lancet 1:923, 1982.
30. Randhawa PS, Yousem SA. Epstein-Barr virus-associated lymphoproliferative disease in a heart-lung allograft. Transplantation 49:126, 1990.
31. Zutter MM, Martin PJ, Sale GE, et al. Epstein-Barr virus lymphoproliferation after bone marrow transplantation. Blood 72:520, 1988.
32. Shapiro RS, McClain K, Frizzera G, et al. Epstein-Barr virus-associated B-cell lymphoproliferative disorders following bone marrow transplantation. Blood 71:1234, 1988.
33. Cleary ML, Warnke R, Sklar J. Monoclonality of lymphoproliferative lesions in cardiac-transplant recipients. N Engl J Med 310:477, 1984.
34. Cleary MJ, Sklar J. Lymphoproliferative disorders in cardiac transplant recipients are multiclonal lymphomas. Lancet 2:489, 1984.
35. Starzl TE, Porter KA, Iwatsuki S, et al. Reversibility of lymphomas and lymphoproliferative lesions developing under cyclosporine-steroid therapy. Lancet 1:583, 1984.
36. Ho M, Miller G, Atchison RW, et al. Epstein-Barr virus infections and DNA hybridization studies in post-transplantation lymphoma and lymphoproliferative lesions: The role of primary infection. J Infect Dis 152:876, 1985.
37. Zanke BW, Rush DN, Jeffery JR, Israels LG. HTLV-1 T-cell lymphoma in a cyclosporine treated renal transplant patient. Transplantation 48:695, 1989.
38. Fahey JL (Moderator). Immune interventions in disease. Ann Intern Med 106:257, 1987.
39. Doyle TJ, Venkatachalam KK, Maeda K, Saeed SM, Tilchen EJ. Hodgkin's disease in renal transplant recipients. Cancer 51:245, 1983.
40. Knowles DM, Chamulak GA, Subar M, et al. Lymphoid neoplasia associated with the acquired immunodeficiency syndrome (AIDS). The New York University Medical Center experience with 105 patients (1981–1986). Ann Intern Med 108:744, 1988.
41. Canioni D, MacKelvie P, Debure A, Nezelof C. Lymphadenopathy in renal transplant patients treated with immunosuppressive antibodies (OKT3 and antithymocyte globulin): A report of nine cases. Am J Surg Pathol 13:87, 1989.
42. Iwatsuki S, Geis WP, Molnar Z, Giacchino JL, Ing TS, Hano JE. Systemic lymphoblastic response to antithymocyte globulin in renal allograft recipients: An initial report. J Surg Res 24:428, 1978.
43. Geis WP, Iwatsuki S, Molnar Z, et al. Pseudolymphoma in renal allograft recipients. Arch Surg 113:461, 1978.
44. Iaochim HL. Neoplasms associated with immune deficiencies. Pathol Annu Part 2:177, 1987.
45. Komorowski RA, Clowry LJ. Porokeratosis of Mibelli in transplant recipients. Am J Cardiovasc Pathol 91:71, 1989.
46. Uumacher C, Myskowski P, Ochoa M, et al. Outbreak of Kaposi's sarcoma in young homosexual men. Am J Med 72:569, 1982.
47. Penn I. Kaposi's sarcoma in organ transplant recipients. Transplantation 27:8, 1979.
48. Safai B. Pathophysiology and epidemiology of epidemic Kaposi's sarcoma. Semin Oncol 14(suppl):7, 1987.
49. Giraldo G, Beth E, Lourilsky F, et al. Antibody patterns to herpes viruses in Kaposi's sarcoma: Serological association of European Kaposi's sarcoma with cytomegalovirus. Int J Cancer 15:839, 1975.
50. Giraldo G, Beth E, Huang E. Kaposi's sarcoma and its relationship to cytomegalovirus III: CMV, DNA and CMV early antigens in Kaposi's sarcoma. Am J Cancer 26:23, 1980.
51. Groopman JE. Biology and therapy of epidemic Kaposi's sarcoma. Cancer 59:633, 1987.
52. Bovi PD, Basilico C. Isolation of a rearranged human transforming gene following transfection of Kaposi's sarcoma DNA. Proc Natl Acad Sci USA 84:5660, 1987.

Index

Note: Page numbers in *italics* refer to illustrations; page numbers followed by t indicate tables; *Plate* refers to the color plate following page 50.

Acquired immunodeficiency syndrome, 247
  Kaposi's sarcoma in, 271
Acyclovir, effect of, on viral inclusions, in lung, 146
  for lymphoproliferative disorder, 269
Adenovirus infection, 246–247
Adhesion molecules, endothelial expression of, 36–39, 37t, 38t
  in coronary vasculopathy, 113–114
  in immune response, 218–219
  in rejection, 13
    of liver, 207–208
  monoclonal antibodies against, for rejection, 45
Adult respiratory distress syndrome, 152
Age, and coronary vasculopathy, 121
AIDS, 247
  Kaposi's sarcoma in, 271
Allografts. See *Transplantation.*
Alpha chains, in major histocompatibility complex, 5, *6*, 7
  of T cell antigen receptors, 7, *8*
Alport's syndrome, kidney transplant for, nephritis after, 182
Alveoli, proteinosis of, in infection, 259, *259*
Angiography, of coronary vasculopathy, 111
Angiopeptin, in prevention of coronary vasculopathy, 124–125
Angioplasty, percutaneous transluminal, for coronary vasculopathy, 124
Antibodies, in coronary vasculopathy, 115–119
  antiendothelial cell, 118
  anti-HLA, 115–116, 126
  panel-reactive, 118–119
  in immune response, 218
  in immunosuppression, antilymphocyte, 222–224, 223t
  engineered, 224
  in rejection, 13–14
  to OKT3, and hemodynamic side effects, vs. microvascular rejection, 106
Anticoagulation, dermatan sulfate proteoglycan–heparin cofactor II pathway in, 56
  heparan sulfate in, endogenous, 56–57

Anticoagulation *(Continued)*
  heparan sulfate proteoglycan–antithrombin III pathway of, 55, 55t, 55–56, *56*, 56t, *Plate*
  in prevention of coronary vasculopathy, 125
  natural pathways of, 49, *49*, 53t, *53–56*, 53–57, 56t, *Plate*
  thrombomodulin–protein C pathway of, *53*, 53–55, *54*, *Plate*
  tissue factor pathway inhibitor in, 57
Antiendothelial cell antibodies, in coronary vasculopathy, 118
Antigens, human leukocyte. See *Human leukocyte antigen.*
  of major histocompatibility complex, 4–7, *5, 6*
  in lung transplant rejection, 138
  recognition of, by B cells, 4
  by T cells, 4, *5*, 7–10, *8–11*
Anti-HLA antibodies, in coronary vasculopathy, 115–116, 126
Antilymphocyte antibodies, in immunosuppression, 222–224, 223t
Antilymphocyte globulin, and lymphoproliferative disorder, 265
Antiplatelet agents, in prevention of coronary vasculopathy, 125
Antithrombin III, in anticoagulation, 55, 55t, 55–56, *56*, 56t, *Plate*
  in coronary vasculopathy, 105, 122
  in microvascular rejection, 93, 94t, 95–97, 99, 104
  binding of, to endothelial cells, 107
Antithymocyte globulin, and vascular rejection, of heart transplant, 116, 117
  rabbit, and lymphoma, 88
  and T cell growth, interleukin-induced, 30
Apheresis, in immunosuppression, 225–226
Arterioles, of kidney, in cyclosporine toxicity, 163, *165, 166*
Arteriosclerosis, in coronary artery, 111–126. See also *Coronary artery, vasculopathy of.*
  transplant-induced, 61–62
Arteritis, necrotizing, after kidney transplant, 161–162, *162*
  obliterative, in liver rejection, 200–203, *200–204*

Aspergillus infection, 240, 254–256, *256*, 258
  of heart, 82
  of lung, 148–150, *148–150*, 150t
Aspiration, recurrent, after lung transplant, 152, *153*
Aspirin, in prevention of coronary vasculopathy, 125
Atherosclerosis, of coronary artery, 111–126. See also *Coronary artery, vasculopathy of.*
  transplant-induced, 61–62
Azathioprine, in immunosuppression, 220
  and lymphoproliferative disorder, 265
  for rejection, 44
  in hepatitis, 230
  toxicity of, after liver transplant, 209
  with heart transplantation, 70, 70t

B cells, antigen recognition by, 4
  in lymphoproliferative disorder, 265, *266*, *268*, 269
    after lung transplant, 155
  in rejection, 10, *11*, 12
Bacterial infection, 239t, 240, 247–250, *249*
  of lung, 143–144, 150–151, 259
Basement membrane, duplication of, in glomerulopathy, 180, *181*
Basic fibroblast growth factor, endothelial production of, 39, 40
  in coronary vasculopathy, 114–115
Beta blockers, for hypertension, cyclosporine-induced, 229
Beta chains, in major histocompatibility complex, 5, *6*, 7
  of T cell antigen receptors, 7, *8*
Beta-2 microglobulin, in cardiac rejection, 71
Bile duct(s), anastomosis of, in transplantation, 186–187
  common, lithiasis of, cyclosporine and, 208
  in rejection, acute, 194, *195–197*, 199t, 199–200
    chronic, 14, 203–207, *205*, *206*
    histology of, 209–210
Biliary cirrhosis, primary, recurrence of, after transplantation, 209
Biopsy, before transplant perfusion, with recipient's blood, 50
  in rejection, cellular changes in, early studies of, 19–20
    diagnostic applications of, 27–30, *29*
    interleukin-2 in, 20–21, *22*
    and major histocompatibility complex antigen expression, 25–27, *26–28*, 28t
    in animal models, 30–32, 31t, *32*
    lymphocyte phenotypes in, 21–25, 24t
  of heart, in children, 88–89
    in coronary vasculopathy, 111–112
    in rejection, complications of, 71–72
      indications for, 72, 72t
      instruments for, 71
      pitfalls in, 84, *84*
      technique of, 72–73, *73*
      vascular, 118
  of kidney, technique of, 159–160
  of liver, after transplant, 186, 186t
    at time of transplant, 187–189, *187–189*
Bladder, reflux from, and nephropathy, 173, 182
Blastomyces infection, after transplantation, 255

Blood cells, red, fragmented, in cyclosporine toxicity, to kidney, 163, *165*
Blood pressure, decreased, and hepatic infarction, 191
  elevated, cyclosporine and, 229
Blood transfusion, for hemophilia, and hepatitis, liver transplant for, 209
Blood vessels, changes in, in allografts, *49*, 49–50
  immunopathology of, 60–61
  endothelium of. See *Vascular endothelium.*
  hemostasis in, 50–53, 53t, *Plate*
  HLA-DR expression in, and lymphocyte proliferation, 26–27, *27*, 28t
  small, in heart transplant rejection, 92–108. See also *Heart, transplantation of, rejection of, microvascular.*
Bone, metabolism of, corticosteroids and, 230
Bone marrow, fibrin ring granuloma in, in cytomegalovirus infection, 244
  suppression of, azathioprine and, 209
Bredinin, in immunosuppression, 220–221
Brequinar sodium, in immunosuppression, 221
Bronchiolitis, herpes simplex virus and, 147, *147*
  in rejection, acute, 134, *135*, 136
  obliterative, 136–141, *137*
    in grading of rejection, 141t, 141–143
    lavage cytology of, 154
Bronchoalveolar lavage, in infection, 258–259
  Pneumocystis, 250–251, *252*, 258
  in rejection, 153–154
Bronchus-associated lymphoid tissue, depletion of, and infection, 144
  vs. rejection, 151
Brunner's gland, in cytomegalovirus infection, *243*, 259

Calcification, dystrophic, after myocardial biopsy, in children, 89
  in renal tubules, in cyclosporine toxicity, 175
Calcineurin, inhibition of, by cyclosporine, 219
Calcium channel, blockers of, for coronary vasculopathy, 124
Cancer. See *Neoplasm(s).*
Candidiasis, 240, 253–255, *256*
  in gastrointestinal tract, 260
Capillaries, in cardiac rejection, 92–108. See also *Heart, transplantation of, rejection of, microvascular.*
Carcinoma, squamous cell, *270*, 270–271
Cartilage, in airways, in lung rejection, 138, 139
Caves-Schulz Stanford bioptome, in heart biopsy, 71
CD3 complex, T cell response to, 7–8, *9*
CD4 complex, in biopsy culture, from murine heart allograft, 31–32, *32*
  in coronary vasculopathy, 112–113
  in rejection, 9–10, *10*, *11*, 13, 41–42, *42*
    and donor HLA specificity, of T cells, 25
    and gamma-interferon regulation, 26, 27
    measurement of, 22–23
    of kidney, 171
  T cell response to, 8, *9*
CD8 complex, in biopsy culture, from murine heart allograft, 31–32, *32*
  in coronary vasculopathy, 112–113
  in rejection, 10, *10*, *11*, 13, 41, 42, *42*
    and donor HLA specificity, of T cells, 25

CD8 complex *(Continued)*
 measurement of, 22–23
 of kidney, 171–172
 T cell response to, 8–9, *9*
CD11a/CD18 complex, expression of, on
  endothelial cells, 38, 39
 monoclonal antibodies against, in treatment of
  rejection, 45
CD28 complex, in coronary vasculopathy, 114
Cervix, cancer of, 271
 condyloma of, 247, *247*
Chemotherapy, phototherapy with, in
   prevention, of anti-HLA antibody
   formation, 116
 of coronary vasculopathy, 125
Childbearing, in transplant recipients, 230
Children, heart transplantation in, pathology of,
  88–89
Cholangitis, after liver transplant, 212, *212*
Cholestasis, after liver transplant, 210
 and jaundice, with preservation injury, 189
 sinusoidal foam cells in, 213, *213*
Cholesterol, blood level of, immunosuppression
  and, 230–231
Chromosome 6, major histocompatibility
  complex on, 5, *6*
Chrysosporium infection, 255, *257*
Cirrhosis, biliary, primary, recurrence of, after
  transplantation, 209
 with transplant rejection, 203, *204*
Coagulation. See also *Anticoagulation.*
 fibrin in, 50–51
 in rejection, 2
 intravascular, in cyclosporine toxicity, to kidney, 166
 tissue factor pathway in, 51–52, 57
Coagulation factors, 2, 51
 and coronary vasculopathy, 122–123
 in microvascular rejection, 95
Coccidioides infection, 255
Complement system, in coronary vasculopathy,
  115
 in inflammation, 2
 in late rejection, 3
Conduction system, after heart transplant, 87
Condyloma, of uterine cervix, 247, *247*
Connective tissue growth factor, in rejection, 39–
  40
Cordis bioptome, in heart biopsy, 71
Coronary artery, vasculopathy of, after heart
   transplant, 14, 43–44, *45*, 104–105, *105*,
   106, 111–126
 antibodies in, 115–119
 cellular rejection and, 120
 coagulation factors and, 122–123
 cytomegalovirus and, 119–120
 diagnosis of, 111–112
 donor age and, 121
 HLA mismatching and, 120
 hyperlipidemia and, 121
 immunopathology of, 112–115
 immunosuppression and, 121–122
 in children, 89
 in long-term survivors, 85–87, *86, 87*
 preoperative ischemia and, 121
 recipient age and, 121
 sex mismatch and, 121
 T cells in, 30, 112–113
 treatment of, 123–125

Coronary artery *(Continued)*
 vascular tone and, 123
Corticosteroids, and lymphoproliferative
   disorder, 265
 effect of, on diabetes, 230
 in immunosuppression, 222
  in rejection, 228
 in treatment of rejection, 44
 resistance to, in cellular rejection, of kidney,
  163
Cough reflex, loss of, and aspiration, after lung
  transplant, 152, *153*
Creatinine, plasma level of, 52, 53t
Cryptococcosis, 252, 255, 257, *258*
Cyclophilin, interaction of, with cyclosporine, 219
Cyclosporine, 219
 absorption of, bile duct obstruction and, 187
 and hypertension, 229
 and lymphoproliferative disorder, 265
 and vascular rejection, 43
 in treatment of rejection, 44
 toxicity of, to kidney, 229–230
  acute, 163–166, *165, 166*
  and glomerular lesions, 180
  and interstitial fibrosis, 177, *178*
  and tubulointerstitial lesions, 173–175,
   174
  chronic, 167–170, *169*
  vs. rejection, 7
 to liver, 208–209, 230
 with heart transplantation, 70, 70t
  and Quilty effect, 81
  infection rate after, 83
Cytokines, in coronary vasculopathy, 113
 in immune response, 219–220
 in rejection, of heart, 71
Cytomegalovirus infection, 239t, *242*, 242–244,
  243
 and coronary vasculopathy, 119–120
 and Kaposi's sarcoma, 271
 in immunosuppression, 228, 229, 240, 241
 in myocarditis, 82, *82, 83*
 in pyelonephritis, 177
 of lung, 138, *144–146*, 144–147, 153
Cytotoxicity, T cell–mediated, in rejection, 13

Deoxyribonucleic acid, effect of azathioprine on,
  220
Deoxyspergualin, in immunosuppression, 222
Dermatan sulfate proteoglycan–heparin cofactor
  II pathway, in anticoagulation, 56
Diabetes, effect of immunosuppression on, 230
Diltiazem, in prevention of coronary
  vasculopathy, 86, 124
Dipyridamole, in prevention of coronary
  vasculopathy, 125
Disseminated intravascular coagulation, tissue
  factor in, 51
DNA, effect of azathioprine on, 220
Duodenum, cytomegalovirus infection in, 242,
  243, 259

Echocardiography, in diagnosis of rejection, 71
ELAM-1, in coronary vasculopathy, 114
 in rejection, 13

Electrocardiography, in diagnosis of coronary
    vasculopathy, 111
  in diagnosis of rejection, 70–71
Electron microscopy, in diagnosis of rejection, of
    heart, 73
Encephalopathy, OKT3 and, 231
Endarteritis, obliterative, in liver rejection, 200–
    203, *200–204*
Endocardium, Quilty effect in, *81*, 81–82
Endocrine system, abnormalities of,
    immunosuppression and, 230
Endothelial leukocyte adhesion molecule-1
    (ELAM-1), in coronary vasculopathy, 114
  in rejection, 13
Endothelium, of blood vessels. See *Vascular
    endothelium.*
Eosinophils, in rejection, of liver, 194, *195*
Epstein-Barr virus infection, 245
  after liver transplant, 209
  after lung transplant, vs. rejection, 152, 154,
    155
  and lymphoproliferative disorder, 262–265,
    266
    after heart transplant, 88
    after kidney transplant, 175–176
  immunosuppression and, 240, 241
E-selectin, and T cell adhesion, to vascular
    endothelium, 37, 37t, 38t
  endothelial expression of, 36
  in hyperacute rejection, 41
Esophagus, candidiasis of, *256*
  herpes simplex infection of, 244, *244*

Factor VII, in coagulation, 51
Factor VIIIra, in microvascular rejection, 95
Factor X, in coagulation, 51
Factor XII, functions of, 2
Fats, blood level of, and coronary vasculopathy,
    113, 121
  immunosuppression and, 230–231
Fatty tissue, of liver, biopsy of, 187–188, *188*, 210
Fetus, immunosuppressive drug effects on, 230
Fibrin, deposition of, in hemostasis, 50–51
  physiology of, 49, *49*
  in cyclosporine toxicity, to kidney, 163, *165*
  measurement of, in hemostasis, 52, *Plate*
Fibrin ring granuloma, in bone marrow, in
    cytomegalovirus infection, 244
Fibrinogen, vs. fibrin, 51
Fibrinolysis, and coronary vasculopathy, 122
  diagnosis of, 60
  in rejection, 2
  in transplant management, 49, *49*, 57–60, *58,
    60, Plate*
Fibroblast growth factor, basic, endothelial
    production of, 39, 40
  in coronary vasculopathy, 114–115
Fibrosis, after heart transplant, in long-term
    survivors, 85
  of kidney, interstitial, 177, 177t, *178*
  of lung, idiopathic, recurrent, 152
  in rejection, *137*, 137–139, *139, 140*
FK506, and Quilty effect, 81
  in immunosuppression, 219
  toxicity of, to kidney, 174–175
Fungal infection, 239t, 240, 252–260, *256–258*
  in myocarditis, 82

Fungal infection *(Continued)*
  of lung, 148–150, *148–150*, 150t, 153
Fusion molecules, in immunosuppression, 224

Gallstones, cyclosporine toxicity and, 208
Ganciclovir, effect of, on viral inclusions, in lung,
    146
Gastrointestinal tract, disorders of, immuno-
    suppression and, 230
  in cytomegalovirus infection, 242, *243*
  infection of, diagnosis of, 259–260
Gender, donor-recipient mismatch of, and
    coronary vasculopathy, 121
Genes, transfer of, for transplant acceptance,
    226–227
Glomeruli. See also *Kidney(s).*
  lesions of, 177–182, 178t, *179, 181, 182*
  reaction of, with thrombomodulin antibody, 55
Glomerulitis, after kidney transplant, de novo,
    181–182, *182*
  recurrent, 180–181
Glomerulopathy, after kidney transplant, acute,
    177–180, *179*
  chronic, 180, *181*
  in rejection, 14
  ischemia and, 160
Glucocorticoids. See *Corticosteroids.*
Graft versus host disease, after liver transplant,
    209
  methotrexate for, 221
Grafting. See *Transplantation.*
Granuloma, in cytomegalovirus infection, 244
  in liver, 210, *210*
  in lung, 152, *153*
    Aspergillus infection and, *149*, 149–150
    Pneumocystis infection and, 148
    sarcoidosis and, 151–152, *152*
Growth factor, connective tissue, in rejection, 39–
    40
  fibroblast, basic, in coronary vasculopathy,
    114–115
    in rejection, 39, 40
  platelet-derived, in coronary vasculopathy,
    114–115
    in rejection, 15, 39–40, *40*

Hageman factor, functions of, 2
Heart, transplantation of, biopsy after, before
      perfusion, with recipient's blood, 50
    culture studies of, lymphocyte growth in,
      21, *22*
    lymphocyte proliferation in, interleukin-
      induced, and donor MHC antigen
      expression, 25–27, *26, 27*, 28t
    T cell growth in, interleukin-induced, in
      mice, 30–32, 31t, *32*
    T cell HLA specificity in, 24t, 24–25
  conduction system after, 87
  coronary artery vasculopathy after, 111–126.
      See also *Coronary artery, vasculopathy of.*
  death after, causes of, 70, 70t
  endothelium in, plasminogen activators in,
      57–58, *Plate*
    reaction of, with thrombomodulin anti-
      body, 55, *Plate*

Heart *(Continued)*
  immunosuppression with, and T cell growth, interleukin-induced, 30
    total lymphoid irradiation in, 225
  infection after, and myocarditis, *82,* 82–84, *83*
    bacterial, 248
  lymphoproliferative disorder after, 87–88, 263
  pathology of, in children, 88–89
    in long-term survivors, 85–89, *86, 87*
  reinnervation after, 87, 112
  rejection of, antibody-mediated responses in, 14
    cellular, 102–103, *103, 104,* 120
    cellular infiltrate in, immunophenotype of, 83–84
    chronic, 43
    diagnosis of, biopsy in, 71–73, 72t, *73*
      echocardiography in, 71
      electrocardiography in, 70–71
      T cell cultures in, 27–29, *28, 29*
    histopathology of, 73–81, 74t, *75–80,* 76t, 77t
    microvascular, and International Society for Heart and Lung Transplantation grading, 99–102, 102t
      as dominant pattern, *103,* 103–104, *104*
      classification of, 95–99, *95–102*
      immunocytochemical determinants of, 93–95, 94t
      pathogenesis of, 107–108
      pathology of, 92–108
      vs. drug-induced processes, 105–107
      with cellular rejection, 102, *103,* 104
    morphology of, 73
      Quilty effect in, *81,* 81–82
    vascular, 14, 42–44, *43, 45,* 82, 116–118
  right ventricular failure after, 74
  survival rates after, 69
Hematopoiesis, after liver transplant, 210, *211*
Hemolytic-uremic syndrome, kidney transplant for, cyclosporine toxicity after, 163
Hemophilia, transfusion for, and hepatitis, liver transplant for, 209
Hemorrhage, in lung rejection, 134–136, *136*
Hemostasis, and coronary vasculopathy, 122
  diagnosis of, 52, *Plate*
  fibrin deposition in, 50–51
  immunopathology of, 61
  systemic manifestations of, 52–53, 53t
  tissue factor pathway in, 51–52
Heparan sulfate, in anticoagulation, 56–57
Heparan sulfate proteoglycan–antithrombin III pathway, in anticoagulation, *55,* 55t, 55–56, *56,* 56t, *Plate*
Heparin, and tissue factor pathway inhibition, 57
  in prevention of coronary vasculopathy, 125
Heparin cofactor II, in anticoagulation, 56
Heparin sulfate proteoglycan, in rejection, 15
Hepatic artery, anastomosis of, in liver transplantation, 186
Hepatitis, biopsy of, 187, 188, *188*
  immunosuppression in, 230
  polymorphonuclear leukocyte clusters in, 210–212, *212*
  recurrent, after transplant, 209
  viral, 240, 245–246
Herpes simplex virus infection, 244, *244*

Herpes simplex virus infection *(Continued)*
  and skin cancer, 262
  of lung, *146,* 146–147, *147*
Herpes viruses, 242–245, *242–245.* See also specific viral infection, e.g., *Epstein-Barr virus infection.*
Histiocytes, foamy, in sinusoids, 213, *213*
Histiocytosis, Langerhans' cell, in lung, 152
Histocompatibility complex, major. See *Major histocompatibility complex.*
Histoplasmosis, 240, 250, 252
HLA. See *Human leukocyte antigen.*
Human immunodeficiency virus infection, 247
  and Kaposi's sarcoma, 271
Human leukocyte antigen, 5, *6,* 7
  antibodies to, in coronary vasculopathy, 115–116, 126
  donor-specific reactivity to, 23–25, 24t
  expression of, and lymphocyte proliferation, 25–27, *26, 27,* 28t
  in lung rejection, 138
  in vascular endothelium, 36
  mismatching of, and coronary vasculopathy, 120
Human papilloma virus infection, 246–247, *247*
Hyaline membranes, in lung rejection, 134–136, *136*
Hyalinosis, of kidney, in cyclosporine toxicity, 167–170, *169*
  in rejection, 167
Hypercholesterolemia, immunosuppression and, 230–231
Hyperlipidemia, and coronary vasculopathy, 121
Hypersensitivity, delayed-type, in coronary vasculopathy, 113
  in rejection, 10, *11,* 12–13
Hypertension, immunosuppression and, 229
Hypoperfusion, and hepatic infarction, 191–193
Hypotension, and hepatic infarction, 191

Immune response, avoidance of, gene transfer in, 226–227
  cell-mediated, 219
  humoral, 116–118, 218
  T cell activation pathways in, 217–218, *218*
Immune system, in liver rejection, 193, 207–208
Immunoadsorption, in immunosuppression, 226
Immunodeficiency virus, human, 247
  and Kaposi's sarcoma, 271
Immunofluorescence, of biopsy samples, myocardial, antibodies for, 93, 94t
  preparation for, 50
Immunoglobulin(s), after heart transplant, in coronary vasculopathy, 115
  in microvascular rejection, 93, 94t
  in vascular rejection, 42
  mouse, effect of, on biopsy culture studies, 20
Immunoglobulin G, in nephritis, after transplant for Alport's syndrome, 182
Immunoglobulin M, in graft failure, 61
Immunoperoxidase, in biopsy sample preparation, 50
Immunophenotyping. See *Phenotyping.*
Immunosuppression. See also specific drugs, e.g., *FK506.*
  and coronary vasculopathy, 121–122
  and endocrine disorders, 230
  and hypertension, 229

Immunosuppression *(Continued)*
 and infection, 228–229, 239–241
 and metabolic abnormalities, 230–231
 and neoplasia, 231, 262, 263t
  in lymphoproliferative disorder, *263*, 263–269, *264, 266–268*
 and neurologic complications, 231
 and survival rates, 69–70, 70t
 and T cell growth, interleukin-induced, 30
 antibodies in, anti-idiotypic, hemodynamic effects of, vs. microvascular rejection, 105–107
  antilymphocyte, 222–224, 223t
  engineered, 224
 cell maturation inhibition in, 222
 cell proliferation inhibitors in, 220–222
 corticosteroids in, 222
 cytokine inhibitors in, 219–220
 for rejection, 44, 228
 fusion molecules in, 224
 gastrointestinal effects of, 230
 immunoadsorption in, 226
 induction phase of, 227–228
 inflammation mediated by, 3
 lymphoid irradiation in, total, 224–225
 maintenance phase of, 228
 photochemotherapy with, in prevention of anti-HLA antibody formation, 116
 photopheresis in, 226
 plasma exchange in, 225–226
 toxicity of, to kidney, 229–230
Infarction, hepatic, 191–193, *192*
Inflammation, in allograft pathology, 1–2
 in late rejection, 2–3
Inosine monophosphate dehydrogenase, inhibition of, in immunosuppression, 220, 221
Insulin-dependent diabetes, effect of corticosteroids on, 230
Integrins, in lymphocyte adhesion, to vascular endothelium, 38, 39
Intercellular adhesion molecule-1, and T cell adhesion, to vascular endothelium, 37t, 38, 39
 endothelial expression of, 36
 in rejection, 13
  monoclonal antibodies against, 45
  of liver, 207–208
Intercellular adhesion molecule-2, and T cell adhesion, to vascular endothelium, 37t, 38, 39
Interferon, and histocompatibility antigen expression, 7
 gamma, antagonists to, 26
  in endothelial cell activation, 36
  in rejection, 12–13, 41, 42, *42*
   in cytotoxicity, 13
   of liver, 207
Interleukin(s), in cytotoxicity, in rejection, 13
 in immune response, 219
 in rejection, 10, *10, 11,* 12, 13, 41–42, *42*
  chronic, 15
Interleukin-1, and thrombomodulin level, 54
 endothelial production of, 39
 in coronary vasculopathy, 113
 in endothelial cell activation, 36
 in liver rejection, 207–208
Interleukin-2, action of, inhibition of, by rapamycin, 219–220

Interleukin-2 *(Continued)*
 and T cell growth, donor MHC antigen expression and, 25–27, *26, 27,* 28t
  immunosuppression and, 30
  in animal models of transplantation, 30–32, 31t, *32*
 in immunoregulation, in rejection, 20–21
 in T cell clone expansion, in biopsy culture studies, 21, *22*
 receptors of, in cardiac rejection, 71
Interleukin-6, in cardiac rejection, 71
Interleukin-10, and suppression of T cell growth, 26
 in immunoregulation, in rejection, 21
International Society for Heart and Lung Transplantation, standardized grading system of, 21, 75–81, 76t, 77t, *77–80*
 for lung rejection, 141t, 141–143
 microvascular rejection related to, 99–102, 102t
Intima, in kidney rejection, hyalinosis of, 167
 proliferation of, 166–167, *168*
Intracellular cell adhesion molecule-1, in coronary vasculopathy, 113–114
Intravascular coagulation, tissue factor in, 51–52
Irradiation, of lymphatic tissue, in immunosuppression, 224–225
Ischemia, and antigen release, 9
 and glomerulopathy, 160
 and inflammation, 1
 in hepatic preservation injury, 191
 myocardial, before transplant, and postoperative vasculopathy, 121
  in rejection, 74–75, *75*
  with coronary vasculopathy, 104–105, *105, 106*
 subcapsular, vs. acute tubular necrosis, 173
Isovolumic relaxation time, in cardiac rejection, 71

Jaundice, cholestatic, with hepatic preservation injury, 189

Kaposi's sarcoma, 271, *271, 272*
Kawai bioptome, in heart biopsy, 71
Kidney(s), cyclosporine toxicity to, 229–230
  acute, 163–166, *165, 166*
  chronic, 167–170, *169*
  tubulointerstitial lesions in, 173–175, *174*
 transplantation of, bacterial infection after, 248
  biopsy after, before perfusion, with recipient's blood, 50
   T cell HLA specificity in, 23–24
   technique of, 159–160
  cyclosporine with, toxicity of, to liver, 208
  glomerular lesions after, thrombomodulin antibody and, 55
   types of, 177, 178t
  glomerulitis after, de novo, 181–182, *182*
   recurrent, 180–181
  glomerulopathy after, acute, 177–180, *179*
   chronic, 180, *181*
  immunosuppression with, total lymphoid irradiation in, 225
  lymphoproliferative disorder after, 263

Kidney(s) *(Continued)*
    tubulointerstitial lesions in, 175–176, *176*
    nephritis after, interstitial, acute allergic, 176
    pathology of, 159–182
        diagnosis of, 159t, 159–161, 160t
    plasminogen activators in, 58–59, *59*
    pyelonephritis after, 176–177
    reflux after, 173, 182
    rejection of, acute cellular, 162–163, *163, 164*
        tubulointerstitial lesions in, 170–173, *171–173*
        antibody-mediated responses in, 13–14
        chronic, 166–167, *167, 168*
            endothelium in, 43
        T cells in, in biopsy culture, 20
        vascular, endothelium in, 42–43
            hyperacute, 161, *161*
            necrotizing, 161–162, *162*
        vasculopathy in, 14
        vs. cyclosporine toxicity, 7
    renal artery disease after, 182
King bioptome, in heart biopsy, 71
Kinin, in inflammation, 2
Koilocytosis, in condyloma acuminatum, 247, *247*
Kupffer cells, in liver rejection, 193, 207, 208

Langerhans' cell histiocytosis, in lung, 152
Lavage, bronchoalveolar, in infection, 258–259
    Pneumocystis, 250–251, *252,* 258
    in rejection, 153–154
Legionella pneumophila infection, in immuno-
    suppression, 229
Leukocyte antigen, human. See *Human leukocyte antigen.*
Leukocyte function-associated antigen-1,
    expression of, on endothelial cells, 38, 39
    monoclonal antibodies against, in treatment of
        rejection, 45
Leukocytes, in adhesion, regulation of, 36–39, 37t, 38t
    in coronary vasculopathy, 114
    polymorphonuclear, after liver transplant, 210–212, *212*
Light, ultraviolet, in immunosuppression, 226
    with chemotherapy, and immunosuppres-
        sion, in prevention of anti-HLA anti-
        body formation, 116
        in prevention of coronary vasculopathy, 125
Lip, cancer of, *270,* 270–271
    herpes viruses and, 262
Lipids, blood level of, and coronary vasculopathy, 113, 121
    immunosuppression and, 230–231
    in hepatic cells, biopsy of, 187–188, *188,* 210
Listeria monocytogenes infection, 248
    in immunosuppression, 229
Lithiasis, of common bile duct, cyclosporine and, 208
Liver, inflammation of. See *Hepatitis.*
    toxicity to, immunosuppression and, 230
    transplantation of, bacterial infection after, 247–248
        biopsy and, at time of grafting, 187–189, *187–189*
        diagnostic uses of, 186, 186t

Liver *(Continued)*
    drug toxicity after, 208–209
    graft versus host disease after, 209
    histology of, 209–213, *210–213*
    immunosuppression after, and T cell growth, 30
    infarction after, 191–193, *192*
    infection after, 209, 259
    lymphoproliferative disorder after, 263, *263, 264*
    pathology of, 186–213
    preservation injury in, 189–191, *190–192*
    primary disease recurrence after, 209
    rejection of, acute cellular, 194–200, *195–198*, 199t
        antibody-mediated responses in, 14
        chronic, 43, *200–206,* 200–207
        hyperacute, *193,* 193–194, *194*
        immunopathology of, 207–208
        vasculopathy in, 14
    vascular anastomotic problems in, 186–187
L-selectin, and T cell adhesion, to vascular
    endothelium, 37–38, 38t
Lung(s), transplantation of, experimental, 133–134
    infection after, 143–151, *144–150,* 148t
        bacterial, 248
        diagnosis of, 258–259, *259*
    lymphoproliferative disorder after, 154–155, 263
    pathology of, 133–155
    rejection of, acute, morphology of, 134–136, *135, 136*
        bronchoalveolar lavage cytology of, 153–154
        chronic, morphology of, 136–141, *137, 139, 140*
        classification of, 141t, 141–143
        differential diagnosis of, 151t, 151–153, *152, 153*
    with heart, survival rates after, 69
Lymphatic system, irradiation of, in
    immunosuppression, 224–225
Lymphocytes. See also *B cells* and *T cells.*
    endocardial infiltration by, in rejection, *81,* 81–82
    in bronchiolitis, 134, *135,* 136
    in bronchoalveolar lavage cytology, 153–154
    in coronary vasculopathy, 112–113
    in liver transplant rejection, acute, 194, *196–198*
        chronic, 201, *201*
Lymphocytolysis, corticosteroid-induced, 222
Lymphoid tissue, bronchus-associated, depletion
    of, and infection, 144
Lymphoproliferative disorder, after
    transplantation, *263,* 263–269, *264, 266–268,* 269t
    immunosuppression and, 231
    of heart, 87–88, 263
        in children, 89
    of kidney, 175–176, *176*
    of lung, 154–155, 263

Macrophages, in *Aspergillus* infection, 149, *149*
    in bronchoalveolar lavage cytology, 153–154
    in coronary vasculopathy, 113

Macrophages *(Continued)*
  in hepatic sinusoids, 213, *213*
  in rejection, 2
  of liver, 201, *201*, 207, 208
Magnetic resonance imaging, in cardiac
      rejection, 71
Major histocompatibility complex, 4–7, *5, 6*. See
      also *Human leukocyte antigen.*
  antigens of, and interleukin-induced lympho-
      cyte proliferation, 25–27, *26, 27*, 28t
  in rejection, 7–10, *10, 11*, 41, *42*
  of liver, 107
  of lung, 138
Malignancy. See *Neoplasm(s).*
Marrow, fibrin ring granuloma in, in
      cytomegalovirus infection, 244
  suppression of, azathioprine and, 209
Metabolism, abnormalities of,
      immunosuppression and, 230–231
Methotrexate, in immunosuppression, 221–222
8-Methoxypsoralen, in photopheresis, 226
Microglobulin, beta-2, in cardiac rejection, 71
  in major histocompatibility complex, 5, *6*, 7
Microscopy, of cardiac rejection, 73, 93, 94t
Microvasculature, of heart, in rejection, 92–108.
      See also *Heart, transplantation of, rejection of,
      microvascular.*
  of kidney, in cyclosporine toxicity, 163–166,
      164, 165
Mitochondria, giant, in cyclosporine toxicity, of
      kidney, 175
Mizoribine, in immunosuppression, 220–221
Monoclonal antibodies, for rejection, 44–45
  in immunosuppression, 222–224, 223t
  OKT3. See *OKT3.*
Mononucleosis, after lung transplant, 154
Mucor infection, after transplantation, 255, 257–
      258
Muscle cells, histology of, in coronary
      vasculopathy, 112
  smooth, cytomegalovirus infection of, 119
    in atherosclerosis, 62
    in coronary vasculopathy, 114–115
    in fibrinolytic system, 57–58, 60, *Plate*
Mycobacterial infection, 240, 248–250
  and pneumonia, 151
Mycophenolate mofetil, in immunosuppression,
      220
Myocardium, biopsy of, in children, 88–89
  in coronary vasculopathy, 111–112
  hypertrophy of, in long-term transplant survi-
      vors, 85
  infection of, *82*, 82–84, *83*
  ischemia of, with coronary vasculopathy, 104–
      105, *105, 106*

Natural killer cells, and graft damage, 12
  in rejection, 42
Neoplasm(s), 262–272
  cervical, 271
  due to malignant cells in allograft, 270
  immunosuppression and, 231
  in Kaposi's sarcoma, 271, *271, 272*
  lymphoproliferative disorder and, 263–269.
      See also *Lymphoproliferative disorder.*
  of liver, 209
  perineal, 271

Neoplasm(s) *(Continued)*
  squamous cell, *270*, 270–271
Neopterin, excretion of, in cardiac rejection, 71
Nephritis, after transplant for Alport's syndrome,
      182
  interstitial, acute allergic, 176
Nephropathy, reflux and, 173, 182
Nervous system, disorders of, immunosuppres-
      sion and, 231
  sympathetic, in transplanted heart, 87, 112
Neutrophils, in pyelonephritis, 177
  in rejection, interaction of, with endothelium,
      39
  of liver, 193, *193*
Nicardipine, in prevention of coronary
      vasculopathy, 124
Nifedipine, in prevention of coronary
      vasculopathy, 124
Nocardia infection, 229, 248, 249, *249*

OKT3, 8
  and lymphoma, 88
  anti-idiotypic antibodies to, and hemodynamic
      side effects, vs. microvascular rejection,
      106
  effect of, on T cell growth, interleukin-in-
      duced, 30
  for rejection, 44–45
    of kidney, acute cellular, 163
  in vascular rejection, allergy to, 42–43
    of heart, 116–117
  mechanism of action of, 224
  mouse immunoglobulin in, effect of, on biopsy
      culture studies, 20
  neurologic effects of, 231
OKT4-A, for rejection, 45
Olympus bioptome, in heart biopsy, 71
Osteoporosis, effect of corticosteroids on, 230

Pancreatitis, immunosuppression and, 230
Panel-reactive antibodies, in coronary
      vasculopathy, 118–119
Papilloma virus infection, 246–247, *247*
Papovavirus infection, 246–247
Parasitic infestation, 240, 250–253, *251–254*
  in immunosuppression, 228–229
  of heart, 82–83
  of lung, 147–148, 148t, 151
Percutaneous transluminal coronary angioplasty,
      for vasculopathy, 124
Perineum, cancer of, 271
Perivascular infiltrates, in lung rejection, acute,
      134, *135*, 136, *136*
  chronic, 137, *140*
Phenotyping, of cellular infiltrate, in cardiac
      rejection, 83–84
  of T cells, from murine heart transplant, 31–
      32, *32*
  in rejection, 21–23
    and donor HLA specificity, 24t, 25
Photochemotherapy, in prevention of coronary
      vasculopathy, 125
  with immunosuppression, in prevention of
      anti-HLA antibody formation, 116
Photopheresis, in immunosuppression, 226

Phycomycosis, 255, 257–258

Plasma, exchange of, in immunosuppression, 225–226
in inflammation, 2

Plasmin, laboratory identification of, 59, *60*

Plasminogen activators, in coronary vasculopathy, 105, 122
in heart transplant, 57–58, *Plate*
in kidney transplant, 58–59, *59*
in microvascular rejection, 93, 94t, 95–97, 99, 104
inhibitors of, laboratory identification of, 59–60

Platelet endothelial cell adhesion molecule-1, 38t, 38–39

Platelet-activating factor, and neutrophil-endothelium interaction, 39
synthesis of, in vascular endothelium, 36

Platelet-derived growth factor, in coronary vasculopathy, 114–115
in rejection, 15, 39

Platelet-derived growth factor–like protein, in rejection, 15, 39–40, *40*

Platelets, in coagulation, 2

Pneumocystis carinii infection, 147–148, 148t, 240, 250–252, *251, 252*
in immunosuppression, 229
in myocarditis, 82

Pneumonia, *Aspergillus* and, 150, *150*
cytomegalovirus and, 144–146, *145*
Legionella pneumophila and, 229
Pneumocystis carinii and, 147–148, 148t
in immunosuppression, 229

Pneumonitis, in cytomegalovirus infection, 242, *242*

Polio, vaccination against, after heart transplant, 229

Polyclonal antibodies, in immunosuppression, 222–224

Polymorphonuclear leukocytes, after liver transplant, 210–212, *212*

Polypeptide chains, in major histocompatibility complex, 5, *6*, 7

Portal vein, anastomosis of, in liver transplantation, 186

Prednisone, and lymphoproliferative disorder, 265

Pregnancy, in transplant recipients, 230

Preservation injury, after liver transplant, 189–191, *190–192*

Pressor agents, and myocardial damage, 75, *76*

Primary biliary cirrhosis, recurrence of, after transplantation, 209

Primed lymphocyte test, T cell HLA specificity in, 24, 24t

Prolactin, in cardiac rejection, 71

Protein A, in immunoadsorption, 226

Protein C, in anticoagulation pathway, *53*, 53–54, *54*, *Plate*

Protein S, in anticoagulation pathway, *53*, 53–54

Proteinosis, alveolar, in infection, 259, *259*

Prothrombin convertase, in coagulation, 51

P-selectin, and neutrophil-endothelium interaction, 39
and T cell adhesion, to vascular endothelium, 37, 37t, 38t
in hyperacute rejection, 41

Pulmonary fibrosis, recurrence of, after transplant, 152

Pyelonephritis, 176–177

Quilty effect, *81*, 81–82, 84

Rabbit antithymocyte globulin, and interleukin-induced T cell growth, 30
and lymphoma, 88

Radionuclide imaging, in cardiac rejection, 71

Rapamycin, and Quilty effect, 81
in immunosuppression, 219–220

Red blood cells, fragmented, in cyclosporine toxicity, to kidney, 163, *165*

Reflux, and nephropathy, 173, 182

Reinnervation, sympathetic, after heart transplant, 87, 112

Rejection, antibody-mediated responses in, 13–14
biopsy culture studies of, 19–32
cellular effectors of, early studies of, 19–20
chronic, vasculopathy in, mechanisms of, 14–15
hyperacute, after heart transplant, 74
interleukin-2 in, 20–21, *22*
major histocompatibility complex in, 4–7, *5, 6*
mechanisms of, 4–15, *5, 6, 8–11*
of heart, 69–108. See also *Heart, transplantation of, rejection of.*
of kidney, 161–173. See also *Kidney(s), transplantation of, rejection of.*
of liver, 193–208. See also *Liver, transplantation of, rejection of.*
of lung, 134–141, 151–154. See also *Lung(s), transplantation of, rejection of.*
T cells in, 7–13, 19–30. See also *T cells.*
therapy for, 44–45
vascular endothelium in, 35–45. See also *Vascular endothelium.*

Renal artery, disease of, 182

Renal pelvis, inflammation of, 176–177

Renal tubules, cyclosporine toxicity to, 173–175, *174*
damage to, in transplantation, 160
in rejection, 170t, 170–173, *171–173*
epithelial cells of, 7

Reticulin, in liver rejection, 201, *203*

Rhizopus infection, 255, 257–258

Right ventricle, failure of, 74

Sarcoidosis, lung transplant for, granuloma in, 151–152, *152*

Sarcoma, Kaposi's, 271, *271, 272*

Scintigraphy, of coronary vasculopathy, 111

Seizures, immunosuppression and, 231

Selectins, and T cell adhesion, to vascular endothelium, 37t, 37–38, 38t

Serine protease, and cytotoxicity, in rejection, 13

Sex, donor-recipient mismatch of, and coronary vasculopathy, 121

Shock, and hepatic infarction, 191

Sinusoids, hepatic, foam cells in, in cholestasis, 213, *213*
in biopsy, at time of transplantation, 187, *188*, 189, *189*
in hepatitis, 210, *211*, 246

Sinusoids *(Continued)*
   in rejection, 201, *202*
Skin, cancer of, 88, 270–271
      herpes viruses and, 262, 270
      immunosuppression and, 231
   grafts of, rejection of, capillaries in, 92
      delayed hypersensitivity in, 13
   infection of, diagnosis of, 259–260
      varicella-zoster, 244–245, *245*
Smooth muscle cells. See *Muscle cells, smooth.*
Staining, of biopsy specimen, in cardiac rejection,
   72–73, *73*
Steroids. See *Corticosteroids.*
Stomach, in cytomegalovirus infection, 242, *243*
Streptococcus infection, 248
Strongyloides stercoralis infestation, 240, 253, *254*

T cells, activation pathways of, 217–218, *218*
   adhesion of, to vascular endothelium, regula-
      tion of, 37t, 37–39, 38t
   and platelet-derived growth factor–like protein
      secretion, 40, *40*
   antigen receptors of, 7–9, *8, 9*
   antigen recognition by, 4, *5*
   growth of, interleukin-induced, in animal mod-
      els, 30–32, 31t, *32*
   in biopsy culture studies, and diagnostic appli-
      cations, 27–30, *28, 29*
      cloning of, interleukin-2 in, 21, *22*
   in coronary vasculopathy, 30, 112–113
   in lymphoproliferative disorder, 265, *266*, 269
   in rejection, 9–13, *10, 11*
      chronic, 43
      donor HLA specificity of, 23–25, 24t
      interaction of, with vascular endothelium,
         41–42, *42*
      interleukin-2 regulation of, 20–21
         donor MHC antigen expression and, 25–
            27, *26, 27*, 28t
      of heart, 83
      of kidney, 171–172
      peripheral blood level of, 19–20
      phenotypes of, 21–23, 83
Thrombin time, increased, in transplant
   recipients, 52–53, 53t
Thrombomodulin, and coronary vasculopathy,
   122
   in microvascular rejection, 107
Thrombomodulin–protein C pathway, of
   anticoagulation, *53*, 53–55, *54*, *Plate*
Thromboplastin, in coagulation, 51–52, 57
Thrombosis, and hepatic infarction, 191
   in cyclosporine toxicity, to kidney, 163, *166*,
      169–170
Thromboxane A2, in cyclosporine toxicity, to
   kidney, 175
Tissue factor, in coagulation, 51–52, 57
Tissue plasminogen activator, in coronary
   vasculopathy, 62, 105, 122
   in heart transplant, 58–59, *Plate*
   in microvascular rejection, 93, 94t, 95–97,
      99, 104
   in kidney transplant, 58
Tolerance, immunologic, to transplantation,
   enhancement of, 227
Total lymphoid irradiation, in
   immunosuppression, 224–225

Toxoplasma infection, 240, 252–253, *253*
   in immunosuppression, 228–229
   in myocarditis, 82–83
   in transplanted lung, 151
Transferrin, receptors of, in cardiac rejection, 71
Transfusion, for hemophilia, and hepatitis, liver
   transplant for, 209
Transplantation, gene transfer in, 226–227
   immunosuppression with, and infection, 228–
      229
     in rejection, 228
     induction phase of, 227–228
     maintenance phase of, 228
     infection after, 239–260. See also specific infec-
      tions, e.g., Pneumocystis carinii *infection.*
      bacterial, 239t, 240, 247–250, *249*
      detection of, 241
      diagnosis of, 258–260, *259*
      fungal, 239t, 240, 252–260, *256–258*
      parasitic, 240, 250–253, *251–254*
      prevention of, 241
      risk of, 239t, 239–241, *241*
      viral, 241–247, *242–245, 247*, 259, 260
   of heart, 69–126. See also *Heart, transplantation
      of.*
   of kidney, 159–182. See also *Kidney(s), trans-
      plantation of.*
   of liver, 186–213. See also *Liver, transplantation
      of.*
   of lungs, 133–155. See also *Lung(s), transplanta-
      tion of.*
   rejection after. See *Rejection.*
   tolerance to, enhancement of, 227
Tuberculosis, 240, 248–250
   and pneumonia, 151
Tumor necrosis factor, and thrombomodulin
   level, 54
   in coronary vasculopathy, 113
   in endothelial cell activation, 36
   in rejection, 12, 13, 15
     of heart, 71
     of liver, 207, 208
Tumors. See *Neoplasm(s).*
Tzanck smear, in diagnosis of varicella-zoster
   infection, 245, *245*

Ultrasonography, of heart, in rejection, 71
Ultraviolet light, in immunosuppression, 226
   with chemotherapy, and immunosuppression,
      in prevention of anti-HLA antibody forma-
      tion, 116
   in prevention of coronary vasculopathy, 125
Umbilical artery, endothelium of, platelet-derived
   growth factor–like protein secretion by, 40,
      40
Umbilical vein, endothelium of, platelet-derived
   growth factor–like protein secretion by, 40,
      40
Uremia, with hemolysis, kidney transplant for,
   cyclosporine toxicity after, 163
Ureterovesical junction, obstruction of, and
   reflux nephropathy, 173, 182
Urokinase, in kidney transplant, 58–59, *59*
Uterine cervix, cancer of, 271
   condyloma of, 247, *247*

Vaccination, after heart transplant, 229
Vanishing bile duct syndrome, in liver rejection, acute, 199, 199t
  chronic, 203, *205*, *206*, 207
Varicella-zoster virus infection, 244–245, *245*
Vascular cell adhesion molecule-1, and T cell adhesion, to vascular endothelium, 37t, 38
  endothelial expression of, 36
  in coronary vasculopathy, 113–114
  in rejection, 13
Vascular endothelium, growth factor production in, 39–40, *40*
  immunoglobulin M absence from, in graft failure, 61
  in coronary vasculopathy, 113–114, 123
    in long-term survivors, 86, *87*
  in rejection, 2, 3, 35–45
    acute cellular, 41–42, *42*
    cell activation in, 35–36
    chronic, 43–44
    hyperacute, 40–41
    in graft vasculopathy, 43–44, *45*
    microvascular, 107, 108
    of kidney, 162–163, *163*, *164*
    of liver, 194–197, *197*, *198*, 199t, 199–200, 210
    of lung, acute, 134, *135*, *136*
      chronic, 139, *140*
    vascular, 42–43, *43*
  leukocyte regulation in, 36–39, 37t, 38t
  morphology of, 35
Vasculopathy, in rejection, 43–44, *45*

Vasculopathy *(Continued)*
  chronic, mechanisms of, 14–15
  of liver, 212–213
    chronic, 200–203, *200–204*
  of coronary artery, after heart transplant, 111–126. See also *Coronary artery, vasculopathy of.*
  transplant-induced, 61–62
Vena cava, stenosis of, after liver transplant, 186
Ventricle, right, failure of, 74
Venules, in rejection, of heart transplant, 92–108. See also *Heart, transplantation of, rejection of, microvascular.*
Verruca vulgaris, 247
Vesicoureteral reflux, and nephropathy, 173, 182
Viral infection, 241–247, *242–245*, *247*, 259, 260. See also specific viral infection, e.g., *Cytomegalovirus infection.*
  and skin cancer, 262, 270
  of liver, 209–213, *211*, *212*
VLA-4, in lymphocyte adhesion, to vascular endothelium, 38, 39
von Willebrand factor, in liver rejection, 208

Yeast infection, 240, 250, 252

Ziehl-Neelsen staining, in diagnosis of lung infection, 151
Zoster virus infection, 244–245, *245*

ISBN 0-7216-4482-1

90038

9 780721 644820